Breast Cancer: New Concepts in Etiology and Control

ACADEMIC PRESS RAPID MANUSCRIPT REPRODUCTION

ORGANIZING COMMITTEE

Marvin A. Rich, Ph.D., Chairman
Comprehensive Cancer Center
of Metropolitan Detroit
and the
Michigan Cancer Foundation
Detroit, Michigan

Pietro Gullino, Ph.D.
National Cancer Institute
Bethesda, Maryland

Francesco Squartini, Ph.D.
Institute of Pathological
Anatomy and Histology
Pisa University Medical School
Pisa, Italy

John B. Moloney, Ph.D.
National Cancer Institute
Bethesda, Maryland

Yoshihiko Tsubura, Ph.D.
Nara Medical College
Kashihara-city, Japan

Louis R. Sibal, Ph.D., Program Coordinator
National Cancer Institute
Bethesda, Maryland

Breast Cancer: New Concepts in Etiology and Control

edited by

MICHAEL J. BRENNAN
Michigan Cancer Foundation
and
Comprehensive Cancer Center of Metropolitan Detroit
Detroit, Michigan

CHARLES M. McGRATH
Department of Tumor Biology
Michigan Cancer Foundation
Detroit, Michigan

MARVIN A. RICH
Michigan Cancer Foundation
and
Comprehensive Cancer Center of Metropolitan Detroit
Detroit, Michigan

ACADEMIC PRESS
A Subsidiary of Harcourt Brace Jovanovich, Publishers
New York London Toronto Sydney San Francisco
1980

ACADEMIC PRESS, INC.
111 Fifth Avenue, New York, New York 10003

United Kingdom Edition published by
ACADEMIC PRESS, INC. (LONDON) LTD.
24/28 Oval Road, London NW1 7DX

Library of Congress Cataloging in Publication Data

Meeting on Mammary Cancer in Experimental Animals and Man, 11th, Detroit, 1978.
Breast cancer, new concepts in etiology and control.

"Held under the auspices of the Michigan Cancer Foundation and the Comprehensive Cancer Center of Metropolitan Detroit."

1. Breast—Cancer—Congresses. I. Brennan, Michael James. II. McGrath, Charles M. III. Rich, Marvin A. IV. Michigan Cancer Foundation, Detroit. V. Comprehensive Cancer Center of Metropolitan Detroit. VI. Title. [DNLM: 1. Breast neoplasms—Congresses. WP870 B8266 1978]
RC280.B8M43 1978 616.99′449 80-13468
ISBN 0-12-131150-3

PRINTED IN THE UNITED STATES OF AMERICA

80 81 82 83 9 8 7 6 5 4 3 2 1

CONTENTS

VIRAL ASPECTS OF BREAST CANCER

IMMUNOLOGICAL ASPECTS OF BREAST CANCER

CONTRIBUTORS

Numbers in parentheses indicate pages on which the authors' contributions begin.

LARRY O. ARTHUR (349), Viral Oncology Program, Frederick Cancer Research Center, Frederick, Maryland

BONNIE B. ASCH (53), Department of Cell Biology, Baylor College of Medicine, Houston, Texas

PETER BENTVELZEN (173), Radiobiological Institute TNO, Rijswijk, The Netherlands

MARIA BISTOCCHI (213), Institute of Pathological Anatomy and Histology, University of Pisa Medical School, Pisa, Italy

MICHAEL J. BRENNAN (3, 29), Michigan Cancer Foundation, Detroit, Michigan

JAN BRINKHOF (173), Radiobiological Institute TNO, Rijswijk, The Netherlands

BILL BRINKLEY (53), Department of Cell Biology, Baylor College of Medicine, Houston, Texas

VIJAYA CHARYULU (387), Department of Microbiology, University of Miami School of Medicine, Miami, Florida

DAVID COLCHER (149), National Cancer Institute, National Institutes of Health, Bethesda, Maryland

EUGENE R. DESOMBRE (69), Ben May Laboratory for Cancer Research, University of Chicago, Chicago, Illinois

ARNOLD S. DION (193), Department of Molecular Biology, Institute for Medical Research, Camden, New Jersey

WILLIAM DROHAN (149), National Cancer Institute, National Institutes of Health, Bethesda, Maryland

DONALD C. FARWELL (193), Department of Molecular Biology, Institute for Medical Research, Camden, New Jersey

CECILIA FENOGLIO (225), Department of Pathology, College of Physicians and Surgeons of Columbia University, New York, New York

DONALD L. FINE (349), Viral Oncology Program, Frederick Cancer Research Center, Frederick, Maryland

ASHER FRENSDORFF (297), Department of Microbiology, The Dr. George S. Wise Faculty of Life Sciences, Tel Aviv University, Tel Aviv, Israel

PHILIP FURMANSKI (243), Department of Biology, Michigan Cancer Foundation, Detroit, Michigan

DAWN G. GOODMAN (269), Division of Cancer Cause and Prevention, Tumor Pathology Branch, National Cancer Institute, Bethesda, Maryland

GEOFFREY L. GREENE (69), Ben May Laboratory for Cancer Research, University of Chicago, Chicago, Illinois

PIETRO M. GULLINO (109), Laboratory of Pathophysiology, National Cancer Institute, National Institutes of Health, Bethesda, Maryland

WILLIAM A. GUYETTE (121), Department of Cell Biology, Baylor College of Medicine, Houston, Texas

JOOST HAAIJMAN (173), Radiobiological Institute TNO, Rijswijk, The Netherlands

PATRICIA H. HAND (149), National Cancer Institute, National Institutes of Health, Bethesda, Maryland

GLORIA H. HEPPNER (317), Department of Immunology, Michigan Cancer Foundation, Detroit, Michigan

KATHRYN B. HORWITZ (89), University of Colorado Medical Center, Department of Medicine, Denver, Colorado

DAVID HOWARD (149), Life Sciences Division, Meloy Laboratories, Springfield, Virginia

JAMES N. IHLE (331), Cancer Biology Program, Frederick Cancer Research Center, Frederick, Maryland

ELWOOD V. JENSEN (69), Ben May Laboratory for Cancer Research, University of Chicago, Chicago, Illinois

IAFA KEYDAR (225), Institute of Cancer Research, Department of Pathology, College of Physicians and Surgeons of Columbia University, New York, New York

DIANA M. LOPEZ (387), Department of Microbiology, University of Miami School of Medicine, Miami, Florida

BISMARCK B. LOZZIO (387), University of Tennessee, Knoxville, Tennessee

MYLES L. MACE (53), Department of Cell Biology, Baylor College of Medicine, Houston, Texas

CHARLES M. McGRATH (243), Department of Tumor Biology, Michigan Cancer Foundation, Detroit, Michigan

WILLIAM L. McGUIRE (89), Department of Medicine, The University of Texas Health Science Center, San Antonio, Texas

RICHARD J. MASSEY (349), Viral Oncology Program, Frederick Cancer Research Center, Frederick, Maryland

ROBERT J. MATUSIK (121), Department of Cell Biology, Baylor College of Medicine, Houston Texas

DANIEL MEDINA (53), Department of Cell Biology, Baylor College of Medicine, Houston, Texas

RICARDO MESA-TEJADA (225), Institute of Cancer Research, Department of Pathology, College of Physicians and Surgeons of Columbia University, New York, New York

ROB MICHALIDES (251), Department of Virology and Genetics, The Netherlands Cancer Institute, Amsterdam, The Netherlands

ANTHONY B. MILLER (17), NCIC Epidemiology Unit, University of Toronto, Toronto, Ontario, Canada

FRED R. MILLER (317), Department of Immunology, Michigan Cancer Foundation, Detroit, Michigan

ROELAND NUSSE (251), Department of Virology and Genetics, The Netherlands Cancer Institute, Amsterdam, The Netherlands

TSUNEYA OHNO (225), Institute of Cancer Research, Department of Pathology, College of Physicians and Surgeons of Columbia University, New York, New York

GABRIEL ORTIZ-MUNIZ (387), Department of Microbiology, University of Miami School of Medicine, Miami, Florida

RAFFAELE PINGITORE (213), Institute of Pathological Anatomy and Histology, University of Pisa Medical School, Pisa, Italy

ANTHONY A. POMENTI (193), Department of Molecular Biology, Institute for Medical Research, Camden, New Jersey

MADHAVA P. RAMANARAYANAN (225), Institute of Cancer Research, Department of Pathology, College of Physicians and Surgeons of Columbia University, New York, New York

MARVIN A. RICH (29), Michigan Cancer Foundation, Detroit, Michigan

JEFFREY M. ROSEN (121), Department of Cell Biology, Baylor College of Medicine, Houston, Texas

WERNER SCHÄFER (331), Max-Planck-Institut für Virusforschung, Germany

JEFFREY SCHLOM (149, 387), National Cancer Institute, National Institutes of Health, Bethesda, Maryland

GERALD SCHOCHETMAN (349), Viral Oncology Program, Frederick Cancer Research Center, Frederick, Maryland

EDWARD M. SCOLNICK (269), Division of Cancer Cause and Prevention, Laboratory of Tumor Virus Genetics, National Cancer Institute, Bethesda, Maryland

M. MICHAEL SIGEL (387), Department of Microbiology and Immunology, University of South Carolina, School of Medicine, Columbia, South Carolina

SOL SPIEGELMAN (225), Institute of Cancer Research, Department of Pathology, College of Physicians and Surgeons of Columbia University, New York, New York

FRANCESCO SQUARTINI (213), Institute of Pathological Anatomy and Histology, University of Pisa Medical School, Pisa, Italy

SCOTT C. SUPOWIT (121), Department of Cell Biology, Baylor College of Medicine, Houston, Texas

YOSHIO A. TERAMOTO (149), National Cancer Institute, National Institutes of Health, Bethesda, Maryland

ROBERTHA VAN NIE (251), Department of Virology and Genetics, The Netherlands Cancer Institute, Amsterdam, The Netherlands

MARTIN L. WENK (269), Microbiological Associates, Bethesda, Maryland

CHARLENE J. WILLIAMS (193), Department of Molecular Biology, Institute for Medical Research, Camden, New Jersey

NING-SUN YANG (243), Department of Biology, Michigan Cancer Foundation, Detroit, Michigan

HOWARD A. YOUNG (269), Division of Cancer Cause and Prevention, Laboartory of Tumor Virus Genetics, National Cancer Institute, Bethesda, Maryland

PREFACE

Breast cancer is a leading cause of cancer deaths in women throughout the world. Epidemiologic studies have identified genetic and endocrine parameters as major determinants in disease onset. Other studies have implicated viruses; and, together with endocrinologic and other immunologic factors, viral antigens serve as aids in diagnosis and prognosis. Current evidence suggests that endocrinologic measurements hold considerable promise for use in selecting treatment modes and predicting disease recurrence rates. Both immunologic and endocrine parameters appear useful in monitoring disease progression and in some cases, effective as therapeutic interventions in achieving disease remission.

Basic research in animal model systems has identified genetic, endocrine, and viral parameters as important factors in the etiology of mammary cancer. Inbred animal strains in which mammary cancer incidence varies and in which the variation can be related to genetic, endocrine, or viral status, permit detailed study of the mechanisms involved in disease onset and progression. Reagents, techniques and concepts derived from the animal models when applied to the human disease have helped us to understand the natural history of breast cancer in man. Conversely, detailed clinical studies in man have delineated more clearly which of the animal models are relevant for study of the disease in man.

The meetings on Mammary Cancer in Experimental Animals and Man began as an updating of information on the murine mammary tumor viruses. Over the years that followed, it has engaged as well the evaluation of new information on endocrinologic and genetic factors, and the realignment of the interface between human and model system investigations. The 11th meeting of the group, was organized in this same tradition and with these same objectives. One hundred fifty scientists met in Detroit to update knowledge and achieve consensus on the best working models to identify genetic, endocrinologic, and virologic factors operative in causality, progression, diagnosis, and treatment of the disease. The scientific presentations and discussions, reflected a substantive evolution of the ideas developed in earlier meetings of the group. Breast cancer viruses are no longer viewed simply as infectious agents, but more as cell genes that in nature have evolved a way to become transposable from their cell and species of origin to other cells in other species. Estrogen and progesterone receptors have become useful, in some cases predicting response to therapy. New molecular reagents combined with new biologic systems and the availability of lines of breast cancer cells have increased our mechanistic understanding of how hormones affect breast cells. Immunologic discussion has focused in the last few years on preventing breast cancer by preventing the growth of malignant cells.

It is our hope that this volume on new concepts in breast cancer research will encourage further research and understanding of all aspects of breast cancer onset and progression. It is directed to all who are eager to understand how breast cancer develops and how it might finally be managed.

Michael J. Brennan
Charles M. McGrath
Marvin A. Rich
Michigan Cancer Foundation
Detroit, Michigan
December 1, 1979

ACKNOWLEDGMENT

The organizing and program committees for the 11th Meeting on Mammary Cancer in Experimental Animals and Man, held under the auspices of the Michigan Cancer Foundation, and the Comprehensive Cancer Center of Metropolitan Detroit, gratefully acknowledge the support of the following in making the meeting possible:

The Breast Cancer Task Force
National Cancer Institute
Bethesda, Maryland

Virus Cancer Program
National Cancer Institute
Bethesda, Maryland

The United Foundation
Detroit, Michigan

Mr. and Mrs. R. Alexander Wrigley
Grosse Pointe, Michigan

Parke-Davis Company
Detroit, Michigan

The Upjohn Company
Kalamazoo, Michigan

ETIOLOGIC AND PROGNOSTIC ASPECTS OF BREAST CANCER

ETIOLOGY AND PATHOPHYSIOLOGY OF BREAST CANCER[1]

Michael J. Brennan

Michigan Cancer Foundation,
110 East Warren Avenue,
Detroit, Michigan

The etiology and pathogenesis of breast cancer in women remains unidentified even though the disease has been under investigation for 75 years. In the early years, genetic and endocrinological aspects of the disease were the major areas of experimental research (Moulton, 1945). Sustained levels of estrogens (Lacassagne, 1936) or of prolactin (Muhlbock, 1956) markedly increase the rate of development and the overall incidence of mammary cancers in many strains of inbred mice and in outbred animals as well. Similar extensive observations have been made in rats (Dao, 1969; Furth, 1953). Human breast cancer is apparently dependent on the presence of estrogen for its development (Bulbrook, 1973; MacMahon and Cole, 1973), but prolactin's role in human mammary cancer formation and hormonal support is not clearly established (Smithline *et al.*, 1975).

The development of inbred mouse strains led to the recognition of a milk-transmitted filterable factor as the cause of the high rate of cancer occurrence in some strains of mice over 50 years ago (Nandi and McGrath, 1973). Extensive work in mammary tumor virology and the development of molecular biological methodology now indicate the viral information complementary to that of the Bittner type mammary tumor agent is present in the somatic cell DNA of many low-mammary-tumor strains. At least three major types of viral related mouse mammary oncogenesis have been defined in inbred mice, differentiated from one another in terms of routes of transmission to progeny, pregnancy dependency of tumor expression, character of focal precancerous mammary gland proliferative alterations, and spectrum of tumor histologies. These three

ISBN 0-12-131150-3

virogenic neoplastic syndromes are thought to be the product of three genetically related viruses which differ from one another antigenically and in host infectivity range for foreign mouse strains. Only one type is strongly dependent on milk transmission for its persistence and oncogenic activity in the progeny of a virus secreting female (Hageman, 1975; Nandi and McGrath, 1973; Schlom *et al.*, 1973 a,b).

In the last five years evidence for the presence of oncornavirus information similar to that encoded in mouse mammary tumor virus RNA has been found in some human breast cancers (Axel *et al.*, 1972; Dmochowski, 1972; Moore *et al.*, 1971; Moore, 1975; McGrath *et al.*, 1974; Schlom and Spiegelman, 1972; Schlom *et al.*, 1973 a,b; Seman and Dmochowski, 1973). 70 S RNA oncornavirus type RNA-dependent DNA transcriptase and oncornavirus-like particles have been found in human milks. In pateints with early breast cancer lesions, macrophage migration inhibition assays have detected immunoresponsiveness to mouse milks containing B-type oncorna particles (Black, 1972). However, no clear evidence for the existence of a human oncornavirus dependent on milk transmission for persistence in progeny has been found, and there has never been described any specific concentration of breast cancer occurrence in children nursed by breast cancer patients decribed in the literature. Indeed since breast cancer is relatively infrequent in women raised in societies where nursing is the predominant mode of infant nurture, as opposed to populations drawn from societies where artificial infant feeding is a dominant custom, it is clearly unlikely that viral transmission via milk will ever be shown to cause human breast cancer (Moore *et al.*, 1971; MacMahon and Cole, 1973). Nevertheless, the exclusion of milk transmission of a cancer-inductive factor does not by any means show that viral dependent mouse mammary oncogenesis is irrelevant to human studies, since viral oncogenesis certainly occurs in the mouse via routes other than milk transmission of the responsible agent.

Infectivity, except for hosts genetically very similar to the host of origin, is generally not demonstrable in oncornavirus systems. Since oncornaviruses of the mouse mammary tumor type do not induce recognizable *in vitro* cell transformations, proof of infectivity and oncogenesis for any candidate human breast cancer oncornavirus will require the discovery either of new animal host systems (e.g., primate), or means of showing the acquisition and multiplication of viral information in target cell cultures which would correlate with tumor formation by these cells in immunodeficient hosts such as the nude mouse.

Existence of a viral etiological component achieving even partial expression in human breast cancer cells would have substantial bearing on immunological prospects in breast cancer research. It could provide opportunity for serological or cell-based immunological detection of a mammary cancer diathesis (Stutman and Herberman, 1976); for blood markers capable of serving as indices of breast cancer burden or growth activity (Heppner *et al.*, 1976); and, finally, as the basis of specific immunoprophylaxis and immunotherapy against breast cancer (Charney *et al.*, 1976; Stutman, 1976; Stutman and Herberman, 1976).

The degree to which it has been possible to exploit these latter two tactical management opportunities in the mouse system remains limited. The implication of these failures should not be that such study is fruitless but rather that more precise and specific methods need to be developed in order to obtain yield from approaches well founded in biological principle but not yet brought to a requisite technical level.

Breast cancer epidemiology and breast cancer genetics likewise have received a strong stimulus from the renewed interest in a potential human mammary cancer virus. In the mouse the outcome of mammary tumor virus oncogenicity is under well-defined genetic governance and determinative gene products involved in susceptibility and resistance to the process have been identified, as they have in the oncornavirus-induced mouse leukemias and sarcomas (Bentvelzen, 1972; Lilly, 1971). Epidemiological studies of the distribution of viral RNA-dependent DNA polymerases and of 70 S-RNA templates for these polymerases in human breast cancers and mammary tissues, with genotyping (including histocompatibility antigens) of patients and their near relatives, would seem to be clearly called for by the murine data on genetic restriction of viral oncogenesis.

Throughout the last decade, during which virological (McGrath *et al.*, 1974) and immunological explorations in mouse and human breast cancer (Baldwin *et al.*, 1973; Edynak *et al.*, 1971; Fossati *et al.*, 1972; McCoy *et al.*, 1974) have been expanding so rapidly, a concomitant and parallel advance has been underway in the endocrinology of mammary cancer (McGuire and Chamness, 1973; Singhakowinta, *et al.*, 1975).

However, whereas immunological, genetic, and virological studies in human breast cancer have taken mouse mammary neoplasia as their major methodological guide and laboratory inspiration, endocrinological breast studies have turned to rat mammary cancer for their principal experimental models (Dao, 1964; Furth, 1967); to epidemiology and endocrine therapeutic oncology for their inspiration (Bulbrook *et al.*, 1960); and to fundamental cellular physiology and biochemical endocrinology for their methods (Jensen *et al.*, 1967; McGuire and Chamness, 1973).

The rat models that have been most important heuristically have been the the dimethylbenzathracene-induced cancers (Dao, 1964) and the breast cancers induced by mammotropin-secreting estrogen-induced transplantable pituitary tumors (Furth, 1967).

Unlike established mouse mammary neoplasms, most rat mammary neoplasms induced by these two methods have proved to be markedly hormone responsive, and to undergo profound regression when either ovarian or pituitary (or mammotropic pituitary tumor) secretions were withdrawn. Resumption of growth in DMBA-induced tumors after ovariectomy is readily obtained with estrogen alone, and ovine prolactin restores growth to pituitary-hormone-deprived mammotropin-induced cancers (Dao, 1967; MacLeod *et al.*, 1964; Pearson *et al.*, 1972). These effects correspond to the clinically established patterns of response of a substantial minority (about 1/3) of metastatic human breast cancers to ovariectomy, hypophysectomy, and adrenalectomy (Atkins *et al.*, 1957). Primary and transplantable DMBA-induced neoplasms also resemble human metastatic breast cancers in their vulnerability to regression or suppression of growth by high doses of exogenous androgens and estrogens (Hilf *et al.*, 1963). However, whereas prolactin deprivation induced by l-dopa and brom-ergocryptine will cause regression of both kinds of induced rat breast neoplasms, these pharmacological agents are uncommonly (and even then only very transiently) effective against human metastatic breast cancer (European Breast Cancer Group, 1972; Heuson *et al.*, 1971/72; Smithline *et al.*, 1975), although both effectively suppress milk secretion by the human mammary gland (Friesen and Hwang, 1973). Consequently, it may fairly be said that, with respect to prolactin dependency, there is a mechanistic discontinuity between the human and rat mammary tumor systems, in spite of the susceptibility of both to disruption by hypophysectomy.

DMBA carcinogenesis is blocked by pregnancy and by pretreatment with large doses of estrogens alone or with progestins (Dao, 1967). This feature of the rat DMBA model assumed even greater importance with the finding that age at first-term pregnancy was the predominant index of relative lifetime breast cancer risk within a number of high- and low-risk breast cancer populations, and that differences in lactation occurrence, frequency, or duration had little or no influence on breast cancer rates in parous women. The effect is strongest for first deliveries prior to age 20. Strangely, after age 28, or 30 at the latest, pregnancy has a reverse effect. The longer time after age 30 a woman waits to deliver her first child, the greater her lifetime breast cancer risk becomes (MacMahon *et al.*, 1970).

There is consequently an implication that breast cancer induction, or at least the cytological or physiological conditions which are necessary to allow it, must occur in late adolescence or early adult life, some 20 to 50 years before the disease surfaces clinically (MacMahon and Cole, 1973). The aggravating effect of first pregnancies occurring at age 30 or later on lifetime breast cancer risk could then be attributed to the endocrine growth stimulus or immunosuppression exerted by the pregnancy on incipient breast cancers.

While the epidemiological discoveries alluded to above have revolutionized breast cancer etiological investigations and reinforced interest in the rat DMBA tumors, clinical endocrine therapeutic experience in metastatic breast cancer over the last 15 years has itself generated an important new focus of mammary cancer endocrinological research. The finding that excretory levels and ratios for dehydro-3-epiandrosterone, etiocholanolone, and corticosteroids, but not for the chemically determined major estrogens, were related to the probabilities of success or failure for adrenalectomy and phpophysectomy in metastatic breast cancer, called attention to adrenal participation in breast cancer pathogenesis (Atkins *et al.*, 1968; Bulbrook *et al.*, 1960).

There followed a series of attempts to correlate the breast cancer risk of apparently healthy women with their adrenal steroid excretory and secretory functions (Brennan *et al.*, 1973; Brooks, 1976; Bulbrook *et al.*, 1971). Because of the influence of thyroid status on DHEA/etiocholanolone excretion ratios, thyroid function in breast cancer also assumed new interest (Kumaoka *et al.*, 1973; Moossa *et al.*, 1973). As serum prolactin assays became available, and as the role of prolactin in DMBA-induced rat mammary cancer was defined (Pearson *et al.*, 1972), prolactin blood levels began to be clinically examined in relation to adrenal steroid secretion and thyroid function (Henderson *et al.*, 1975; Mittra and Hayward, 1974). These lines of investigation began to converge when the sensitization of the mammary gland to prolactin stimulation at physiologic blood levels in thyroprivic animals was recognized (Mittra, *et al.*, 1974; Mittra, 1974), calling forth renewed appreciation that more than the absolute serum levels and secretory rates of a given family of hormones need to be known in order to understand the trophic stimulus being experienced by the mammary epithelium in any given setting.

Presence of estrogen receptor, estrogen-induced alpha-one-lactalbumin production, and casein synthesis have now been shown to be preserved in many breast cancers. Among other uses, these properties have served to identify with certainty the differentiated mammary epithelial component in cell cultures established from experimental and clinical breast cancers (Brooks *et al.*, 1973; Horwitz *et al.*, 1975; Lippman and Bolan, 1973; Rose and McGrath, 1975; Soule *et al.*, 1973), a capability necessary for arriving at regularly reliable methods for the culture of breast cancers on a routine basis, and therefore an important contribution to breast cancer science and potentially to treatment planning.

The finding that the breast cancer process is multicentric (Fisher *et al.*, 1975; Gallager and Martin, 1969; Wellings and Jensen, 1973), points to a generalized rather than a focal process of neoplastic transformation in the gland. In 20 to 30% of cases, additional microscopic loci of neoplasia can be demonstrated in the opposite, clinically non-cancerous breast at the time of mastectomy for breast cancer even though only a small portion of mammary epithelium had been taken for study. If the causative factor were viral, it would seem likely that the entire mammary epithelium must be generally harboring virus information. That might be taken to connote entry into the mammary tree at a time prior to its arborization, since it would imply that the growing end of each of the several primitive ducts from which the gland develops must have contained the viral information before it branched out from the anlage of the organ in order for the entire epithelium to be involved. Therefore only genetic, congenital, or (at the latest) prepuberal, timing of viral information acquisition, prior to extensive arborization of the gland, would seem to be competent to allow a universal involvement of the entire mammary epithelium such as is demonstrable in the mouse.

A generalized ultrastructural change in the duct epithelia of cancerous human breasts has recently been described (Spring-Mills and Elias, 1975). This finding, and the multicentric character of human mammary neoplasia demonstrated by whole-organ pathological studies, certainly point away from causation by duct stasis, mutation, or other directly localized events, although they do not distinguish between early exogenous (e.g., congenital or neonatal) viral infection of the budding anlage of the gland and other generalized oncogenic processes such as can be induced by systemically administered hydrocarbon carcinogens or by strong endocrine stimulation in young virgin female rats in the absence of demonstrable viral participation.

However, while a universalized (Spring-Mills and Elias, 1975), or at least multitudinous discrete alteration (Fisher *et al.*, 1975; Gallager and Martin, 1969; Wellings and Jensen, 1973) of the mammary epithelium commonly characterizes the breast cancer oncogenic process in man, it is probable that many microscopic foci of histologically malignant microneoplasia in the human breast are incapable of forming progressively growing clinical cancers. Standard surgical therapy over the last 100 years has been unilateral mastectomy. Thousands of women have survived 20 years or more after unilateral mastectomy without developing new cancers in the residual breast, although we have strong reason to believe from recent studies that at least 1/5 of these breasts contained microcancers at the time of diagnosis of clinical cancer in the contralateral gland (Urban, 1969; Wellings and Jensen, 1973). In fact the rate of occurrence of new cancers in residual breasts is known not to exceed one new cancer per 100 woman-years (McCredi *et al.*, 1975). Were all the multiple microinvasive cancers present in such breasts actually capable of clinical cancer formation, a much higher rate of presentation of new clinical cancers should certainly have to be expected.

These considerations have led to the contention that all breast cancer foci may not grow continuously or autonomously. The fact that median survival after recognition of clinically recurrent disease in 1,400 patients was not substantially different for women with short, as opposed to long, disease-free intervals between primary therapy and recurrence in hormonally nonresponsive cases (Brennan and McMahan, 1976) was brought forward in support of a disease-process model in which transition to a final rapidly progressive terminal phase of the disease becomes the determinative event for lethality. Prior to this event the disease is visualized as existing in a chronic, essentially nonprogressive, or very slowly progressive and well-tolerated phase, in which tumor burden remains static or only gradually increases, but death attributable to cancer rarely occurs.

A disease-process hypothesis of this kind connotes only an indirect dependency of survival probability on post-mastectomy tumor burden. It may be thought of as finding the paradigm for breast cancer in chronic myelogenous leukemia rather than, as has been implicit in current adjuvant chemotherapy design, using acute leukemia models for this purpose (Fisher and Wolmark, 1975); Skipper and Schabel, 1973).

If long periods of essentially zero cell-population growth can occur naturally in human breast cancer, as they apparently can during the natural history of RIII mouse mammary tumors and some DMBA-induced rat mammary tumors, as well as after endocrine ablations, or during hormonal treatment in human breast cancer, long survivorship need not be a direct function of residual tumor burden after primary treatment. In this setting, neither tumor burden nor growth rate during periods of new growth (e.g., primary tumor growth rate or growth rate of clinically demonstrable metastases in the terminal phase of the disease) would be as important in determining survivorship as the duration of "dormancy" intervals in the two sets of patients.

Should there be long periods of near dormancy during which the growth fraction is actually low in metastatic deposits, cytotoxic cycle-specific drugs would do very little harm to the tumor-cell population during such intervals. Consequently, this process model would call for a somewhat different approach to adjuvant therapy than is presently being tried. Optimal results, especially with cycle-specific cytotoxic drugs, would depend upon the development of marker systems for sensitively determining the time of onset of higher rates of proliferation and the reservation of intensive cytotoxic therapy until that had occurred. Alternatively, means for temporarily increasing growth fraction in metastatic deposits prior to chemotherapy (e.g., endocrinological stimulation) might have to be employed early in the disease in chemotherapeutic attempts to eradicate or markedly reduce residual tumor burden.

A concept of the breast cancer process calling for long periods during which cytokinesis is depressed, and the growth fraction is very small in micrometastases would allow for the known therapeutic outcomes and the established temporal characteristics of breast cancer recurrence. However, "dormancy," in the sense of absence of net increase of tumor cell population over long periods, could also be explained even in the presence of a continuously high growth fraction in micrometastases if high compensating rates of cell loss were simultaneously occurring during such zero-growth periods (Silvestrini *et al.*, 1974).

In any event, it seems probable that the overall kinetics of micrometastases may undergo a change of state at some point in the course of the disease in order to allow for transition from a long quiescent to a rapidly progressive tumor growth condition.

The general observation that mitotic indices and thymidine labeling indices correlate well and directly with rates of net tumor mass increase in many tumor systems can be taken as supporting the argument that variances in growth fraction rather than variances in rates of cell loss are most apt to underline alterations in rates of new tumor mass increase (Mendelsohn and Dethlefsen, 1968). Consequently, the hypothesis that during periods of breast cancer "dormancy" growth fractions may in fact be very low, probably deserves preference and active investigation. The practical importance of this possibility is reinforced by the notorious general resistance of indolent, slowly growing neoplasms to cytotoxic chemotherapy.

The accumulation of total tumor burden in metastatic breast cancer is the summation of the growth produced over time at a large number of individual metastatic loci, which are out of synchrony with one another in their time-course toward attainment of individually preset maximal masses. That these individual loci of growth represent clones of tumor cells derived from some original stemline subject to substantial genetic instability seems well established (Hauschka, 1961). Thus genetic differences between the cell populations of individual metastatic foci are an additional source of disease process complexity.

Given all these circumstances, it would be expected that prognostication in metastatic breast cancer should be extremely difficult. Yet there is a remarkable degree of predictability in the course of metastatic breast cancer once clinical metastatic disease has become manifest, and the duration of the clinically disseminated phase of the disease process is notably similar in women with short, as opposed to long, "disease-free" intervals between first treatment and the appearance of metastases (Brennan and McMahan, 1976).

It is relevant in this regard that the survival pattern of breast cancer populations is more consistent with a lethality mechanism based upon constant risk of the occurrence of some critical random state-transition toward progressive growth than it is with any lethality mechanism rooted directly in the *continuous exponential growth* of a tumor cell population from the time of diagnosis to the attainment of some final large and mortal tumor burden. The probability of death from metastatic breast cancer occurring in any given future time interval was found to remain constant for members of surviving postmastectomy populations over a span of many years (Jones, 1956). This probability does not increase with elapsed time from diagnosis as it should were death due directly to the continuous growth of cancer deposits.

Transplantable animal tumors and leukemias kill as the direct result of continuous cell multiplication. These tumors need not adapt to new microenvironments and induce new supporting vasculature at many discrete anatomical sites in order to cause death. Characteristically, in such experimental systems a plot of death risk per unit future time after clinical appearance of tumor rises steeply to a maximum of such severity that the entire tumor-bearing population is quickly extinguished. In contrast, disease-specific breast cancer death rate per 1,000 postmastectomy survivors per year is essentially the same for women presenting with a given stage of operable disease in the first three years after diagnosis as it is in the tenth or fifteenth years after surgery (Jones, 1956).

These considerations regarding the general characteristics of the human breast cancer lethality process and their implication that metastatic proliferation may require additional "progression" (in Foulds' sense of that term [Foulds, 1949]) call to mind the paucity of information on the comparative properties of cancer cell populations of individual primary breast neoplasms vis-a-vis the cell populations of the metastatic lesions derived from them. They reveal the need for longitudinal clinical studies comparing detailed cytogenetic, kinetic, cytoendocrine, metabolic, cell, and organ culture, vascular inductive and immunologic characterizations of tumor-cell populations sampled at various phases of the breast cancer process in order to identify specific cell-population adaptations which may be critical for successful proliferation at metastatic sites.

But the pursuit of such clinical studies, while certainly to be recommended, will be fraught with difficulty and their success will require exceptionally strong administrative coordination of demanding clinical and laboratory procedures over long time periods. They can be successful only in specially organized interdisciplinary cancer research centers with large clinical breast cancer services and stable long-term support. At the same time, the understanding of the metastatic process which may be achieved through such efforts will have relevance for all cancer work, and not merely for breast cancer science and treatment. The Michigan Cancer Foundation Breast Cancer Prognostic Study is an example of such a long-term multidisciplinary program and is described in a subsequent chapter of this volume.

To provide experimental guidance for these efforts and accelerate progress in the understanding of the breast cancer metastatic process, emphasis should be given to finding suitable animal models for its study (Kim *et al.*, 1975).

The precedent of the mouse system for studies of virus participation in human breast cancer etiology, for work in breast cancer pathogenesis, and for *in vitro* biological studies of mammary tumor, has been central to the progress of human breast cancer research in the last decade. The precedents given by studies in rat mammary tumor systems have been correspondingly important for endocrinological studies in human mammary carcinogenesis, pathogenesis, and therapeusis. Even though these models probably have only a segmental complementariness to the full informational description of the human breast cancer process, they have served as useful sources of methodology and theoretical guidance in human breast cancer research. Workable comparative breast tumor models specifically useful for studying the metastatic process in autochthonous and transplantable hormone-responsive mammary tumor systems should be able to make comparable contributions toward the theory and methodology of clinical studies of the human breast cancer metastatic process (Kim *et al.*, 1975; Gullino, *et al.*, 1975).

[1]ACKNOWLEDGMENTS

Supported in part by a research grant (P01-CA-16175) awarded by the National Cancer Institute, DHEW, and an institutional grant from the United Foundation of Detroit.

REFERENCES

Atkins, H. J., Falconer, M. A., Hayward, J. L., and MacLean, K. S. (1957). *Lancet 1*, 489.

Atkins, H. J., Bulbrook, R. D., Falconer, M. A., Hayward, J. L., MacLean, K. S., and Schurr, P. H. (1968). *Lancet 2*, 1255.

Axel, R., Schlom, J., and Spiegelman, S. (1972). *Nature (London) 229*, 611.

Baldwin, R. W., Embleton, M. J., Jones, J. S., and Langman, M. J. (1973). *Internat. J. Cancer 12*, 73.

Bentvelzen, P. (1972). *Internat. Rev. Exp. Pathol. 11*, 259.

Black, M. M. (1972). *Natl. Cancer Inst. Monogr. 35*, 73.

Brennan, M. J., Bulbrook, R. D., Deshpande, N., Wang, D. Y., and Hayward, J. L. (1973). *Lancet 1*, 1076.

Brennan, M. J., and McMahan, C. A. (1976). Analysis of recent breast cancer treatment studies. *In* "The Physiopathology of Cancer" (F. Homburger, ed.), Vol. II. S. Karger, Basel.

Brooks, S. C., Locke, E. R., and Soule, H. D. (1973). *J. Biol. Chem. 248*, 6251.

Brooks, S. C. (1976). The metabolism of steroid hormones in breast cancer, a reappraisal. *In* "Steroid Hormone Action and Cancer" (K. M. Menon and J. R. Reel, eds.). Plenum Press, New York.

Bulbrook, R. D., Greenwood, F. C., and Hayward, J. L. (1960). *Lancet 1*, 1154.

Bulbrook, R. D., Hayward, J. L., and Spicer, C. C. (1971). *Lancet 2*, 395.

Bulbrook, R. D. (1974). Hormonal factors in mammary carcinogenesis. *In* "Proceedings of the Fifth International Symposium on the Characterization of Human Tumors." Bologna, (W. Davis, ed.). Elsevier, New York (1974).

Charney, J., Holben, J. A., Cody, C. M., and Moore, D. H. (1976). Further immunization studies with mammary tumor virus. Symposium on Immunological Control of Virus-associated Tumors in Man: Prospects and Problems, held at National Institutes of Health, Bethesda Maryland, April 7-9, 1975.

Dao, T. L. (1964). *Prog. Exp. Tumor Res. 5*, 157.

Dao, T. L., (1967). Endocrine environment and neoplasia. *In* "Endogenous Factors Influencing Host-Tumor Balance" (R. W. Wissler, T. L. Dao, and S. Wood, eds.). University of Chicago Press, Chicago.
Dao, T. L., (1969). *Prog. Exp. Tumor Res. 11,* 235.
Dmochowski, L. (1972). *Triangle 12,* 37.
Edynak, E. M., Lardis, M. P., and Vrana, M., (1971). *Cancer 28,* 1457.
European Breast Cancer Group (1972). *Eur. J. Cancer 8,* 155.
Fisher, E. R., Gregorio, R., and Fisher, B. (1975). *Cancer 36,* 1.
Fisher, B., and Wolmark, N., (1975). *Cancer 36,* 627.
Fossati, G., Canevari, S., Della Porta, G., Balzarini, G. P., and Veronesi, U. (1972). *Internat. J. Cancer 10,* 391.
Foulds, L., (1949). *Brit. J. Cancer 3,* 345.
Friesen, H., and Hwang, P., (1973). *Ann. Rev. Med. 24,* 251.
Furth, J. (1953). *Cancer Res. 13,* 477.
Furth, J., (1967). *In* "Endogenous Factors Influencing Host-Tumor Balance" (R. W. Wissler, T. L. Dao, and S. Wood, eds.), p. 49. University of Chicago Press, Chicago.
Gallager, H. D., and Martin, J. E., (1969). *Cancer 23,* 855.
Gullino, P. M., Pettigreur, H. M., and Grantham, F. H., (1975). *Natl. Cancer Inst.* (USA) *54,* 401.
Hageman, P. C., (1975). *Internat. Union Cancer Tech. Rep. Ser. 20,* 98.
Hauschka, T. A., (1961). *Cancer Res. 21,* 957.
Henderson B. E., Gerkins, V., Rosario, I., Casagrande, J., and Pike, M. C. (1975). *New Engl. J. Med. 293,* 790.
Heppner, G. H., Kopp, J. S., and Medina, D. (1976). Microcytotoxicity assay of immune responses to non-mammary tumor virus-induced, pre-neoplastic, and neoplastic mammary lesions in BALB/c mice. Symposium on Immunological Control of Virus-associated Tumors in Man: Prospects and Problems, held at National Institutes of Health. Bethesda Maryland, April 7-9, 1975.
Heuson, J. C., Waelbroeck, C., Legros, N., Gallez, G., Robyn, C., and L'Hermite, M. (1971/72). *Gynecol. Invest. 2,* 130.
Hilf, R., Johnson, M. M., Breuer, C., Greeman, J. J., and Borman, A. (1963). *J. Natl. Cancer Inst. 31,* 541.
Horwitz, K. B., Costlow, M., and McGuire, W. L., (1973). *Steroids 26,* 785.
Jensen, E. V., DeSombre, E. R., and Jungblut, P. W. (1967). Estrogen receptors in hormone-responsive tissues and tumors. *In* "Endogenous Factors Influencing Host-Tumor Balance" (R. W. Wissler, T. L. Dao, and S. Wood, eds.), p. 15. University of Chicago Press, Chicago.
Jones, H. B. (1956). *Trans. N. Y. Acad. Sci. 18,* 298.
Kim, U., Baumler, A., Carruthers, C., and Bielat, K. (1975). *Proc. Natl. Acad. Sci. 72,* 1012.

Kumaoka, S., Abel, O., Utsunomiya, J., Bulbrook, R. D., Hayward, J. L., and Swain, M.D. (1973). Plasma oestradiol and urinary oestrogen metabolites in normal Japanese and British women. Host-Environment Interactions in the Etiology of Cancer in Man, Proceedings. International Agency for Research on Cancer, Lyon.
Lacassagne, A. (1936). *Am. J. Cancer 28*, 735.
Lilly, F. (1971). H-2, membranes, and viral leukemogenesis. *In* "Cellular Interactions in the Immuno Response" (S. Cohen, G. Cudkowicz, and R. T. McCluskey, eds.), p. 103. S. Karger, Basel.
Lippman, M., and Bolan, G. (1973). *Nature (London) 256*, 592.
Mendelsohn, M. L., and Dethlefsen, L. A. (1968). *In* "The Proliferation and Spread of Neoplastic Cells," p. 197. Williams and Wilkins, Baltimore.
Mittra, I., and Hayward, J. L. (1974). *Lancet 1*, 885.
Mittra, I., Hayward, J. L., and McNeilly, A. S. (1974). *Lancet, 1*, 889.
Mittra, I. (1974). *Lancet 248*, 525.
Moore, D. H., Charney, J., Kramarsky, B., Las Fargues, E. Y., Sarkar, N. H., Brennan, M. J. Burrows, J. H., Sirsat, S. M., Paymaster, J. C., and Vaidya, A. B. (1971). *Nature (London) 229*, 611.
Moore, D. H. (1975). *In* "Cancer" (F. F. Becker, ed.), p. 131. Plenum Press, New York.
Moossa, A. R., Price-Evans, D. A., and Brewer, A. C. (1973). *Ann. R. Coll. Surg. 53*, 178.
Moulton, F. R. (1945). Mammary Tumors in Mice, A Symposium. American Association for the Advancement of Science, Washington.
Muhlbock, O. (1956). *Adv. Cancer Res. 4*, 371.
MacLeod, R. M., Allen, M. S., and Hollander, V. P. (1964). *Endocrinology 75*, 249.
MacMahon, B., Cole, P., Lin, T. M., Lowe, C. R., Mirra, A. P., Ravnihar, B., Salber, E. J., Valaoras, V. G., and Yuasa, S. (1970). *Bull. World Health Org. 43*, 209.
MacMahon, B., and Cole, P. (1973). *J. Natl. Cancer Inst. 50*, 21.
McCoy, J. L., Jerome, L. F., Dean, J. H., Cannon, G. B., Alford, T. C., Doering, T., and Herberman, R. B. (1974). *J. Natl. Cancer Inst. 53*, 11.
McCredi, J. A., Inch, W. R., and Alderson, M. (1975). *Cancer 35*, 1472.
McGrath, C. M., Grant, P. M., Soule, H. D., Glancy, T., and Rich, M. A. (1974). *Nature (London) 252*, 247.
McGuire, W. L., and Chamness, G. C. (1973). *Adv. Exp. Med. Biol. 36*, 113.

Nandi, S., and McGrath, C. M. (1973). *Adv. Cancer Res. 17,* 353.

Pearson, O. H., Molina, A., Butler, T. P., Llerena, L., and Nasr, H. (1972). *In* "Estrogen Target Tissues and Neoplasia" (T. L. Dao, ed.), p. 287. Univ. of Chicago Press, Chicago.

Rose, H. D., and McGrath, C. M. (1975). *Science 190,* 673.

Schlom, J., and Spiegelman, S. (1972). *Science 175,* 542.

Schlom, J., Michalides, R., Kufe, D., Hehlmann, R., Spiegelman, S., Bentvelzen, P., and Hageman, P. (1973a). *J. Natl. Cancer Inst. 51,* 541.

Schlom, J., Colcher, D., Spiegelman, S., Gillespie, S., and Gillespie, D. (1973b). *Science 179,* 696.

Seman, G., and Dmochowski, L. (1973). *Cancer 32,* 822.

Silvestrini, R., Sanfilippo, O., and Tedesco, G. (1974). *Cancer 34,* 1252.

Singhakowinta, A., Mohindra, R., Brooks, S. C. Vaitkevicius, V. K., and Brennan, M. J. (1975). *In* "Estrogen Receptors in Human Breast Cancer" (W. L. McGuire, P. P. Carbone, and E. P. Vollmer, eds.), p. 131. Raven Press, New York.

Skipper, H. E., and Schabel, F. M. (1973). *In* "Cancer Medicine" (J. F. Holland and E. Frei, eds.), p. 629. Lea and Febiger, Philadelphia.

Smithline, F., Sherman, L., and Kilodny, H. D. (1975). *New Engl. J. Med. 292,* 784.

Soule, H. S., Vasquez, J., Long, A., Albert, S., and Brennan, M. J. (1973). *J. Natl. Cancer Inst. 51,* 1409.

Spring-Mills, E., and Elias, J. J. (1975). *Science 188,* 947.

Stutman, O., and Herberman, R. B. (1976). Immunological control of breast cancer: discussion. Symposium on Immunological Control of Virus-associated Tumors in Man: Prospects and Problems, held at National Cancer Institutes of Health, Bethesda, Maryland, April 7-9, 1975.

Stutman, O. (1976). Correlation of in vitro and in vivo studies of antigens relevant to the control of murine breast cancer. Symposium of Immunological Control of Virus-associated Tumors in Man: Prospects and Problems, held at National Institutes of Health, Bethesda, Maryland, April 7-9, 1975.

Urban, J. A. (1969). *Surg. Clin. N. Am. 49,* 291.

Wellings, S. R., and Jensen, H. M. (1973). *J. Natl. Cancer Inst. 50,* 1111.

BREAST CANCER ETIOLOGIC INFLUENCES

A.B. Miller

NCIC Epidemiology Unit
University of Toronto
Canada

Breast cancer is commonly regarded as influenced largely by hormonal factors. Indeed, it is the cancer which first comes to mind when one considers hormonally associated tumors. This has arisen largely because of the obvious association with a number of reproductive factors, all of which appear to point to the importance of ovarian activity. MacMahon *et al.* (1973) pointed to the importance of early age at menarche, late age at menopause, a low frequency of artificial menopause, nulliparity, and delayed age at first pregnancy as being risk factors for breast cancer. However, not all these factors are found to be operative even when carefully sought in well-designed case control studies. A number of investigators, including ourselves, (Choi *et al.* 1978) have, for example, had difficulty in confirming that early age at menarche is a risk factor.

In their international study, MacMahon *et al.* (1970) demonstrated that age at first pregnancy was the most important risk factor and that this accounted for most of the effect of parity. However, although most have been prepared to accept age at first pregnancy as the most important risk factor, not all have been able to confirm that it explains the parity association. In a recent study in Finland (Soini, 1977), the parity effect persisted even if age at first pregnancy was accounted for, while we in two studies have with some difficulty demonstrated a parity effect, but been unable to demonstrate an age at first pregnancy effect. As I have recently discussed these and other discrepant findings, I shall not repeat the arguments here (Miller, 1978). Suffice it to say that it is by no means certain that age at first pregnancy should be regarded as the

ISBN 0-12-131150-3

major risk factor for breast cancer and that maybe it is only a reflection of another possibly more important risk factor, which under certain circumstances may confound the age at first pregnancy effect. However, before leaving this topic it is well to recall that for some time it has been accepted that age at first pregnancy does not explain international variation of breast cancer (MacMahon *et al.*, 1973) and what is more fails to explain the changing rates of breast cancer in Iceland, on which I shall comment further later (Bjarnason *et al.*, 1974).

It is, I believe, now well recognized that one of the outstanding features of the epidemiology of breast cancer is the substantial variation in international incidence. Table I summarizes this, taking data from "Cancer Incidence in Five Continents" (Waterhouse *et al.*, 1976).

TABLE I. International Variation in Incidence of Breast Cancer[a]

Ages standardized rate per 100,000[b]	*Number of registries*
80 or more	2
60 - 79	11
40 - 59	36
20 - 39	19
Less than 20	12

[a] *From Waterhouse et al (1976).*

[b] *"World" population as standard. Range: 11.0 per 100,000 in Israel, non-Jews to 80.3 per 100,000 in Hawaii, Caucasians.*

Although there is some evidence when one compares registries contributing to the three volumes of "Cancer Incidence in Five Continents," (Doll *et al.*, 1966; Doll *et al.*, 1970; Waterhouse *et al.*, 1976) that incidence of breast cancer may be increasing in some areas (Table II) it is a little difficult to distinguish increases largely due to increasing efficiency of registration from real increases. Further, in some countries, and Canada is a prime example, reports of increasing incidence of breast cancer (Cutler *et al.*, 1971; Grace *et al.*, 1977) have to be interpreted by recognizing that there has been a substantial change in the approach to diagnosis of the disease. Not only have women been more willing to take lumps to be examined but also pathologists have been more prepared to examine material in greater detail. The fact that

TABLE II. Change in Incidence of Breast Cancer, Registries Contributing to Volumes I (1960-1962) and III (1968-1972), "Cancer Incidence in Five Continents"[a]

Number of registries	*Percentage change in age standerdized rate*[b]
2	More than 100%
0	75 - 99%
1	50 - 74%
7	25 - 49%
16	0 - 24%
2	- 1 -- 10% Decrease
Median change	16.8%

[a]*From Doll et al. (1966) and Waterhouse et al. (1976).*

[b]*Range: Decrease of 8.9% in Nigeria, Ibadan to increase of 142.5% in Singapore, Chinese.*

increases in incidence have been reported could still be a diagnostic artifact, especially in the light of the fact that breast cancer mortality has remained stable in technically advanced countries over the last 30 years (Wigle, 1977).

In the light of the acknowledged association between breast cancer and a positive family history (Anderson, 1974), one of the favored explanations for international variation of incidence and mortality is genetic factors. However, in spite of reports of families in which breast and colon cancer are inherited, possibly by some dominant process (Lynch *et al.*, 1973), it is recognized that such occurrences are extreme. Indeed, population studies suggest that they may contribute little to the overall problem of breast cancer (Lynch *et al.*, 1974). Furthermore, studies of migrant populations suggest that genetic differences are not important, if time is given for acculturation. A well-known example is the study of Buell (1973) in which he showed that although first generation Japanese migrants had a much lower breast cancer mortality than the white population of California, the second generation showed a substantial increase particularly in more recent years, though only time will tell whether the rates for second or even third generation Japanese migrants will eventually reach those of the host population.

Nevertheless, this evidence is now being supplemented with

evidence from Japan itself where, particularly since the last war, breast cancer incidence has begun to rise particularly in those age groups and areas where acculturation to western habits has been the greatest (Hirayama, 1977). Even more impressive evidence of changes has been noted in Iceland, where the changes in the age-specific curves for breast cancer have been elegantly domonstrated to be due to increasing rates in different birth cohorts, the most recent birth cohorts having the highest risk (Bjarnason *et al.*, 1974). Thus in Japanese migrants, in Japan itself, and in Iceland the changes that appear to have followed acculturation to western lifestyles appears to have been responsible for substantial increases, admittedly after some delay, in the risk of breast cancer. The genes of course have not changed, reminding us that increased familial risk may not only be due to genetic factors but to common environments and lifestyle. This does not mean that genetic factors cannot make some contribution, but their study would be enormously improved if one could identify a genetic marker (Petrakis and King, 1977). A number of investigators are pursuing the search for genetic markers and it is possible that success may eventually reward them. At the moment, however, it has to be accepted that such markers have not yet been reported.

If then we are prepared to accept the possibility that breast cancer like most other cancers is largely influenced by external environmental mechanisms, using the environment in its widest sense, we have to look for evidence as to what these influences could be, keeping in mind the fact that they are likely to exert their effect after a substantial delay period and maybe a lifetime, in contradistinction to the evidence for large intestine cancer which suggests that environmental influences have a much more rapid effect and are therefore possibly much more easy to demonstrate. It was pointed out some time ago that international temperature differences seem to correlate well with differences in breast cancer mortality (Lea, 1965), but subsequently differences in dietary practices were much more highly favored (Drasar and Irving, 1973; Hems, 1970; Lea, 1966; Stocks, 1970).

Three separate lines of evidence serve to support the importance of dietary factors. The first derives from animal experimental studies which have demonstrated that both in the presence and absence of mammary carcinogens, the feeding of high fat diets substantially increases the incidence of mammary cancer in rats (Carroll, 1975). The second comes from population correlation studies which have been performed by a number of investigators, but which all appear to indicate the importance of correlation between breast cancer incidence or mortality and total dietary fat intake (Armstrong and Doll, 1975; Knox, 1977). Carroll (1975) demonstrated that the correlation persists when animal fat intake is considered but seems to almost disappear when vegetable fat intake is considered. However, in considering such studies it is well to remember that there is a substantial correlation between individual food items, and this extends to a number of factors of relevance to the environment including, as it happens, gross national product (Armstrong and Doll, 1975). Nevertheless, positive correlations have been noted not only between countries but also within countries, at least from Japan. Hirayama (1977) has found a strong correlation between dietary fat intake and breast cancer adjusted mortality rates in twelve districts in Japan, a similar correlation being observed with dietary pork intake but not with any other nutritional element. He comments that dietary fat intake appears to have shown the most striking increase of all the nutritional changes that have been noted in Japan in recent years.

A disadvantage of population correlation studies is that they tend to be based on data on national food practices which quantify food disappearance rather than food consumption, and that they tend to relate recent dietary data with the most recent incidence or mortality data. This in spite of the fact that from other evidence it would seem that an interval of 30 or more years might be more appropriate.

The third line of evidence relates to data demonstrating that certain risk factors, which one might suspect to be nutritionally related, are important in breast cancer. Much of the work in this area has been done by deWaard, who has shown an association with both height and weight acting independently in postmenopausal women (de Waard and Baanders Van Halewijn, 1974). He has followed his original study in general practice with a further study which demonstrates similar findings in Japan as well as the Netherlands (de Waard *et al.*, 1977). Although in de Waard's studies both height and weight seem to act independently, height accounted for most of his findings, pointing to the importance of lean body mass. This has caused him to modify his own hypothesis of induction of breast cancer suggesting that overnutrition is of primary importance in relation to breast cancer occurring in post menopausal women, whereas in breast cancer occurring in premenopausal women an endocrine imbalance is responsible in which possibly ovarian hormones are involved (de Waard, 1975). However, de Waard still hypothesizes a mechanism through estrogens partly on the basis of data indicating that estrogen production after the menopause takes place in peripheral tissues, especially adipose tissue. He has pointed out that height correlates well with lean body mass and that several endocrine and metabolic functions seem to correlate better with body surface area than body weight. As in his data, weight has no independent effect if there is an adjustment for its correlation with height, this suggests that if nutritional factors are relevant, these must operate in infancy and childhood and throughout the menarchial years rather than in adult life.

Nevertheless, this emphasis on height as well as weight has not been supported in our own studies in which hardly any effect for height was noted, but an effect of weight, both twelve months before diagnosis and at the time of the menopause in postmenopausal women (Choi *et al.*, 1978). The difference was particularly striking in women aged 70 or more, less important in other postmenopausal women, and completely absent in premenopausal women.

Although we recognized the problem of dietary assessment, sometime ago we decided that indirect assessment of the importance of dietary factors was unsatisfactory and that we should instead attempt some sort of direct assessment using the case control approach. After careful evaluation of available dietary instruments, we eventually decided to use three methods, a 24-hr recall, which was mainly used as a training instrument for a four-day record and a detailed dietary questionaire which was directed to the period two months before interview (time I) and to the two month period six months prior to the time of interview (time II). In administering these instruments, we used food models which permitted an estimate of the volume of all food items normally consumed. This with a detailed data bank based on U.S. and Canadian food tables enabled us to derive a quantitative estimate of the intake of the nutrients of interest, which were total calories, total fat, saturated fat and oleic acid, linoleic acid, and cholesterol (Morgan *et al.*, 1978).

The results of this study were first reported in summary form about a year and a half ago in which was presented estimates derived from a mean of the two major methods used the four day diary and the dietary history (Miller, 1977). For all respondents the mean difference for the matched pairs was statistically significant for total calories, total fat, and saturated fat, and although no longer significant when we considered premenopausal and postmenopausal groups separately, the general direction was similar in both groups as for all respondents, though with possibly a greater difference for post-menopausal women.

Subsequently, in preparing our results for more definitive publication, we decided that it may well have been a mistake to have presented a mean of the findings for the two major methods. One of the difficulties we faced was that we were not certain which method represented the true intake. Although in most circumstances when we used both the means of methods and the individual methods separately the direction

TABLE III. Simple Correlation Coefficients Between Dietary Methods For Total Fat Intake in Controls[a]

	Dietary method		
Dietary method	*History at time I*	*History at time II*	*Four-day record*
24 hour record	0.29	0.24	0.25
History at time I		0.92	0.36
History at time II			0.31

[a]*From Morgan et al. (1978).*

of the differences was the same, there were some discrepancies and indeed the correlation between the different methods except for the two compenents of dietary history though significant was not substantial, as is shown for total fat intake in Table III. In addition, we have two concerns over the four-day record. The first is that it was made during the period following the diagnosis of breast cancer, a time when both the fact of the diagnosis and the results of treatment for cancer could have influenced the amount of the food intake, even though we were careful to restrict our interviewing to periods when all treatment had been completed. Second, the response to the four-day record was far less satisfactory than from the questionnaires, all of which were completed at the time of the initial interview. The record was left for completion with women and a number did not complete the task, many in fact being the controls who possibly had less reason to collaborate with us than the cases. This resulted in an overall nonresponse to the four-day record of 23% of the 400 case-control pairs. The 24 hr recall suffers from a similar disadvantage to the four-day record in that it also was directed to a period following the diagnosis while it has the additional disadvantage that it depends not only on recall but on one day's intake and this, for various reasons, might have been highly atypical.

Intuitively, therefore, we have more confidence in the detailed dietary history. This has the advantage that a section of the questionnaire directed our respondents' attention to an earlier time period prior to the diagnosis of breast cancer. This may well have avoided the physical and/or psychological impact of the diagnosis and treatment of breast cancer on the responses given. In practice, the instrument collects information on usual intake as conceived by the respondent. They are presented with a detailed list of dietary food items and asked to estimate with the aid of the food models what their normal intake is. We have, unfortunately, no evidence as yet that estimates of intake using this instrument are valid, mainly because attempts at validation are likely to interfere with actual intake. We are, however, attempting to develop approaches to the validation of the instrument as, in practice, we have gone on to use it in further cancer studies.

In using this method, we found the most informative analysis based on risk ratios though we had to dichotomize fat intake at different levels for pre- and postmenopausal women because the premenopausal group as a whole consumed more than the postmenopausal group. A dichotomy level at 90 gr for premenopausal women resulted in a risk ratio for total fat intake of 1.6 and for postmenopausal women with a dichotomy level at 50 gr the risk ratio was 1.5 (Miller *et al.*, 1978). In neither group could we find evidence of a dose-response relationship. In premenopausal women controlling for the other nutrients if anything strengthened the assocation for total fat, in postmenopausal women the association with other nutrients was almost nonexistent.

We thus have direct evidence of an association between total fat intake and breast cancer in both pre- and postmenopausal women, in contradistinction to the findings from the indirect approaches, which suggested an effect only in postmenopausal women. The association is admittedly weak, but this could have been anticipated in the light of the fact that our inquiry was directed to a time period probably several decades after the actual effect was likely to have operated.

It is of course possible that none of the dietary methods we used were sufficiently accurate nor may they sufficiently reflect lifetime dietary experience to be relevant in relation to the etiology of breast cancer. Further, our use of neighborhood controls in an endeavor to control for socioeconomic status may have contributed to a difficulty in demonstrating real differences in dietary intake that may in fact have been present. Indeed, we noted that one result of neighborhood matching was the tendency to result in relatively few discordant pairs in the risk ratio analysis. Nevertheless, if we can accept the risk ratios at their face values as being the best evidence we currently have for the effect of dietary fat intake as a risk factor for breast cancer, by an appropriately weighted average over pre- and postmenopausal women, we have calculated an attributable risk percent for total fat intake of 27% (Miller, 1978). Although relatively low, this is still the most important risk factor for breast cancer found in our data, as the only other factor which comes anywhere near it is family history of breast disease, which seems to be largely independent of other factors with a risk ratio in our study of 2.4 resulting in an attributable risk of 20%, a lower proportion because of the lower proportion in the population who do in fact have the factor. As already indicated, age at first pregnancy did not show any evidence of an effect in our data though in practice if we were to use other people's estimate of the appropriate risk ratio, which seems to approximate to 1.7, and use the data from our controls for the population estimate we can calculate a possible attributable risk of 25%.

If we are to accept that dietary factors and particularly, as the evidence suggests, total fat intake is relevant to the etiology of human breast cancer, it is necessary to consider the mechanism through which they may operate. Although Cole and Cramer (1977) suggest that dietary factors operate through a hormonal mechanism, there is no particular evidence, other than the possible indirect effect of nutrition on age of menarche (Frisch and McArthur, 1974) as to how such a factor could indeed operate. Rather, there seems to be accumulating evidence that the effect could be through some sort of direct carcinogenic effect upon the breast, possibly mediated through intestinal bacteria as first postulated by Hill *et al.*, (1971). Another hypothesis is that differences in cholesterol metabolism may be relevant and both the latter possibilities are being considered for investigation by the Breast Cancer Task Force. Another possibility is that diet may operate directly through some sort of mechanism which affects circulating carcinogens, maybe through breast cancer fluid, as postulated by Petrakis (1977).

Studies supported by the Breast Cancer Task Force are also evaluating the importance of diet in both Hawaii and Israel. If they confirm the importance of a high fat diet, then we may be in a position to advocate a reduction of dietary fat as one means for controlling breast cancer. However, in view of the relatively slow change that occurs in migrant populations, it seems likely that such dietary modification as may be appropriate would have to be made early in life in order to have a full effect in line with the apparent importance of hormonal factors in relatively early life. Fortunately, the sort of dietary modification that will be recommended on present evidence is similar to that advocated in an attempt to reduce the frequency of occurrence of cardiovascular disease, namely, the "Prudent Diet" which seeks to avoid the evils of nutritionally associated cancers and cardiovascular disease by promoting the intake of moderate amounts of animal protein, fat, and cholesterol, and avoiding obesity. It is perhaps reassuring that these measures are likely to be encouraged for economic reasons because of the world food shortage and the high cost of production of fat and protein from animal sources.

REFERENCES

Anderson, D. E., (1974). *Cancer 34*, 1090-1097.

Armstrong, B., and Doll, R., (1975). *Internat. J. Cancer 15*, 617-631.

Bjarnason, O., Day, N., Snaedal, G., and Tulinius, H., (1974). *Internat. J. Cancer 13*, 689-696.

Buell, P., (1973). *J. Natl. Cancer Inst. 51*, 1479-1483.

Carroll, K. K., Gammal, E. B., and Plunkett, E. R., (1968). *Can. Med. Assoc. J. 98*, 590-594.

Carroll, K. K., (1975). *Cancer Res. 35*, 3374-3383.

Choi, N. W., Howe, G. R., Miller, A. B., Matthews, V., Morgan, R. W., Munan, L., Burch, J. D., Feather, J., Jain, M., and Kelly, A., (1978). *Am. J. Epidemiol. 107*, 510-521.

Cole, P., and Cramer, D., (1977). *Cancer 40*, 434-437.

Cutler, S. J., Christine, B., and Barclay, T.H.C. (1971). *Cancer 28*, 1376-1380.

de Waard, F., and Baanders-Van Halewijn, E. A., (1974). *Internat. J. Cancer 14*, 153-160.

de Waard, F., (1975). *Cancer Res. 35*, 3351-3356.

de Waard, F., Cornelis, J. P., Aoki, K., and Yoshida, M., (1977). *Cancer 40*, 1269-1275.

Doll, R., Payne, P., and Waterhouse, J., (eds.) (1966). Cancer Incidence In Five Continents, International Union Against Cancer, Springer-Verlag, Berlin.

Doll, R., Muir, C., and Waterhouse, J., (eds.) (1970). Cancer Incidence in Five Continents, Volume II. International Union Against Cancer, Springer-Verlag, Berlin.

Drasar, B. S., and Irving, D., (1973). *Brit. J. Cancer 27*, 167-172.

Frisch, R. E., and McArthur, J. W., (1974). *Science 185*, 949-951.

Grace, M., Gaudette, L. A., and Burns, P. E., (1977). *Cancer 40*, 358-363.

Hems, G., (1970). *Brit. J. Cancer 24*, 226-234.

Hill, M. J., Goddard, P., and Williams, R.E.O. (1971). *Lancet 2*, 472-473.

Hirayama, T., (1977). *In* "Origins of Human Cancer" pp. 55-75. Cold Spring Harbor Laboratory.

Knox, E. G., (1977). *Brit. J. Prev. Soc. Med. 31*, 71-80.

Lea, A. J., (1965). *Brit. Med. J. 1*, 488-490.

Lea, A. J., (1965). *Lancet 2*, 332-333.

Lynch, H. T., Krush, A. J., and Guirgis, H., (1973). *Am. J. Gastroenterol. 1*, 31-40.

Lynch, H. T., Guirgis, H., Albert, S., and Brennan, M. (1974). *Cancer 34*, 2080-2086.

MacMahon, B., Cole, P., Lin, T. M., Lowe, C. R., Mirra, A. P., Ravnihar, B., Salber, E. J., Valoras, V. G., and Yuasa, S. (1970). *Bull World. Health Org. 34*, 209-221.

MacMahon, B., Cole, P., and Brown, J., (1973). *J. Natl. Cancer Inst. 50*, 21-42.

Miller, A. B., (1977). *Cancer 39*, 2704-2708.

Miller, A. B., (1978). *Cancer Res. 38*, 3985-3990.

Miller, A. B., Choi, N. W., Matthews, N., Morgan, R. W., Munan, L., Burch, J. D., Feather, J., Howe, G. R., and Jain, M., (1978). *Am. J. Epidemiol. 107*, 499-509.

Morgan, R. W., Jain, M., Miller, A. B., Choi, N. W., Matthews, V., Munan, L., Burch, J. E., Feather, J., Howe, G. R., and Kelly, A., (1978). *Am. J. Epidemiol. 107*, 488-498.

Petrakis, N. L., (1977). *Cancer 39*, 2709-2715.

Petrakis, N. L., and King, M. C., (1977). *Cancer 39*, 1861-1866.

Soini, I., (1977). *Internat. J. Epidemiol. 6*, 365-373.

Stocks, P., (1970). *Brit. J. Cancer 24*, 633-643.

Waterhouse, J., Muir, C., Correa, P., and Powell, J., (eds.) (1976). Cancer Incidence In Five Continents, Vol. III, IARC Scientific Publication No. 15, International Agency for Research On Cancer, Lyon.

Wigle, D. T., (1977). *Am. J. Epidemiol. 105*, 428-438.

THE BREAST CANCER PROGNOSTIC PROGRAM: A STUDY OF THE METASTATIC PROCESS

Marvin A. Rich
Michael J. Brennan
and
the Scientific, Pathology and Surgical Associates of the MCF Breast Cancer Prognostic Study

Michigan Cancer Foundation
110 E. Warren Ave
Detroit, Michigan

The long-term survival of the breast cancer patient is directly determined by the probability of metastatic spread of the disease. The majority of women surgically treated for breast cancer ultimately die with disseminated disease. Were it not for the recurrence of tumors at local or distant sites, breast cancer would be readily controllable.

The metastatic progression of a breast carcinoma is not likely the result of random colonization. Metastasis occurs following the release of cells from a primary tumor; the process of cell separation allowing their release in single or multiple units. It has been suggested (Folkman, 1974) that the extent of vascularization of the primary tumor may play an important role in this process.

The process of dissemination of the cancer cells, which leads to their arrest at some hospitable site, depends on their entry into normal tissue or into circulatory channels and to their subsequent ability to survive the mechanical trauma of transport and to attach to the vascular endothelium and thus escape the bloodstream (Weiss, 1977).

During the stages which follow, the surface properties of the metastasizing tumor cells undoubtedly influence their interaction with blood cells, with other tumor cells, and with the vascular endothelium. Their surface properties likewise influence the interaction with hormones and with immunological reactants.

As the tumor grows beyond the mass where its nutritional

ISBN 0-12-131150-3

needs can be met by diffusion, and it is likely that this occurs with a tumor mass which exceeds a few millimeters in diameter, or about a million cells, the tumor's survival depends on the development of a vascular apparatus. Since tumors probably do not make their own vessels, but induce them in the surrounding normal tissue (Cavallo *et al.*, 1972), the tumor's angiogenic potential is another important determinant in both the establishment of the disseminated tumor, and in turn the establishment of a metastatic cascade.

It is at this point in the metastatic process that susceptibility to immunological attack is an especially important consideration. Since cancer cells express novel antigens, which, especially in the case of new and vulnerable *micrometastases,* should lead to their detection and destruction by host immune reaction, we must conclude that effective means to evade immune surveillance mechanisms are in effect.

It is unlikely that all of these are random events and even a simplistic view of the complexities of the metastatic process would suggest that the successful colonization of a metastatic tumor depends on *specific* and *predeterminable* characteristics of a patient and her tumor.

Increasingly, therapeutic research in breast cancer has been concerned with the development of systemic treatment methods involving cytotoxic agents, endocrine maneuvers, and immunological stimulation, with the intent to develop effective interventions aimed at the metastases which are responsible for the high lethality of the disease.

Since all of the therapeutic modalities for breast cancer, developed to date, are rigorous and generally hazardous, an increasing need for improved prognostic discrimination at the time of first diagnosis is increasingly evident (Carbone, this volume).

The Breast Cancer Prognostic Study was organized to identify those characteristics of individual breast tumors and their hosts which are associated with early recurrence of metastatic disease. Success in this effort would permit the identification of patients under greatest threat, and it is indeed with these patients that the most aggressive modes of therapy and the most frequent and intensive follow-up procedures should properly be employed.

If it were possible to select with a high degree of accuracy, those patients otherwise doomed to early disease recurrence and death, questions as to the efficacy of prophylactic and adjuvant chemotherapy in breast cancer could be addressed more vigorously, with fewer women needlessly exposed to the hazards of these trials. Further, the ability to identify the groups at uniformly high risk of recurrence would enhance the ability to detect incremental improvements in clinical response and thus would further expedite such clinical trials.

A further incentive for the study arose from the fact that as researchers we were convinced that breast cancer offered the opportunity for the systematic characterization of a primary tumor and its capacity to metastasize and thus offered a human research system for the study of the metastatic process.

With the active participation of our clinical community, we undertook a systematic study aimed at the detailed biological characterization of large numbers of human, primary breast tumors and of those host factors which may be correlated with the tumor's development and metastatic progression. Our initial approach to the development of prognostic markers considered the fact that human breast cancers comprise a heterogeneous group of tumors, whose malignancy could be approximated by pathologic criteria, which with varying degree of certainty could predict a tumor's aggressiveness.

As early as the 1890s, the relationship between the malignant behavior of cancers and their degree of differentiation was described. Greenough (1925) and Scarff and Patey, (1928) described grading systems for mammary carcinomas, dividing tumors into three grades of malignancy based on degree of tubule formation, size of cell and nuclei, degree of hyperchromatism, and number of mitoses.

Utilization of these grading methods was stimulated by the work of Bloom (1950), and by Black and his associates (1956, 1958), who emphasized the importance of nuclear grade and evidence of sinus histiocytosis.

The grading method of Bloom and Richardson (1957), was adapted and modified for our study.

It may be seen in Table I, from data reported by Bloom and Richardson (1957) and by Schiodt (1966), that breast cancer is indeed a heterogeneous disease. Five years after surgery, 75-85% of those patients whose tumor was histologically graded as type I, were still alive. In contrast, among those patients whose tumors were graded as type III only 35% were alive five years post surgery.

It may be seen, however, that grade II, which comprises about half of all of the tumors, is not prognostic. It may well be that grade II is not a bonafide subgroup, but rather represents those tumors that are not clearly members of grade I or III.

In any case, it is evident that while morphological grading divides breast cancer patients into two groups, one with good prognosis and limited risk for early recurrent disease, and the other in which recurrence and early death are more likely, morphological grading alone is not sufficient to establish prognosis for a large proportion of individual breast cancer patients.

TABLE I. Correlation of Tumor Grade and Prognosis

	Tumor grade		
	I	II	III
Five year survival[a] (%)	75	47	32
Number of cases[a]	362	640	407
Five year survival[b] (%)	87.5	66	37
Number of cases[b]	129	358	153

[a]From Bloom and Richardson (1957).
[b]From Schiodt (1966).

In view of the fact that simple morphological criteria can be used to predict the probability for the development of metastatic disease, it appeared reasonable to expect that the detailed characterization of breast tumors and their hosts, with respect to the pathophysiological factors which underlie the expression of metastatic disease, would demonstrate even greater and more precise prognostic potential.

The design of many clinical trials is based on the concept that metastatic deposits grow continuously from their time of establishment in all patients. Yet there is impressive evidence which suggests a considerable heterogeneity in tumor growth (Brennan and McMahan, 1978). If the concept of a uniform and constant tumor growth rate is incorrect, or applicable only to a minor subset of cases, one might predict that gains from current adjuvant chemotherapy trials would be modest and confined only to an early superiority in the treatment group.

A critical factor in the design of optimum screening strategies for the early detection of breast cancer is an estimate of the growth rate of breast tumors. It should be noted that the estimates currently employed, which are from diffuse and indirect sources, range from cell doubling times of 20 to over 200 days.

It appeared reasonable that those tumor, or host characteristics which could be correlated with high metastatic potential, could also provide effective, quantitative markers for tumor burden if systematically assayed from the time of primary surgery through the appearance of clinically detectable recurrent disease and that these in turn could provide useful approximations of tumor growth kinetics.

ORGANIZATION OF THE STUDY

In the planning process we solicited from a wide range of clinical and laboratory scientists a battery of questions or characterizations (Fig. 1) which could be posed to a series of breast tumors of high and low potential for metastatic progression. The questions to be directed at the primary tumors, and to their hosts, fell into the fields of immunology---are there, for example, grade-specific antigens, or are there grade-specific immunological host responses? We asked whether the presence of hormone receptors were related to early recurrence of breast cancer. The disciplines of cell kinetics, cell surface characteristics, biochemistry, and markers for cellular invasiveness were similarly canvased.

To undertake such a venture required the cooperation and active participation of large numbers of our clinical colleagues especially in community hospitals where the majority of primary breast tumors are diagnosed and treated.

Two large clinical associate groups were organized for this purpose. With the assistance of our cancer registry, we identified and recruited into this research program, a group of practicing surgeons at 14 hospitals who operate on 70% of the breast cancer patients in the metropolitan Detroit area. To insure complete patient follow-up in the study, the surgical associates group developed a series of clinical procedures (Fig. 2) to be carried out at regular intervals following surgery.

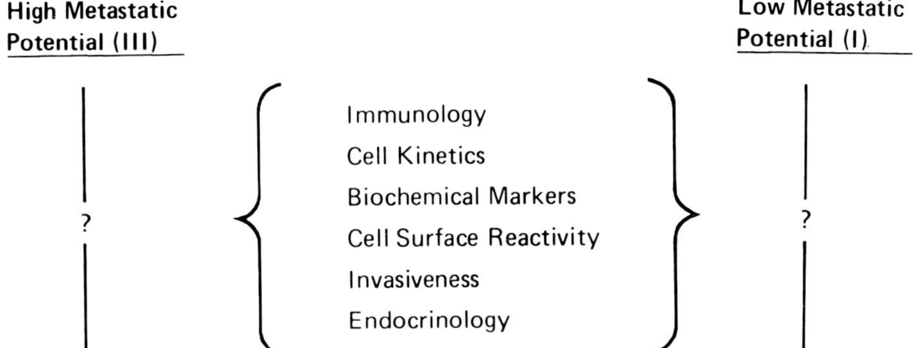

FIGURE 1. Charateristics that may be associated with the potential for metastasis of human breast cancers.

A parallel effort organized the region's clinical pathologists. The objectives of this group were first to provide in a large number of patients, a substantial portion of the breast tumor in a state suitable for its biological and biochemical characterization, and second to establish a pathology panel which would carry out a detailed histopathological analysis on each tumor entered into the study.

At present more than 70 practicing surgeons, pathologists, and medical oncologists are actively involved in this program.[1]

CLINICAL FOLLOW-UP PROTOCOL

Every 3 Months -

Physical Examination
Blood Sample (20cc.)

Every 6 Months -

Physical Examination
Blood Sample (20cc.)
Chest X-Ray
Pelvic X-Ray
(performed once/year at the 6 month interval)

Every 9 Months -

Physical Examination
Blood Sample (20cc.)

Every 12 Months -

Physical Examination
Blood Sample (20cc.)
SMA - CBC
Bone Scan or Bone Survey
Chest X-Ray
Mammogram

FIGURE 2. Clinical follow-up procedures for monitoring patients entered into the Breast Cancer Prognostic Study.

[1] *As of December, 1979, more than 110 practicing surgeons, pathologists and medical oncologists are actively involved in this program, and more than 615 patients have been entered into the study.*

Our Cancer Center has long been associated with the study of breast cancer in man and in experimental animals. Our laboratories had been engaged in various aspects of breast and other cancer research. The plan for the implementation of this study was predicated on the expectation that it would be possible to bring to bear the interests and expertise represented in these laboratories on a single type of malignancy, indeed to focus them where possible on single tumor specimens.

Rather than creating a new set of laboratory and administrative units for these research activities, we superimposed this program onto our existing research structure. Individuals specifically responsible for the conduct of these studies, were placed in laboratories with preexisting expertise and active programs in related areas. This research plan provided both flexibility in design and direct access to state of the art expertise for each of the study's components.

SUPPORT GROUPS

A fundamental requirement for the implementation of this program was a workable mechanism to coordinate the collection and dissemination of the tumor specimens, to standardize the pathological characterization of the tumors, and to assist in the evaluation and correlation of the data obtained in our various research and clinical components. Ultimately, our ability to determine the factors involved in the metastatic potential of human breast cancers is heavily dependent on the program support units which are responsible for the implementation of these services. The units comprising this group are: the Biological Resources Unit, the Pathology Core Unit, and the Biostatistical and Data Processing Unit.

BIOLOGICAL RESOURCES

The Biological Resources Unit is responsible for (1) the collection of breast tumor specimens; (2) the delivery of fresh breast tumor collection kits to the participating hospitals; (3) the transport of tumor specimen slides and evaluation forms to and from the Pathology Panel Members; and (4) the distribution of tumor segments to the appropriate research units.

A most critical element in the implementation of the research programs has been the development of the logistics for the rapid and systematic collection of specimens and their distribution to the appropriate laboratory units. In consultation with the participating surgeons, pathologists, and research scientists, a protocol and collection kit were developed by the Biological Resources Unit.

The kit (see Fig. 3) contains: a dissection protocol sheet and report form, a sterile specimen container for operating room collection, sterile gloves, scalpels, an instrument tray that includes a teflon cutting board, scissors, forceps, and a ruler for measuring the specimen and slices, and a rack with sterile scintillation vials containing the various fluids into which the tumor slices are placed.

The rack containing the vials is placed in a styrofoam basket with ice. The pathologist fills out a Gross Pathology Form to describe the tumor. The specimens, the report, associated blood samples and the used materials are returned to our laboratories.

An efficient method for transporting the tumors from the hospitals to the Michigan Cancer Foundation was developed. After evaluation of Emergency Medical Service, our own drivers, and taxicabs, we decided on the latter. A single taxi company, which had indicated a willingness to cooperate was employed and provides priority service and central billing.

When the tumor arrives at our laboratories, it is assigned

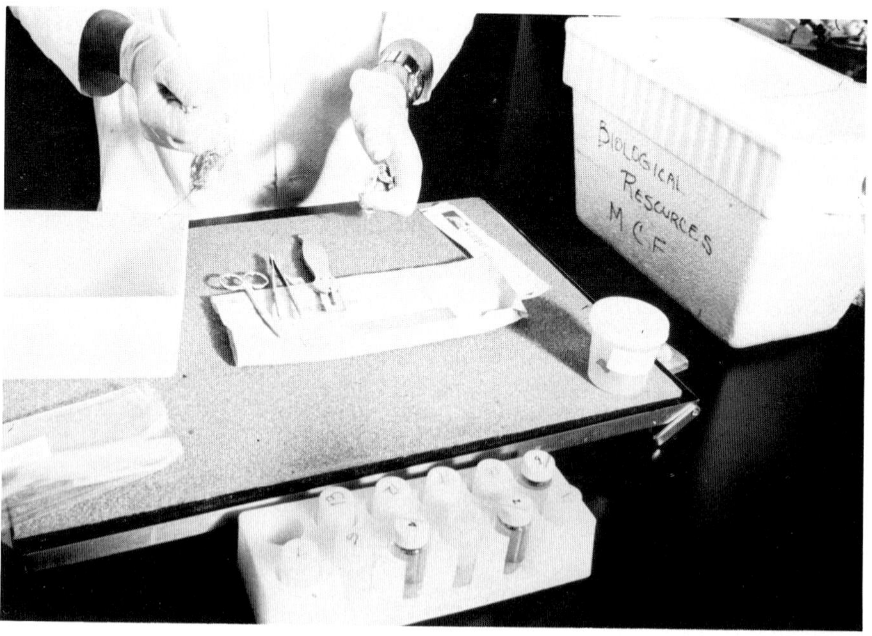

FIGURE 3. Tumor kit used in the Breast Cancer Prognostic Study.

a code number, and the tumor samples are distributed to the appropriate laboratory units. The tumor specimens are generally available to the Research Units within one to two hours after surgery.

The specimens designated for use by our Pathology Panel are fixed, embedded, sectioned and stained, and distributed to the panel members for evaluation (see Pathology Core Unit, below). The Biological Resources Unit is responsible for the distribution of the specimens, collection of the relevant data, and the organization of panel meetings for the purpose of establishing consensus diagnoses and grades.

Pathology Core Unit

While the prognostic efficacy of the tumor and host characteristics will ultimately be determined by the incidence of recurrent tumors in the patient population under study, intermediate evaluation for purposes of monitoring and experimental design depends on pathological criteria such as nuclear and histological grade, which can be provisionally correlated with a tumor's ultimate aggressiveness.

The responsibilities of the Pathology Core Unit include the establishment of the diagnosis, grade, and pathological characterization for each of the tumors entered into the study. This involves the processing of tumor and lymph node specimens, the evaluation of panel reports, and the development of consensus diagnosis and grades for correlation with other clinical and laboratory data.

The laboratory and clinical studies which comprise this program are heavily dependent on this complete pathological characterization of each of the tumors entered. These pathological data establish that the tissue under study is indeed from a malignant breast cancer, the histopathological type of the tumor, that each slice of tumor for experimental use indeed contains malignant tissue, and a reasonably accurate estimate of the prognosis for the patient based on cytological grade. Those determinations are dependent, for the most part, on subjective criteria. We have, therefore, enlisted five clinical pathologists from our associated hospitals, who have had extensive experience with breast cancers, to form a Pathology Panel responsible for establishing those characteristics with each tumor. The members of this panel are shown in Table II.

One slide from each of three different segments/tumor (six slides in all) are sent out to the five panel members once a week. Evaluation forms accompany the slides.
Each pathologist establishes the diagnosis and grades the speci-

TABLE II. Breast Cancer Prognostic Study

Pathology panel
Gerald Fine, M. D. (Chairman), Division Head, Department of Anatomic Pathology, Henry Ford Hospital
Mujtaba Husain, M. D., Department of Pathology, Sinai Hospital of Detroit
Herbert I. Krickstein, M. D., Associate Pathologist, Department of Pathology, St. John Hospital
Thomas O. Robbins, M. D., Assistant Director, Department of Anatomic Pathology, William Beaumont Hospital
Barbara F. Rosenberg, M. D., Associate Pathologist, Department of Anatomic Pathology, William Beaumont Hospital

men without knowledge of the preliminary clinical diagnosis or the scores of the other panel members. The completed report forms are then returned to the Biological Resources Unit.

The pathological diagnosis and evaluation of each tumor by each panelist is compared and differences are resolved at regularly held panel workshops. Thus a consensus diagnosis or calculated average score is determined for all of the histopathologic characteristics of the tumor for correlation with laboratory and other clinical determinations.

The histopathological classification of Foote and Stewart (1946), used as a starting point, proved inadequate for the tumor types in this study. Therefore, a new classification system was designed (Table III).

The grading of the tumors is based primarily on the systems of Bloom and Richardson (1957), and Black *et al.* (1956), as modified by our Pathology Panel. The degree of tubule formation and nuclear pleomorphism, as well as the frequency of mitoses, are considered in the establishment of grade (Table IV). The nuclear grade is based on the classification developed by Black (1957), in which grade I is the least differentiated (worst prognosis) and grade III is the most differentiated (best prognosis). To conform to the other grading systems, the designation of nuclear grade is reversed in our system. The area for grading, based on agreement reached by the panel members is

TABLE III. Tumor Classification

1. *Infiltrating ductal carcinoma*
   A. *N.O.S. (not otherwise specified)*
   B. *Tubular*
   C. *Cribriform*
2. *Intraductal* in situ
   A. *Comedo*
   B. *Papillary or cribriform*
   C. *Other*
3. *Mucoid*
4. *Lobular*
   A. *Invasive*
   B. In situ
5. *Medullary*
   A. *Typical*
   B. *Atypical*
6. *Tubular*
7. *Adenocystic*
8. *Other*

considered to be the least differentiated area of the section in contrast to the system of Bloom and Richardson (1957), which uses a hypothetical average over the entire section.

Lymph Node Analysis

Lymph node involvement, while a strong indicator of probable dissemination and poor prognosis, is now absent in at least half of the women presenting with breast cancer in urban regions of the United States. Yet it is known that at least 15 to 25% of even these favorable cases will have died of metastatic breast cancer within 10 years of diagnosis. At the same time, a corresponding fraction of women with more than four positive nodes will be alive and well 10 years after radical mastectomy.

At least 30% of women having operable cancers (Columbia Stage A and B) with clinically negative axillary nodes will have positive nodes when these nodes are examined microscopically after a radical mastectomy. In major clinical trials, simple mastectomy (which leaves such involved nodes *in situ*) has given clinical results indistinguishable from those obtained with radical operations, which routinely remove at least the great majority of such cancerous nodes.

These contradictions suggest that much remains to be

TABLE IV. Tumor Grading

	Histological grade	Nuclear grade	Mitotic grade
Grade I	Well developed tubules	Most differentiated; uniform size, shape and chromatin staining	0–10/hpf[a]
Grade II	Moderate tubule	Moderate variation	11–20/hpf
Grade III	Slight to no differentiation of tubules; cells in sheets or strains	Marked pleomorphism with great variation in size and shape	$\geq$21/hpf

[a]High power field.

learned about the role of lymph node involvement in the development of metastatic breast disease. It is of great importance to determine if the fundamental postulate of adjuvant chemotherapy is correct, i.e., is it necessary to destroy all microscopic foci of cancer cells to provide the long survivorships which are taken as cure?

The lymph node has been considered not only as a station of metastasis in the spread of breast cancer, but also as an indicator of the immune response of the host to metastatic progression. Numerous studies (Hirschl *et al.*, 1976; Humber *et al.*, 1975; Patt, 1975) have proposed modifications in the architecture of the lymph node as indicators of disease progression. One of these parameters is the reaction of nodal sinus histiocytes (Hirschl *et al.*, 1976) and their relationship with the degree of tumor anaplasticity. On the basis of such reports, we have initiated studies to determine the relationship between the degree of sinus histiocytosis present in axillary lymph nodes of patients in whom breast cancer has been diagnosed and graded by our Pathology Panel using the criteria shown in Table V.

Follicular prominence has also been reported (Humber *et al.*, 1975; Patt, 1975) to be an indicator of the immunological reaction of the host to the neoplastic process. Follicular promi-

TABLE V. Lymph Node Evaluative Criteria

1. *Number of lymph nodes*
   - A. *Hospital report count*
   - B. *Panelist count*
2. *Positive lymph nodes*
   - A. *Hospital report count*
   - B. *Panelist count*
3. *Largest metastasis observed*
   - A. *Under 2 mm*
   - B. *Over 2 mm*
4. *Pericapsular invasion*
5. *Sinus histiocytosis*
   - A. *Minimal with degenerative*
   - B. *Minimal*
   - C. *Moderate*
   - D. *Marked*
6. *Follicular prominence*
   - A. *Minimal*
   - B. *Moderate*
   - C. *Marked*

nence is determined by evaluating the follicular reaction in all of the lymph nodes and scoring according to the number and intensity of germinal centers in the lymph node with the greatest degree of follicular prominence.

Biostatistics and Data Processing Unit

This unit is responsible for the computer storage and processing of all clinical, pathological, and laboratory data. The data processing for the Breast Cancer Prognostic Study utilizes the services and equipment of the Wayne State University Computer Center equipped with IBM 360/67 and Amdahl 470 central processors. The operation of these computers is controlled by the Michigan Terminal System (MTS) supervisory program. MTS allows operation in batch mode or a highly interactive terminal mode.

A separate computer file is maintained for each data form which allows for updating the files as the data come in. The data storage and retrieval system has been designed to meet the special needs of the Prognostic Study. This system has the capabilities for periodic routine report generation. In addition, because of the need for intensive statistical analyses, efficient interface with established statistical software was necessary. With these factors in mind, TAXIR was chosen as an appropriate system.

TAXIR is a information storage and retrieval system developed at the University of Michigan. The system is based on set theory which allows for data retrieval by boolean calculation, which is much more rapid than a comparison search. This logical basis also allows for merging of files, selecting only those cases meeting certain criteria, with the merging dependent on up to 10 keys. Building a file, updating, querying, and merging are further simplified by the high-level language capacity.

TAXIR has report-generating capabilities allowing ordered, labeled, formatted output including N-way cross tabulation, totals, and subtotals, in addition to simple lists. Due to the logical structure incorporated into this system, selection of cases to be outputted is relatively simple. This system has an interface to the Michigan Interactive Data Analysis System (MIDAS), a powerful statistical analysis system.

Clinical Coordination

A critical element in the clinical segment of this program is the standardization of the diagnostic and follow-up procedures for each of the patients entered. The Nurse-Coordinator is an essential component in the implementation of this standardized clinical protocol, the collection of data and the organization of follow-up activities. Two or three days after mastectomy, the patient is visited by the nurse and any additional medical history not initially obtained is recorded. In consultation with the surgeon and pathologist, she diagrams the involved breast and describes the status of the breast and lymph nodes. All of the data are recorded on standardized forms to facilitate computer entry.

In addition to hospital patient visits to obtain primary disease data, the Nurse-Coordinator working closely with the patient, her physician, and the Laboratory Research Group, arranges for appropriate tests and specimen collection at the appropriate follow-up intervals.

During the past year, to increase the number of participating surgeons and hence the rate of entry of patients, the Clinical Coordinator (Dr. Gerald Wilson, a senior practicing surgeon) has arranged meetings with eighteen surgeons in five participating hospitals. Topics discussed were patient introduction to the program, presurgical studies, specimen preparation, and follow-up protocols. As a result, ten new surgeons have been added to the roster of MCF Surgical Associates, with the organization of three additional contributing hospitals in the community.

Since a number of the patients entered into the study have their follow-up visits with Medical Oncologists, it has become essential to elicit the cooperation of these physicians to enable the continuation of all follow-up observations. This has been organized under the aegis of our Center's Community Cancer Control Program (Metropolitan Detroit Community Cancer Control Program) and its demonstration hospitals and medical advisory panels.

Operation of the Study

A Pathology Resident at each participating hospital under the direction of the hospital's Chief of Pathology, is assigned to the study and is responsible for the implementation of the tumor processing protocol.

Alerted by a participating surgeon, the tumor is obtained and processed by the Hospital's Pathology Resident. After collection, the Resident slices the tumor into 1 - 2-mm sections and places them into consecutively numbered vials in the collection kit. The contents and sequence of the vials (Table VI) were developed with full consideration for the variation in tumor size, cellular heterogeneity and the needs of the various research units.

TABLE VI. Contents of the Vials in the Tumor Collection Kit

Slice number	Purpose	Slice number	Purpose
1	Cell culture	8	Hospital pathology (frozen section)
2	Pathology panel		
3	Immunology	9	Biochemical studies
4	Pathology panel	10	Pathology panel
5	Hospital pathology (permanent)	11	Tissue culture
		12	Storage at -80°C
6	Estrogen receptor	13	Storage at -80°C
7	Invasion (enzyme studies)		

To control the influence of tumor heterogeneity, the protocol for tumor segment distribution ensures that alternate segments are used for procedures involving morphological examination of the tumor material. The nature of the material in segment 3, for example (see Table VI), to be used for immunological tests, can be approximated by the material examined in segments 2 and 4. The protocol also establishes priority of testing for small tumors entered in the study.

We attempt to culture the cells from each tumor in the study, to determine if a series of growth characteristics of these cells can be correlated with the tumor's malignant potential in the patient and for other *in vitro* tests. At present, we are able to prepare useful cultures of epithelial cell from 70% of the tumors entered.

To date more than 350 patients, at a current rate of three to five per week, have been entered into the prognostic study and are being followed at three month intervals following surgery. The grades of the first 217 tumors entered in the study are shown in Table VII. It may be seen that the distribution of tumors is similar to that reported by others (see Table I) with approximately 50% of the tumors in grade II. It may also be seen that the relationship between tumor grade and malignancy as measured by early tumor recurrence is very impressively confirmed. As shown here, of the 37 patients whose cancer has already recurred following surgical removal of the primary tumor, only one had been diagnosed with a grade I tumor.

The tests being carried out on the tumor and host material (Table VIII) were choices drawn from a large group of candidate tests. The choices drawn from a theoretical consideration of the metastatic process are based on:

(1) The probability that a test would yield information useful to the characterization of the tumor's malignant

TABLE VII. Recurrence of Human Breast Cancers as a Function of Tumor Grade

Grade	*I* 31 (14%)	*II* 104 (48%)	*III* 82 (38%)	n 217 (100%)
	1	*19*	*17*	*37*
Percent of recurrent tumors	*3%*	*51%*	*46%*	
Percent recurrent in each grade	*3%*	*18%*	*21%*	

potential. This was based on our own studies, and those of other investigators, in appropriate human and animal systems.
(2) Consideration for a test's applicability to small amounts of heterogeneous breast tissue.
(3) The possible use of the test for continuous monitoring of tumor burden in follow-up clinical studies.

Some determinations have been discontinued because they showed no discernible prognostic potential. The priority of others has been altered as a result of the outcome of the preliminary tests. Still others have already demonstrated a clear association with grade and prognosis. The study, in its biostatistical structure, is designed for maximum flexibility for the introduction of new pathophysiological characterizations of the tumor and its host.

In addition to characterizing the primary tumors, the lymph nodes, and patient material at three month intervals following surgery, the study will similarly characterize the metastatic tumors as they recur. If those primary tumor cells with high metastatic potential constitute only a subpopulation of the tumor, then it is the successful metastases that warrant special attention.

Results obtained to date and to be developed during the course of the study (it is anticipated that 1,000-1,200 patients will be studied) will be published in the appropriate current literature and in a series of Annual Progress Reports, prepared for study participants and interested investigators.

An example of the data obtained to date is that on the presence of estrogen receptor in primary breast tumors as a function of that tumor's metastatic potential.

TABLE VIII. Host and Tumor Characteristics Which May Influence Prognosis for Recurrent Breast Cancer

Immunological markers	*Enzymatic markers*
Leucocyte migration inhibition (host vs. MCF-7)	*Fucosyltransferase*
Leucocyte adherence inhibition (host vs. MCF-7)	*Prolylhydroxylase (collagen synthesis)*
Serum immunofluorescence (host vs. autologous tumor)	*Dipeptidase activity*
C-reactive protein	*Cathepsin activity*
CEA	
Mouse mammary tumor virus antigens	
Other markers	In vitro *growth characteristics*
Fibrinolysis	*Saturation density*
Lectin reactivity	*Serum requirement*
	Anchorage dependence
	Three-dimensional growth
Hormonal markers	
Hormone receptors	

The work by DeSombre and Jensen and their colleagues (1972), on the receptor mechanism for the stimulation of target tissue by steroid hormones led to the observation by McGuire and his associates (1975), that breast tumors which do not contain adequate levels of estrogen receptor are more likely to be refractory to hormonal therapy.

Singhakowinta and Brooks, with our own clinical group (1976), have reported that patients with estrogen receptor-containing tumors live longer, respond better to treatment and appear to experience a longer disease-free period than patients with estrogen-receptor negative tumors.

Since the prognostic study offered an opportunity to quantitate this phenomenon systematically under controlled laboratory and clinical conditions, all tumors entered into the Breast Cancer Prognostic Study were tested in the laboratory of Samuel Brooks for the presence of estrogen-binding protein.

It may be seen from Table IX, that 56% of the first 300 tumors in the study contained detectable estrogen receptor. The relationship between axillary node involvement and probability of recurrent disease while not absolute, is considered a prominent prognostic indicator. It was of interest to note, therefore, that so far a correlation between node positivity and estrogen-receptor positivity has not been observed (Table X).

Since it is the duration of disease-free period which we will be measuring in our study, it was of interest to plot the time to recurrence for patients with estrogen-receptor positive and negative tumors. In Fig. 4, of the 121 patients with estrogen-receptor positive tumors, only five have suffered a recurrence to date, with 93% of the patients disease free after 21 months. During this same period in the 164 estrogen-receptor negative cases, 27% of these patients had early recurrent tumors.

These studies, carried out in a system where laboratory, diagnostic, and follow-up procedures are well standardized and controlled, support the preliminary observations of our own

TABLE IX. Estrogen Receptor Content of Primary Breast Tumors

Total number of specimens	*Femto-mole E_2R/10mg Tissue wet weight (% of total)*		
	<1	*1-3*	*>3*
297	*129 (43.4%)*	*38 (12.7%)*	*130 (43.7%)*

TABLE X. Relationship between Estrogen-Receptor Content of the Tumor and Lymph Node Status in Patient with Breast Cancer

Tumor infiltrated auxilliary nodes	*Number of patients*	E_2R^+ (>3 Fmole/10 mg)
0	*143*	*43%*
1-3	*56*	*36%*
4	*50*	*40%*

clinical group and the recent report by Knight and McGuire and their associates (1977), that estrogen-receptor negativity in breast cancer is associated with early recurrence and metastatic disease, and that this appears to be independent of some other prognostic indicators. While a preliminary report of this work has been published (Rich *et al.*, 1978) the specific biological significance of these observations remains to be determined.

Other segments of the Prognostic Study in progress so far suggest that the immunologic reactivity of tumor cells, and of the patient's response to her tumor, appear to be *greatest* in those study patients whose tumors are most likely to metastasize and recur.

Glycosyltransferases, the group of enzymes which add specific sugars to glycoprotein acceptors, are elevated in the sera of tumor-bearing animals and man (Bernacki and Kim, 1977; Allen and Kessel, 1975). In a study just completed, we have demonstrated a striking correlation between likelihood of tumor recurrence and serum levels of fucosyltransferase (Kessel *et al.*, unpublished). High levels of enzyme were associated with high metastatic potential.

In a series of collaborative studies with scientists at other cancer centers, we are providing our controlled materials to investigators with promising leads for metastatic indicators.

Currently in progress are collaborative studies with Spiegelman and his associates on the presence of mouse mammary tumor virus antigen in human breast tumors. In those studies we are determining if and how the presence in the tumor cells of an antigen related to that of the MuMTV gp52 is related to prognosis (Spiegelman, this volume).

Another collaborative study, on cytologic elastosis as a prognostic marker, is being developed with John Masters at St. Paul's Hospital in London.

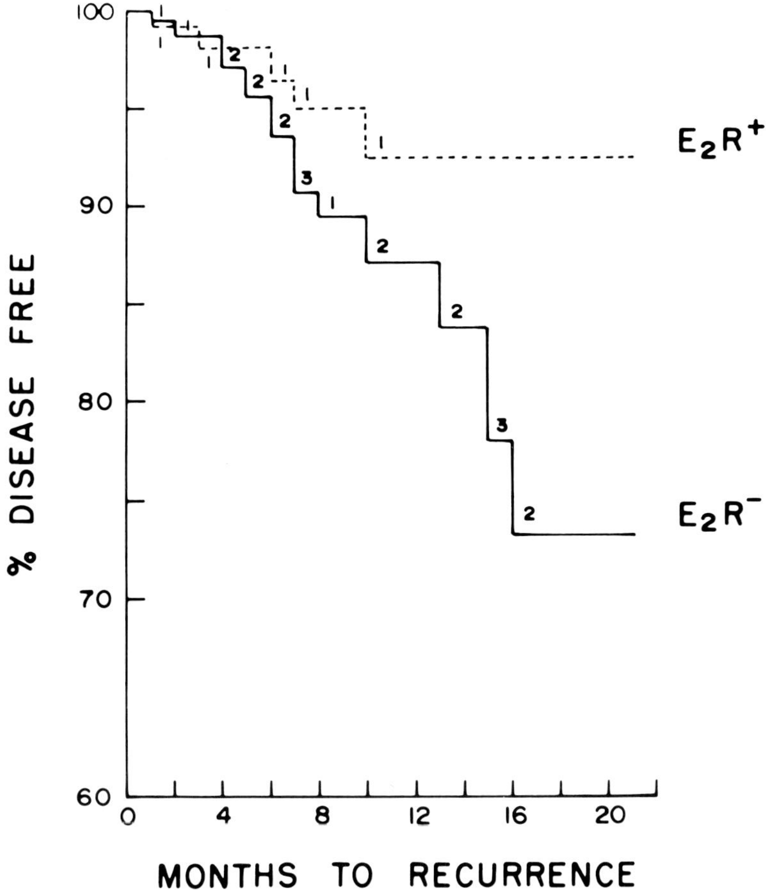

FIGURE 4. Recurrence of cancer in patients whose primary breast tumors were estrogen-receptor positive (>3 fmoles/10 mg wet weight, E_2R^+) or negative (E_2R^-).

A collaborative study with Ken Cutroneo at the University of Vermont Cancer Center indicates that elevated collagen synthesis, as had been suggested by animal studies (Cutroneo *et al.*, 1972), may be associated with early metastatic recurrence of human breast cancer.

SUMMARY

The metastatic process is a complex one whose mechanisms we are just beginning to approach. It is the objective of our prognostic study to measure a series of pathophysiological characteristics, many in the same tumors and all under controlled laboratory and clinical conditions; thus to elicit a pattern of decipherable interrelationships that will bring us closer to an understanding of this vital biological process.

We believe the system we have developed is a powerful one, capable of responding quickly and thoroughly, to evaluate new insights developed in our own and collaborating laboratories. The system has attracted considerable attention which in turn has provided us with expert guidance and consultation by many students of the metastatic process.

The Breast Cancer Prognostic Study will involve the detailed characterization of over a thousand tumors and their hosts. It has linked the operations of our cancer center with the medical community responsible for the care and management of breast cancer.

We are developing a family of tumor and host characteristics which by their prognostic information can provide a vastly improved capability for the management of the breast cancer patient. In addition, a broad systematic approach to the study of a single neoplastic disease offers an unprecedented opportunity to understand the mechanisms which may underlie the metastatic process for all cancers.

ACKNOWLEDGMENTS

Supported in part by a research grant (P01-CA-16175) awarded by the National Cancer Institute, DHEW, and an institutional grant from the United Foundation of Detroit. Principal segments of this Study are being carried out in the Suzanne Korman Morton Research Laboratory, and the Isabelle K. Albachten Memorial Laboratory.

REFERENCES

Allen, J., and Kessel, D. (1975). *Cancer Res. 35*, 670.

Bernacki, R., and Kim, U. (1977). *Science 195*, 577.

Black, M. M., and Spear, F. (1958). *Surg. Gynecol. Obstet. 105*, 97.

Black, M. M., Spear, F. D., and Opler, B. R. (1956). *Am. J. Chim. Path. 26,* 250.
Bloom, H.J.G. (1950). *Brit. J. Cancer 4,* 259.
Bloom, H.J.G., and Richardson, W. N. (1957). *Brit. J. Cancer 11,* 359.
Brennan, M. J., and McMahan, C. A. (1978). *In* "The Physiopathology of Cancer" (F. Hamburger, ed.), Vol.2. S. Karger. Basel.
Carbone, P. This volume.
Cavallo, T., Sade, R., Folkman, J., and Cotran, R. S. (1972). *J. Cell Biol. 54,* 408.
Cutroneo, K. R., Guzman, N. A., and Liebolt, A. G., (1972). *Cancer Res. 32,* 2828.
DeSombre, E. R., and Jensen, E. V. (1972). *In* "Biochemical Action of Hormones" (G. Litwalk, ed.). Academic Press, New York.
Folkman, J. (1974). *Advances in Cancer Res. 19,* 331.
Foote, F. W., and Stewart, F. W. (1946). *Surgery 19,* 74.
Greenough, R. B. (1925). *J. Cancer Res. 9,* 453.
Hirschl, S., Black, M., and Kwon, C. S. (1976). *Cancer 36,* 807.
Humber, R. L., Ferguson, D. J., and Coppleson, W. L. (1975). *Cancer 36,* 528.
Kessel, D., Chou, T. H., Furmanski, P., and Rich, M. A. (unpublished).
Knight, W. A., Livingston, R. E., Gregory, E. J., and McGuire, W. L. (1977). *Cancer Res. 37,* 4669.
McGuire, W. L., Carbone, R. P., and Volfmer, R. P. (1975). *In* "Estrogen Receptor in Human Breast Cancer." Raven Press, New York.
Patt, D. J. (1975). *Cancer 35,* 1388.
Rich, M. A., Furmanski, P., and Brooks, S. C. (1978). *Cancer Res. 38,* 4296.
Scarff, R. W., and Patey, D. N. (1928). *Lancet i,* 801.
Schiodt, T. (1966). "Breast Carcinoma." Munksgaard, Copenhagen.
Singhakowinta, A., Potter, H. G., Buroker, T. S., Samal, S., Brooks, S. C., and Vaitkevicius, V. (1976). *Ann. Surgery 183,* 84.
Sommers, S. C. (1969). *Cancer 23,* 822.
Spiegelman, S. This volume.
Weiss, L. (1977). "Fundamental Aspects of Metastasis." North-Holland, Amsterdam.

IN VIVO AND *IN VITRO* MODELS FOR TRANSFORMATION OF BREAST CELLS

Daniel Medina
B. B. Asch
B. Brinkley
and
M. L. Mace

Department of Cell Biology
Baylor College of Medicine
Houston, Texas

I. INTRODUCTION

Over the past two decades, evidence has indicated that mammary neoplasia, like most epithelial neoplasias, evolves from an initially altered cell or cell population that subsequently progresses through sequential changes in cellular and behavioral characteristics (Medina, 1976, 1978). The factors that contribute to the progression of neoplasms from their initial emergence were outlined by Leslie Foulds in his theory of neoplastic progression (Foulds, 1964). Basically, Foulds stated that neoplastic cell populations are continually progressing to a more anaplastic and simplified state, even after the neoplastic transformation. The basic mechanism that explains the phenomena of progression was outlined by the Kleins in a series of experiments on ascites conversion and antigenic variation of tumor cells (Klein and Klein, 1955; Klein *et al.*, 1960). They demonstrated that progression of neoplastic populations was due to the appearance of cell variants within the neoplastic populations and the subsequent selection for variants with a particular set of properties.

A similar concept can be invoked at the level of the initial alteration of normal mammary cells and their sequential progression through hyperplastic and eventually neoplastic states. This concept implies that hyperplasias can be populations comprised of multiple clones of altered cells, as well

ISBN 0-12-131150-3

as being mixtures of altered and normal cells. Furthermore, the pathogenesis of mammary neoplasia is not limited to two stages but is a continuum from normal to neoplasia. It is our intent to illustrate two points: (1) the multiple-stage character of the neoplastic transformation of the mammary gland, and (2) the basic proposition that much research on the neoplastic transformation has ignored the implication of neoplastic progression and thus has led to concepts that may have no application to primary neoplasms.

II. *IN VIVO* MODELS

A. *Induction of Mammary Precursor Lesions*

The current model of murine mammary cancer is shown in Fig. 1 and suggests that the pathogenesis involves multiple stages and multiple pathways. The major pathways progress through either alveolar hyperplasias (HAN) or ductal hyperplasias (DH). The keratinized nodules (KN) are conceived as being a specialized form of HAN that have a tremendous propensity for squamous metaplasia. Alveolar hyperplasias that subsequently produce mammary tumors can be selected from these KN. Plaques, which are found in GR and related strains of mice, are derived from ducts and are conceived to be benign tumors, not analogous to HAN or DH.

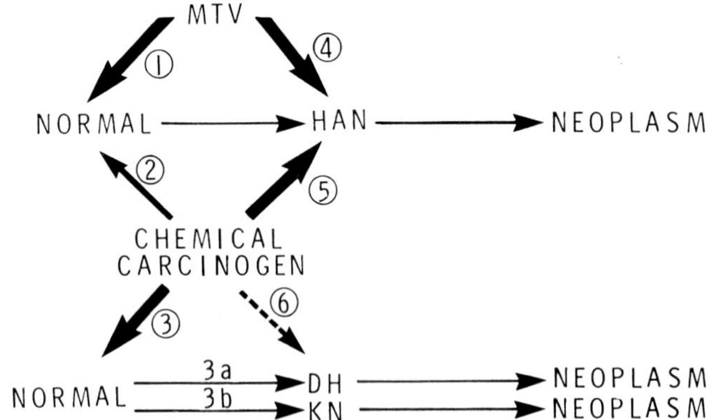

FIGURE 1. Scheme for mammary tumorigenesis in BALB/c mice. MuMTV induces primarily HAN (1) and chemical carcinogens such as DMBA induce primarily DH (3a), although DMBA can induce HAN (2) rarely and KN (3b) under special conditions. Both agents markedly enhance the HAN to tumor transformation (4) (5), but the effects of either of these agents on the progression of DH (6) is unknown.

The pathway through which the normal cell progresses is determined by the etiological agents and/or the differentiative state of the target cell. The MMTV (murine mammary tumor viruses) give rise primarily to HAN, whereas chemical carcinogens give rise to DH. Both MMTV and chemical carcinogens can enhance the nodule to tumor transformation, although it is not known whether this is a direct or indirect effect on the part of these carcinogens. Some data to support this concept are given in Table I. Mice of strains BALB/c, C57BL, and C3H/StWi exposed to DMBA, (7,12-dimethylbenzanthacene) develop predominately DH, whereas similar mice infected with MMTV develop predominately HAN. Exceptions to this general rule are seen in the occasional induction of HAN by DMBA in virgin mice, the presence of HAN in old retired breeders, the high frequency of KN in hormone-stimulated BALB/c mice treated with DMBA, and the presence of plaques, presumably ductal-derived in MMTV-positive GR mice. Whether the presence of HAN under these rare conditions is a consequence of the induction of endogenous MMTV by DMBA or hormones remains an interesting and unanswered question.

Both the alveolar and ductal hyperplasias have been demonstrated to give rise to mammary tumors upon transplantation into the cleared mammary fat pads of syngeneic mice. The results are shown in Table II. Since they give rise to tumors more frequently than normal mammary gland transplants, the hyperplasias are considered high risk or "preneoplastic" lesions.

In view of the preceding concepts, it is not surprising that the most frequent and tumorigenic precursor in chemical carcinogen-treated rat mammary gland is of ductal origin. The experiments by Sinha and Dao (1974), Haslam and Bern (1977), and Russo *et al.* (1977) have clearly demonstrated that rat mammary tumors arise from ducts, whereas HAN are weakly tumorigenic and probably represent a minor pathway. Several interesting questions however still remain to be answered with respect to the tumorigenic potential of HAN in rats. For instance, what frequency of primary HAN gives rise to hyperplastic outgrowths of tumors? Are tumors that do arise hormonally dependent or independent? Do HAN contain cells that have the potential for ductal proliferation? Can the technique of enzymatic dissociation enhance the rate of tumor formation or select out cell populations with different developmental potentials?

B. HAN to Tumor Progression

The recent work by Miyamoto *et al.* (1975) has shown clearly that in MMTV-positive systems, cells with the potential for producing HAN outgrowths are present by two months of age, at least six months before HAN can be detected *in situ*. This result raises questions regarding the type of factors involved in

TABLE I. Effect of Chemical Carcinogens and MuMTV on Mammary Dysplasias

Strain	Carcinogen (Mg)	Incidence of Dysplasias[a] HAN	%	DH	%	Reference
BALB/c	MMTV	14/61	23	0/61	0	Medina et al., 1970
BALB/c	DMBA (6)	0/30	0	16/30	53	Medina, unpublished
C3H/StWi	MMTV	11/12	92	0/12	0	Medina, unpublished
C3H/StWi	DMBA	0/15	0	11/15	73	Smith et al., 1978
C57BL	MMTV	19/22	86	N.D.		Nandi et al., 1966
C57BL	DMBA (6)	1/5	20	3/5	60	Medina, unpublished
C57BL	Urethan (200)	0/12	0	9/12	75	Medina and Warner, 1976

[a]Incidence = number of mice with dysplasias over the total number of mice examined by observation of stained whole mount preparations of the mammary glands.

TABLE II. Tumor Potential of Mammary Outgrowth Lines Established from HAN and DH

Line	Type outgrowth	No. tumors / No. transplants	%	TE_{50} (weeks)[a]
D1	Alveolar	21/109	19	--
D2	Alveolar	46/85	57	46
CD-8	Ductal	47/65	72	18
HD-7	Ductal	88/133	66	35

[a]*Time for 50% of the transplants to produce mammary tumors after transplantation into the mammary fat pads.*

the regulation of the expression of HAN and the progression of HAN to tumors. One would predict that the hormonal milieu of the host is important in the expression of HAN and their progression to tumors, but the nature of this effect is unknown. Also, since the mammary gland is comprised of a heterogeneous cell population, one might speculate that normal mammary epithelial or myoepithelial cells might regulate the expression and progression of HAN or DH. Slemmer (1974) has proposed that the progression of premalignancy to malignancy is associated with the loss of normal cells in the progressing tumor cell population. Experiments to demonstrate the potential role of normal cells on progression of HAN are shown in Table III. The data were interpreted to demonstrate that normal mammary cells can inhibit the neoplastic progression in HAN cell populations. In retrospect, this result is not overly surprising since it was demonstrated by Faulkin and DeOme (1960) that the growth and progression of HAN can be inhibited by adjacent normal mammary gland cells. Is HAN a mixture of neoplastic and normal cells; a mixture of altered, nonneoplastic cells and normal cells; or a mixture of several different populations of altered, nonneoplastic cells with various morphological, biological, and neoplastic potentials? In order to answer this question, stage-specific markers need to be available to analyze the different cell populations.

TABLE III. *Effect of Normal Mammary Cells on Tumor Potentials of Nodule Lines D2 and D1*

Type of normal tissue	Ratio of (nodule/normal)	No. tumors / No. transplants	%	TE_{50} (months)
---	Control (10^5 D2 cells)	14/14	100	3.8
Pregnant	1:1	13/23	57	8.0[a]
---	Control (10^5 D2 cells)	11/16	69	7.0
Lactating	1:3	6/20	30	---[b]
---	Control (10^5 D2 cells)	15/20	75	5.8
Virgin	1:3	7/19	37	---[a]
---	Control (10^5 D1 cells)	10/17	59	9.0
Lactating	1:3	2/15	14	---[b]
---	Control (10^5 D1 cells)	8/18	44	---
Virgin	1:3	3/17	18	---[b]

[a]Data were calculated nine months after cells were transplanted.
[b]Data were calculated ten months after cells were transplanted.

III. *IN VITRO* STUDIES

One way to approach the analysis of different cell populations is to examine and compare normal, HAN and neoplastic cells in primary monolayer cell cultures. The comparison of these cell populations against each other and against established *in vitro* mammary tumor cell lines affords the opportunity to characterize unique properties of neoplastic or HAN cells. In particular, the use of primary tumors rather than established cell lines avoids the pitfalls of looking at cell characteristics that may be present in a minority cell population or that are present as a result of cell adaptation to prolonged exposure to atypical environmental constraints.

Table IV shows some characteristics of *in vitro* transformed cells that are often associated with neoplastic cells. Almost without exception, these characteristics were developed using

TABLE IV. Properties of Transformed Cells In Vitro

Morphological
Changes in cell size and appearance[a]
Changes in staining properties[a]
Growth
Loss of parallel orientation[a]
High saturation density[a]
Different (usually reduced) serum requirements[a]
Acquisition of anchorage independent growth[a]
Growth on monolayers of other cells[a]
Loss of contact inhibition of cell division and movement[a]
Tumor formation in vivo
Surface
Increased agglutinability by plant lectins
Changes in composition of glycoproteins and glycolipids
Loss of cell surface proteins (LETS)
Absence of tight junctions
Reappearance of fetal proteins
Increased rate of transport of nutrients
Appearance of tumor-specific antigens
Chromosomal
Heteroploid chromosome complement

[a]*Indicates markers used to select or identify* in vitro *transformed cells.*

cells of mesenchymal or embryonic origin. In contrast, mammary epithelial cells show few differences in *in vitro* growth characteristics (Hosick, 1974; Das *et al.*, 1974; Voyles and McGrath, 1976), morphological characteristics (Pickett *et al.*, 1975), and certain cellular characteristics (Asch, 1977; Asch *et al.*, 1978). In a series of experiments, normal, HAN, and neoplastic cells in primary monolayer cell culture were compared with respect to light microscopy, surface topography, lectin agglutination, and cytoskeletal organization. Figure 2 shows light microscopy of the three cell populations as well as a culture of fibroblasts from cleared fat pads. No differences in saturation density, cell orientation, shape, size, and nuclear number, were seen in the three types of epithelial cell cultures. The culture of epithelial cells were clearly different from that of fibroblast cells. Scanning microscopy of the three cell populations (Fig. 3) revealed extensive similarities in surface topography, type and distribution of microvilli, and flatness of cells as compared to the unusual and complex surface topography seen in established mammary tumor cell lines. Indirect immunofluorescence staining for microtubule and actin-containing filaments using antibodies against tubulin and actin, respectively, demonstrated that the distribution of positive and negative cells was similar for the three cell types (Fig. 4), indicating that epithelial cells from primary mammary tumors did not behave like transformed fibroblasts. Finally, the ability of the three cell populations to exhibit concanavalin A(Con A)-mediated hemadsorption was the same for the three cell populations and much less than for the established mammary tumor cell lines (Table V).

The above data are consistent with the results of others (Hosick, 1974; Das *et al.*, 1974; Voyles and McGrath, 1976; Pickett *et al.*, 1975; Anderson and Hosick, 1977) who have reported that normal and transformed mammary cells in monolayer culture exhibit similar growth characteristics, production of plasminogen activator, and maintenance of specialized cell junctional complexes. Furthermore, Table VI demonstrates that the three different cell culture populations retain their developmental and morphogenetic potentials when transplanted back into the cleared mammary fat pads of syngeneic mice. Normal cells in culture produced ductal outgrowth. HAN cells produced hyperplastic alveolar outgrowth and, subsequently, mammary tumors at the same rate as dissociated uncultured cells, and tumor cells produced rapidly growing invasive tumors by three weeks after transplantation.

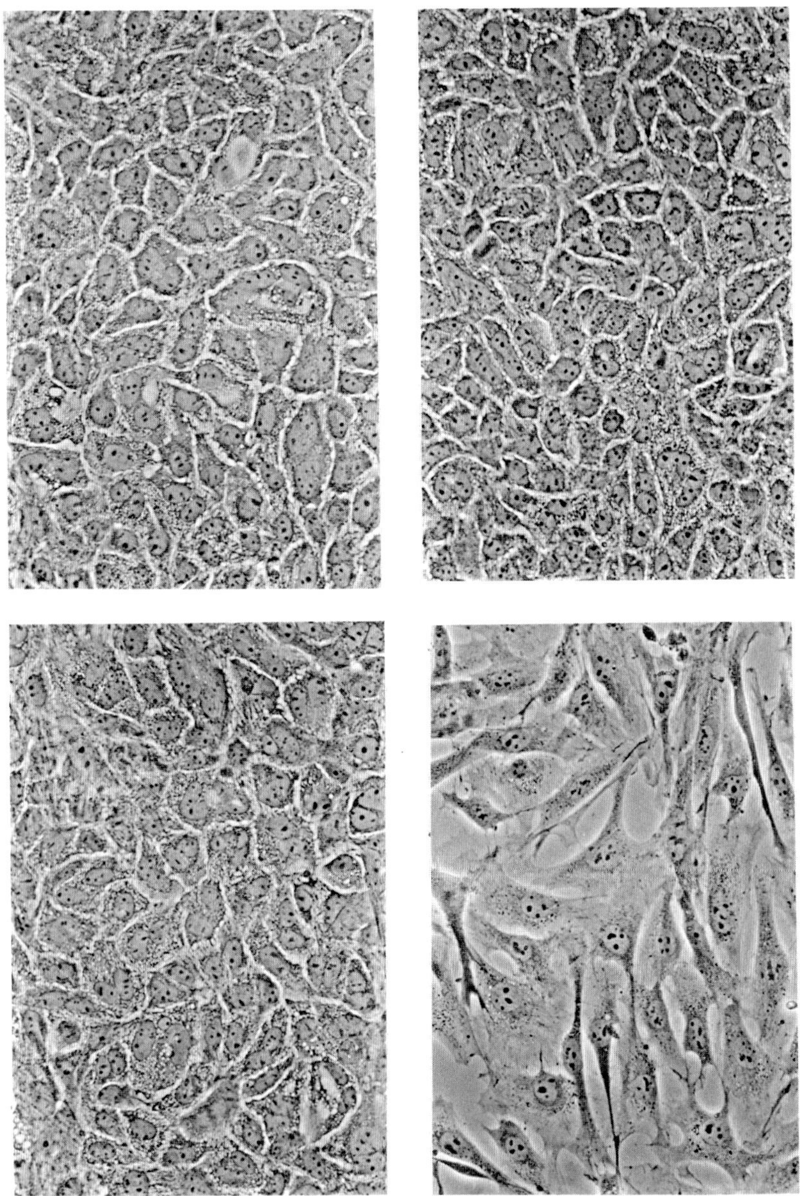

FIGURE 2 Light microscopy of mammary cells in primary cultures. Figure 2a shows mammary epithelial cells from normal (a), D2 HAN outgrowth (b), and D2 tumor (c), and fibroblasts from a cleared mammary fat pad (d). All cell cultures were four days postseeding. X190. From Asch et al., *1979, by permission of Waverly Press, Inc., and Cancer Research, Inc.*

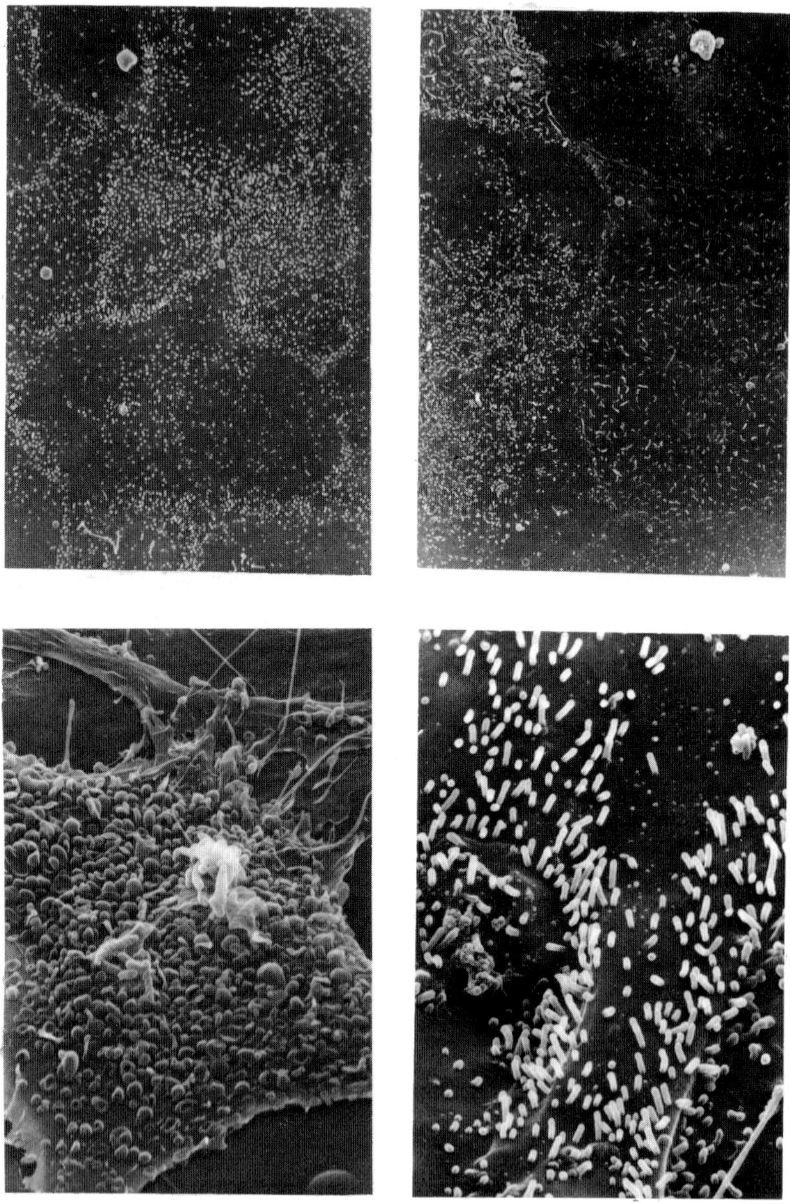

FIGURE 3. Scanning electron microscopy of mammary cells in primary cultures. Shows surface topography of normal cells (a: X1933), D2 tumor cells (b: X1933), an established cell line (c: X2677), and a higher magnification or normal cells (d: X7436).

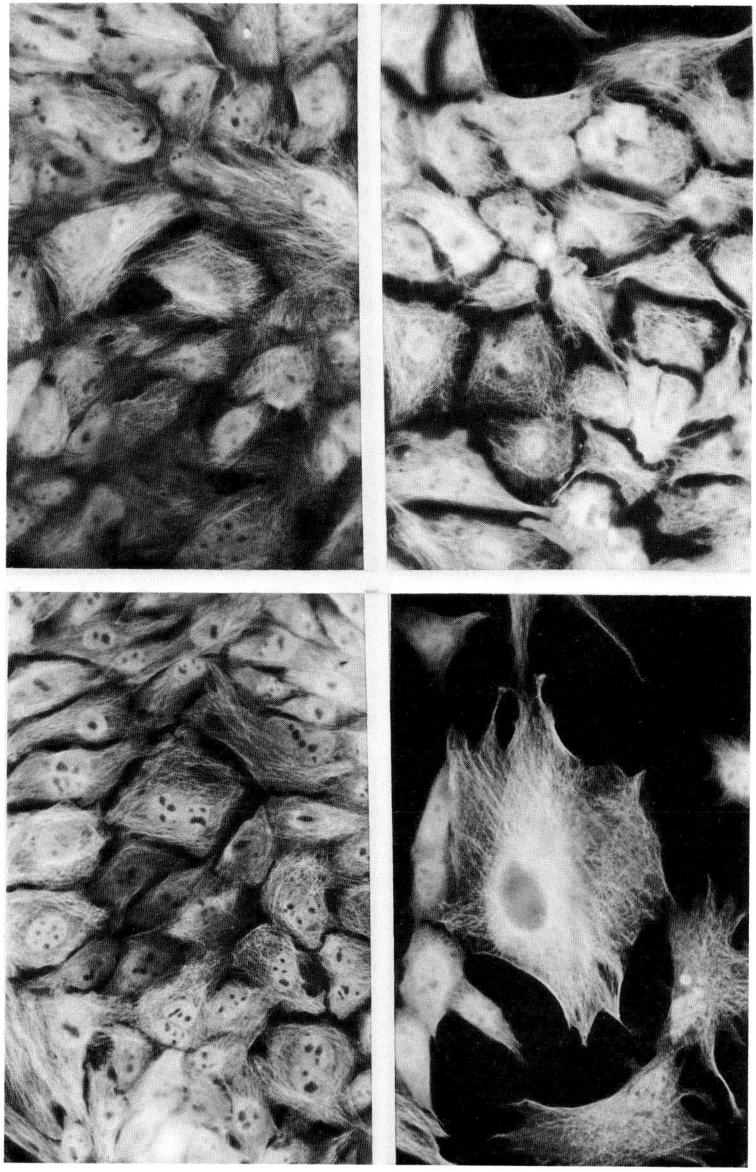

FIGURE 4. Indirect immunofluorescent staining for microtubules. Shows presence of intact and abundant microtubules in mammary cells from normal (a), D2 Han (b), D2 tumor (c), and an established mammary tumor cell line (d). X380. From Asch et al., 1979, by permission of Waverly Press, Inc., and Cancer Research, Inc.

TABLE V. Agglutinability of Normal, Preneoplastic and Neoplastic Mouse Mammary Cells by Concanavalin in A[a]

Cell type	Lectin concentration (μg/ml required for agglutination)		
	Threshold	1/2 Maximal	Maximal
Normal	25	500	>500
D2HAN	50	500	>500
D2 Tumor	25	500	>500
BESD/C13	12.5	50	≤200
MTV-L/C12	≤12.5	25	100
DMBA/BALB	6	6	100

[a]The hemadsorption procedure developed by Furmanski et al. (1972) as modified by Asch and Medina (in press) was used to determine Con A agglutinability of mammary cells.

TABLE VI. Tumorigenic Potential of Mammary Epithelial Cells Grown as Primary Monolayer Cell Cultures

Tissue	*Outgrowth* in vivo	*No. tumors* / *No. transplants*	*%*	$\overline{X}$ *time of tumor appearance (weeks)*
Normal	*Ductal*	*0/20*	*0*	---
HAN	*Hyperplastic alveolar*	*23/28*	*82*	*26*
Neoplastic	*Tumor*	*10/10*	*100*	*3*

IV. CONCLUSION

Several important points emerge from the above results that deserve further comment. First, it is clear from a variety of reports, as well as those mentioned, that transformed mammary epithelial cells *in vitro* do not show the same morphological, cellular, and growth characteristics as do transformed cells of mesenchymal or embryonic origin. Secondly, the use of established *in vitro* cell lines, like serially transplanted tumors *in vivo*, may yield results and concepts on the nature of the neoplastic cell that have little bearing on the characteristics of the neoplastic cell in the primary tumor. The characteristics of the neoplastic cells in established cell lines may be due to selection by environmental pressures and/or to neoplastic progression of cells with a unique set of characteristics. It becomes important then to attempt to validate on cells from primary tumors and appropriate normal controls those observations pertaining to the neoplastic state that were developed from studies on established cell lines. One would predict that the closer to the primary tumor observations are made, the more applicable the observations will pertain to unique characteristics of the neoplastic state. Finally, it is clear that the task of developing stage specific markers to examine the types of cells in the preneoplastic cell population is going to be difficult and time consuming. However, the elucidation of the cellular nature of the "preneoplastic" state promises a better understanding of the pathogenesis of mammary neoplasia.

REFERENCES

Anderson, L. W., and Hosick, H. L. (1977). *J. Cell Biol. 75,* 2, 85a.
Asch, B. B. (1977). *Proc. Am. Assoc. Cancer Res. 18,* 96.
Asch, B. B., and Medina, D. (1978). *J. Natl. Cancer Inst. 61,* 1423-1430.
Asch, B. B., Brower, M. E., and Brinkley, B. R. (1978). *Proc. Am. Assoc. Cancer Res. 19,* 267.
Das, N. K., Hosick, H. L., and Nandi, S. (1974). *J. Natl. Cancer Inst. 52,* 849-861.
Faulkin, L. J., Jr., and DeOme, K. B. (1960). *J. Natl. Cancer Inst. 24,* 953-969.
Foulds, L. (1964). *In* "Cellular Control Mechanisms and Cancer" (P. Emmelot and O. Mühlbock, eds.), pp. 242-258. Elsevier, Amsterdam.
Furmanski, P., Phillipo, P. G., and Lubin, M. (1972). *Proc. Soc. Exp. Biol. Med. 140,* 216-219.
Haslam, S. Z., and Bern, H. A. (1977). *Proc. Natl. Acad. Sci. 74,* 4020-4024.
Hosick, H. L. (1974). *Cancer Res. 34,* 259-261.
Klein, G., and Klein, E., (1955). *Exp. Cell Res. Suppl. 3,* 218.
Klein, E., Klein, G., and Hellstrom, K. E. (1960). *J. Natl. Cancer Inst. 25,* 271.
Medina, D. (1976). *Cancer Research 36,* 2589-2595.
Medina, D. (1978). *In* "Experimental Breast Cancer" Vol. II (W. L. McGuire, ed.). Plenum Press, New York.
Medina, D., and Warner, M. R. (1976). *J. Natl. Cancer Inst. 57,*331-337.
Medina, D., Young, L., and DeOme, K. B. (1970). *J. Natl. Cancer Inst. 44,* 167-174.
Miyamoto, M. J., DeOme, K. B., and Osborn, R. C. (1975). *Proc. Am. Assoc. Cancer 66,* 57.
Nandi, S., Handin, M., Robinson, A., Pitelka, D. R., and Webber, L. E. (1966). *J. Natl. Cancer Inst. 36,* 783-801.
Pickett, P. B., Pitelka, D. R., Hamamoto, S. T., and Misfeldt, D. S. (1975). *J. Cell Biol. 66,* 316-332.
Russo, J., Saby, J., Isenberg, W. M., and Russo, I. H. (1977). *J. Natl. Cancer Inst. 59,* 435-445.
Sinha, D., and Dao, T. L. (1974). *J. Natl. Cancer Inst. 53,* 841-846.
Slemmer, G. (1974). *J. Invest. Dermatol. 63,* 27-47.
Smith, G. H., Pauley, R. J., Socher, S. H., Medina, D. (1978). *Cancer Res. 38* (in press).
Voyles, B. A., and McGrath, C. M. (1976). *Int. J. Cancer 18,* 498-509.

ENDOCRINOLOGIC ASPECTS OF BREAST CANCER

ESTROGEN RECEPTORS AND THE HORMONE DEPENDENCE OF BREAST CANCER

Eugene R. DeSombre
Geoffrey L. Greene
and
Elwood V. Jensen

Ben May Laboratory for Cancer Research
University of Chicago
Chicago, Illinois

I. INTRODUCTION

Evidence for the hormone dependence of human breast cancer spans more than three-quarters of a century, but it is only in the last decade that basic knowledge about the features of hormone-dependent tissues and appropriate laboratory techniques for characterizing them have become available. In the late nineteenth century, Beatson (1896) reported the remission of premenopausal breast cancer following oophorectomy. The modern age of endocrine treatment for breast cancer commenced with the classic report of the efficacy of adrenalectomy in the treatment of postmenopausal breast cancer patients (Huggins and Bergenstal, 1952). This was followed by reports showing the benefits of hypophysectomy (Luft *et al.*, 1958; Ray and Pearson, 1958) in similar breast cancer patients. Breast cancer response rates to both types of ablative endocrine surgery in the postmenopausal patients are about 25 to 30% and appear to be of similar magnitude to the response rates to oophorectomy in the premenopausal breast cancer patients. A number of more recent trials of endocrine additive therapy with various agents indicate similar proportions of patients respond to this type of endocrine therapy. Therefore, it is evident that while endocrine therapy is a very useful and effective treatment for those patients who respond, fewer than one-third of all metastatic breast cancer patients will receive objective benefit from such treatment. Hence, a practical laboratory method for

ISBN 0-12-131150-3

differentiating hormone-dependent and hormone-independent breast cancer has been a goal for the last several decades. As knowledge of the nature of the estrogen interaction with its target tissues expanded, the sophistication and accuracy of assay methods improved. The original data from our laboratory (Jensen *et al.*, 1971) has subsequently been extended and supported by work in a number of laboratories throughout the world (for a compilation see McGuire *et al.*, 1975) and attests to the usefulness of the assay of estrogen receptors as a guide to the selection of patients for endocrine therapies for breast cancer. This chapter will briefly review the scientific basis for the estrogen receptor assay, discuss our most recent clinical correlations of response showing the importance of the quantitative levels of cytosol estrogen receptor, summarize data concerning the use of the estrogen receptor assay in the primary tumor, and, finally, present information about the use and specificity of our recently obtained antibody to the estrogen receptor protein.

II. INTERACTION OF ESTROGENS WITH TARGET TISSUES

Investigations of the last two decades have led to the recognition of the principal characteristics of the interaction of estrogens with target cells (Jensen and DeSombre, 1973; O'Malley and Means, 1974; Gorski and Gannon, 1976). The general features of this interaction are shown in Fig. 1. Estrogen (E) enters the cell, apparently by passive diffusion, and readily associates with its receptor protein, called estrophilin (Jensen *et al.*, 1974), (R_C) present in excess in the cytoplasm. The association of hormone with receptor endows the resulting complex with an important new property, namely, its ability to undergo a temperature-dependent, steroid-specific activation. Such an activation step has now been identified in a number of different steroid hormone-receptor systems. In the case of estrogens, the receptor activation can be identified by the change in sedimentation rate of the estrogen receptor complex (ER_N); in high salt sucrose gradients, the activated cytosol complex, in similarity with the receptor complex extracted from the nucleus, moves with a sedimentation coefficient of about 5S, clearly distinguished from the native cytosol 4S complex (Jensen *et al.*, 1968). A second important new characteristic of the activated, or nuclear-type, estrogen-receptor complex is its ability to enter the nucleus and bind to acceptor sites of the chromatin. In some as yet not clearly understood process, the nuclear uptake and binding of the estrogen-receptor complex leads to increased biosynthetic activity of the hormone-dependent cell. It has been found that the

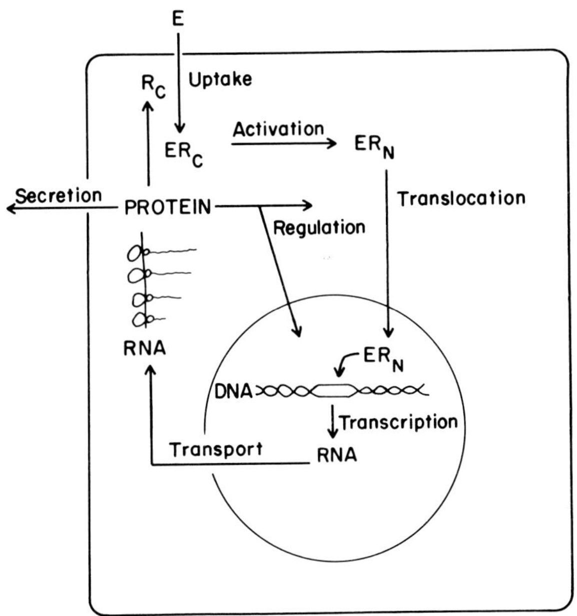

FIGURE 1. General representation of estrogen interaction pathway and biochemical responses in target cells.

activated estrophilin complex can effect a target-tissue specific increase in RNA polymerase I activity *in vitro* (Jensen *et al.*, 1974). While the effect, if any, of estrophilin on the processing and transport of RNA in the target cell is not known, *in vivo* the hormone leads to increased protein synthesis. Some of these newly synthesized proteins, such as glycolytic enzymes, are required for the increased metabolic activity of the growing tissue. Others, such as the steroid receptor proteins themselves, are directly involved in the further hormonal regulation of the target cells. Thus in the target cell, both normal and neoplastic, the cytosol estrophilin appears to be the major determinant for the activity of estrogen on the genome. Nonetheless, cytosol estrophilin, while necessary for estrogen action, is not an unfailing indicator of hormone dependence, at least in tumor cells. With DMBA-induced rat mammary tumors, some, but not all, hormone-independent tumors may contain substantial amounts of cytosol estrophilin, capable of estrogen-dependent, nuclear transmigration (Boylan and Wittliff, 1975). It appears that despite the nuclear uptake of the estrophilin complex by such hormone-independent tumors, the nuclei do not respond with the increased RNA synthesis seen with the hormone-dependent tumors (Arbogast and DeSombre, 1974).

III. HORMONE DEPENDENCY OF HUMAN BREAST CANCER

A. *Sedimentation Assay for Estrogen Receptors*

Although the first reported uptake of tritiated estrogen by human breast cancer tissue involved administration of the labeled estrogen *in vivo* prior to ablative surgery (Folca *et al.*, 1961), it indicated the potential of studying the uptake of labeled estrogen by the cancer tissues. A more practical *in vitro* assay, based on the uptake of tritiated estradiol in the presence or absence of an antiestrogen by slices of the breast cancer tissue in physiological buffer, also appeared to provide useful results (Jensen *et al.*, 1971) but also suffered from several disadvantages, in particular, requiring substantial amounts of fresh tumor.

After recognition that the basis for the *in vivo* and *in vitro* uptake and retention of estrogen in target tissues was the cytoplasmic estrogen receptor, more sensitive and reliable methods based on actual assay of cytosol estrophilin were developed. In 1966, Toft and Gorski had reported the application of sedimentation analytical methods to characterization of the cytosol receptor of rat uterus. We found that sedimentation analysis of breast cancer cytosols for specific estradiol binding components was a sensitive and reliable technique to identify estrogen receptors in human breast cancer tissue (Jensen *et al.*, 1971). Furthermore, since only small amounts of tissue were required and, under proper conditions, the tissue could be stored frozen prior to analysis, this method overcame the two major limitations of the earlier uptake technique. For sedimentation analysis, aliquots of the cytosol fraction of a breast cancer homogenate are incubated at 2°C with tritiated estradiol in the presence or absence of a competitor of receptor binding, such as CI628, diethylstilbestrol, or estradiol itself and, after layering on 10-30% sucrose gradients, subjected to centrifugation for about 16 hr at 250,000 x g. Following sedimentation, the sucrose gradients are fractionated and the tritium profile in the gradients determined by scintillation counting (DeSombre *et al.*, 1974). Inhibitable DPM in the 8S and 4S regions of the gradient correspond to the H^3 estradiol-estrophilin complex.

Although a number of simpler, less expensive analytical techniques have been developed in recent years for the detection of breast cancer cytosol estrophilin, sucrose gradient techniques have provided the most consistent correlation of estrophilin with clinical response (McGuire *et al.*, 1975). There was an early suggestion that the sedimentation nature of the cytosol estrophilin, whether 8S or 4S, may be of prognostic significance (Wittliff and Savlov, 1975) even though both sedimentation forms show the same affinity and steroid specificity. Data from our laboratory however, have not confirmed any such prognostic differences as related to sedimentation rate of estrophilin (DeSombre and Jensen, 1978).

B *Quantitative Clinical Correlations*

Early attempts to correlate the clinical response to endocrine therapy both in our laboratory (Jensen *et al.*, 1971, 1972, 1973; DeSombre *et al.*, 1974) and elsewhere (Maass *et al.*, 1973; Leung *et al.*, 1973; McGuire *et al.*, 1975) did not appreciate the possible significance of the quantitative level of cytosol estrophilin in breast cancer tissue. Despite the relative insensitivity of the earliest techniques for assay of estrophilin, the early clinical correlations showed that most, but not all, of the patients with estrophilin-containing cancers responded to endocrine therapy while very few patients whose tumors lacked estrophilin responded. With the widespread use of more sensitive analytical techniques such as sedimentation analysis and dextran-coated charcoal assays with Scatchard plots of the data, and in particular with the availability of tritiated estradiol of substantially higher specific activity, it became possible to detect smaller amounts of estrophilin. This changing situation took on added relevance when in 1974 investigators attending the Breast Cancer Task Force workshop on estrogen receptors in human breast cancer reported that a higher percentage of human breast cancers contained detectable estrophilin (McGuire *et al.*, 1975) than was previously evident. While the proportion of estrophilin-positive breast cancers reported at that workshop ranged up to over 80%, it was still evident that only 25 to 30% of the patients overall responded to endocrine therapy. Therefore with the increased detectability of estrophilin, the accuracy of the prediction of clinical response to endocrine treatment appeared to suffer.

We had been impressed with the large range of the estrophilin concentration in breast cancer, and at that workshop reported that those patients with low, but clearly detectable, levels of cytosol estrophilin did not in general respond to endocrine therapy (Jensen *et al.*, 1975). The relationship between the quantitative level of tumor cytosol estrophilin and endocrine response rate is particularly evident with postmenopausal patients as shown in Fig. 2. As expected, the 37 patients whose tumors have no cytosol estrophilin or barely detectable amounts (<100 fmole/g) do not have a significant response rate to endocrine therapy. What is more impressive is that the patients whose tumors contain low but distinct levels of estrophilin (100-750 fmole/g) have no better chance of remission than the estrophilin-poor cancer patients. Moreover, while a tumor estrophilin content of more than 750 fmole/g

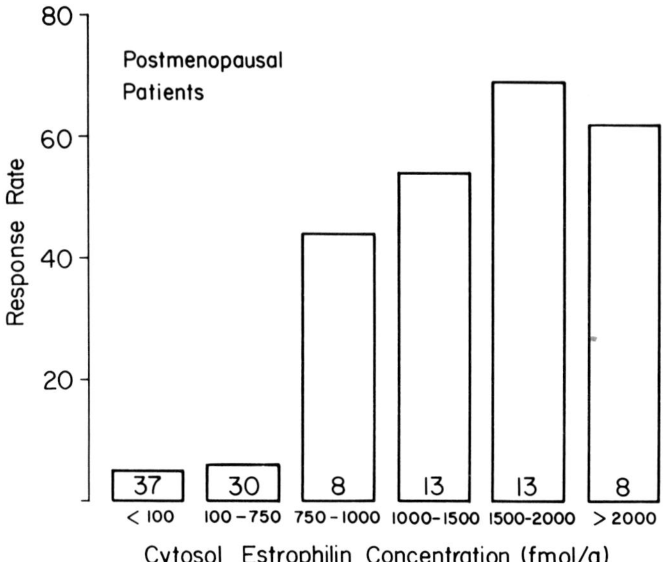

FIGURE 2. Relation of quantitative breast cancer cytosol estrophilin content and postmenopausal patient response rate to endocrine therapy. The number inside each bar shows the total number of patients in that group. (DeSombre et al., *1978).*

would seem to presage a better chance for response, the trend seen in Fig. 2 suggests that in general the response rate improves with increasing concentration of estrophilin. It is interesting that studies on the presence of progesterone receptors in human breast cancer, suggested by Horwitz *et al.* (1975), as a biologic indicator of an active estrogen receptor pathway and hence a predictor of endocrine response, have shown an increasing proportion of progesterone receptor-positive tumors with increasing tumor estrophilin content (McGuire *et al.*, 1977).

When one examines the cytosol estrophilin levels in the breast cancers of the 160 patients for whom we have evaluable clinical data on response to endocrine therapy (Fig. 3), it is apparent that the estrophilin content of the tumors in premenopausal patient tends to be significantly less than that of the postmenopausal or castrate patient. Concomitantly, the apparent critical level of estrophilin separating the group of endocrine-responsive patients from the nonresponders appears also to be less in premenopausal patients (300 fmole/g vs. 750

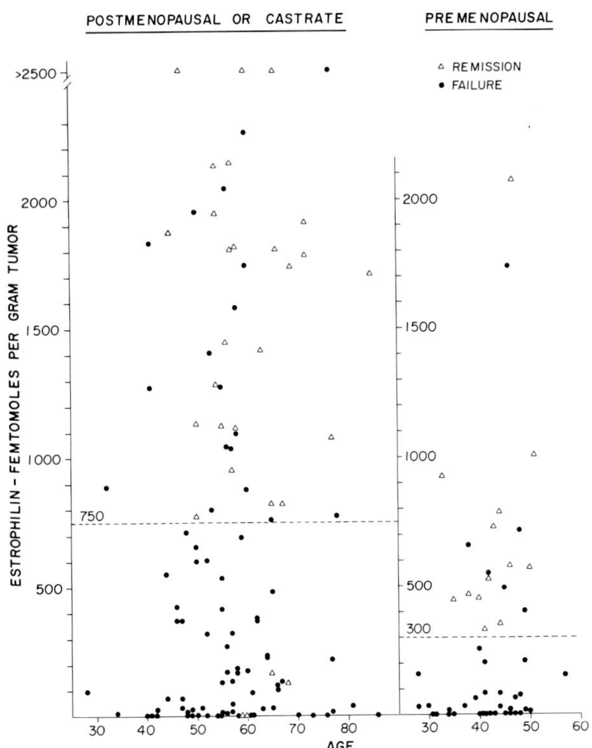

FIGURE 3. Correlation of tumor cytosol estrophilin content with response to endocrine therapy for 160 patients with metastatic breast cancer. Estrophilin assay by sedimentation analysis of tumor cytosol with 0.5 nM tritiated estradiol. (From DeSombre et al., *1978).*

fmole/g in postmenopausal patients). It is possible that, due to endogenous estrogen in the premenopausal patient, a significant proportion of the cytosol estrophilin may have been translocated to the nucleus and thus not measured by the assay methods employed. Of most importance, however, is the empirical observation that for both premenopausal and postmenopausal patients one can define an apparent critical level of estrophilin, separating the tumors into estrophilin-rich and estrophilin-poor categories, thereby improving the predictability of endocrine response and hence the usefulness of the assay. In the four years since our original suggestion at the Estrogen Receptor Workshop that one could empirically define a critical level of estrophilin to improve the usefulness of the assay

TABLE I. Remissions to Endocrine Therapy

	ER-rich[a]	ER-poor[a]
Ablation		
Adrenalectomy	4/6[b]	0/20[b]
Adrenalectomy + oophorectomy	14/19	1/17
Hypophysectomy	2/4	0/9
Oophorectomy	9/12	1/30
Total ablation: 117	29/41 (71%)	2/76 (3%)
Hormone		
Androgen	0/1	0/4
Estrogen	4/5	1/9
Estrogen + Progestin	5/13	1/18
Antiestrogen	1/2	0/1
Total hormone: 53	10/21 (48%)	2/32 (6%)
Total cases: 170	39/62 (63%)	4/108 (4%)

[a]*Based on the critical estrophilin levels shown in Fig. 3.*
[b]*Objective remissions/total cases.*

(Jensen *et al.*, 1975), the number of evaluable patients has increased from 98 to 170 while the concept of the critical level has not changed.

Up to the present, 170 patients, whose breast cancers have been analyzed for estrophilin content, have been treated by endocrine therapies and evaluated for objective response. The data from these patients are presented in Table I. Of the 170 patients, 43 experienced objective remission to various types of endocrine therapy, a response rate of about 25%, similar to the general experience of the last 20 yr where patients were unselected for endocrine therapy of metastatic breast cancer. In the group treated by ablation all but two of the patients experiencing objective remissions were in the estrophilin-rich category. The probability of response to ablative therapy for patients with estrophilin-rich tumors was found to be 71% and, considering the relatively small numbers of patients in some of the groups, there did not appear to be any significant differences in response rates among the various ablative procedures. The overall accuracy of response prediction to endocrine ablation based on the critical level of estrophilin was 88% (29 + 74 of 117). Fifty-three patients were treated by hormone additive therapy and, although the overall response rate (12/53 or 22.6%)

and the prediction accuracy (10 + 30 of 53 or 75%) were somewhat lower in this group than in the patients treated by ablation, the remissions also were largely restricted to the patients with estrophilin-rich cancers.

The foregoing results clearly indicate that patients with estrophilin-poor tumors have little chance (4%) for objective benefit from endocrine therapy while nearly two-thirds of patients with estrophilin-rich tumors will experience remissions. The overall utility of the critical level of estrophilin for prediction of response to a variety of endocrine treatments is suggested by the 84% prediction accuracy for the 170 patients evaluated in this way.

C *Use of Mastectomy Specimens*

Since in most cases a sufficient quantity of the primary breast cancer is available for estrophilin assay whereas samples of the metastatic lesions may be hard to obtain at time of recurrence, it is of considerable importance to determine how well the estrophilin assay of the mastectomy specimen would predict response to endocrine therapy at time of recurrence, often up to several years later. While a large number of assays are now being performed on mastectomy samples for this purpose, there is little published information documenting how useful such assays are. Our study, which has accumulated 34 evaluable patients, is presented in Table II. These results are encouraging since they show that the cytosol estrophilin assay of the primary tumor predicted the correct clinical response to endocrine therapy in 29 of the 34 patients. Nine of the 13 patients with estrophilin-rich primary tumors (69%) responded to endocrine therapy, even though the interval between mastectomy and treatment of recurrent disease was quite long in some cases. The correlation with ablative therapy (six of seven) was especially good. Only one of the 21 patients with estrophilin-poor primary breast cancer later responded to endocrine therapy. Interestingly, the single responding patient had the longest time to recurrence, over 5 1/2 yr.

It has been pointed out earlier that patients with estrophilin negative or estrophilin-poor tumors tend to show an earlier recurrence than those whose tumors are estrophilin-rich (Knight *et al.*, 1977; DeSombre *et al.*, 1978). The data from the patients presented in Table II are consistent with such a finding; the median time to recurrent disease for the patients with estrophilin-rich tumors (24 mos.) was twice as long as the median recurrence time for the estrophilin-poor group (11 mos.). In view of the fact that not all stage I and II breast cancer patients treated by mastectomy will recur, there has been an understandable reluctance to enter all such

TABLE II. Use of Estrophilin Assay of Mastectomy Specimen for Predicting Response after Recurrence

ER rich 9/13			ER poor 1/21		
Rx[a]	Months[b]	Response	Rx[a]	Months[b]	Response
O	49	R	E	67	R
O	46	R	O	60	F
Ord	36	F	An	31	F
Ad	29	R	EP	27	F
EP	26	R	EP	25	F
EP	26	F	EP	18	F
E	24	F	Ord	16	F
E	24	R	Ord	15	F
O	23	R	AdO	12	F
AdO	14	R	H	12	F
E	9	F	O	11	F
AdO	5	R	An	10	F
E	1	R	AdO	8	F
			Ord	8	F
			Ord	7	F
Ablation 6/7			O	7	F
			EP	7	F
Hormone 3/6			E	4	F
			E	1	F
			EP	0[c]	F
			E	0[c]	F

[a]AdO, adrenalectomy plus oophorectomy; An, androgen; E, estrogen; EP, estrogen + progestin; H, hypophysectomy; O, oophorectomy; Ord, radiation castration.

[b]Time between mastectomy and treatment of recurrent disease.

[c]Patients had evidence of distant metastases at time of mastectomy so treatment was started immediately. The patients progressed from stage III to IV on treatment.

patients onto adjuvant chemotherapy, especially with possibly leukemogenic agents. If the data on the relation of estrophilin to recurrence rate hold up in a large series of patients, it would allow one to delineate a subgroup of the mastectomy patients with a higher risk, i.e., the node-positive patients with estrophilin-poor tumors, who might be better candidates for adjuvant chemotherapy than simply unselected node-positive patients.

IV. ANTIBODY TO ESTROGEN RECEPTOR

A. *Background*

Although, as summarized earlier in this chapter, a critical level of estrophilin appears to be necessary for breast cancer hormone response, the biologic basis for the empirically determined critical levels is not yet clear. Since small amounts of estrophilin have been detected in classically estrogen-independent cells (Jensen and DeSombre, 1972), it is possible that a minimum or critical, cellular concentration of receptor is necessary for hormone dependence. Alternatively, in analogy to the transplantable, hormone-responsive GR mouse mammary tumor system, where the decrease in estrogen receptor content from generation to generation correlates with increasing hormone independence and appears to reflect a decrease in the proportion of hormone-responsive cells in the tumor (Sluyser *et al.*, 1976), the quantitative estrophilin content in a human breast cancer specimen may simply relate to the proportion of hormone-dependent cells in the specimen. To provide evidence relative to these two alternatives, it would be of considerable value to be able to detect estrophilin in individual cells or pathologic sections. Such capability could be provided by antibody to estrophilin, one goal of our research for several years. Furthermore, estrophilin antibody could be the basis for an estrophilin radioimmunoassay, which should readily detect estrogen receptor whether or not it complexed with hormone.

For preparation of antibody, the nuclear estrophilin-tritiated estradiol complex was purified from calf uterus by salt extraction, ammonium sulfate precipitation, gel filtration, and polyacrylamide gel electrophoresis as previously described (DeSombre and Gorell, 1975; Greene *et al.*, 1977). The estrophilin complex used in the immunizations contained from 10 to 30% of the tritiated estradiol expected for the binding of one estradiol per receptor protein of 70,000 daltons. The immunization of 6-month old New Zealand white rabbits with the purified nuclear estrophilin complex was by the intradermal procedure of Vaitukaitas *et al.*, (1971).

B. *Reactivity and Specificity*

The initial evidence for antibody to estrophilin was obtained with serum from a rabbit that had received six booster injections over the course of almost one year after the initial immunization. In subsequent animals, which received estrophilin of higher purity, antibody was seen earlier. Evidence for specific antibody to estrophilin has been obtained from four approaches (Greene *et al.*, 1977). For each of these studies the estrophilin complex has been quantitated by virtue of the tritiated estradiol associated with it. The techniques used are double antibody precipitation, adsorption of estrophilin complexes by immunoglobulin bound to Sepharose, binding of estrophilin complex to immobilized *Staphylococcus aureus* protein A in the presence of immune globulins, and immune globulin-induced changes in sedimentation rate and gel elution volume of the estrophilin complexes.

Because the interaction of antibody with estrophilin forms a nonprecipitating complex, investigations on the characteristics of the antibody can conveniently be carried out by sedimentation analysis. The interaction of the immunoglobulin of the estrophilin-immunized rabbit with calf uterus nuclear estrophilin-tritiated estradiol complex is shown in Fig. 4. This estrophilin complex, in the original nuclear extract, is essentially an unrefined version of the antigen used to immunize the rabbit. As is apparent from Fig. 4, while the 5S receptor complex is essentially unaffected by incubation with immunoglobulin from a normal rabbit, after incubation with the immunoglobulin from the estrophilin-immunized animal all the tritiated estradiol sediments further down the gradient. These faster sedimenting moieties apparently represent ternary complexes of estrophilin-estradiol with the antibodies. The antibody to estrophilin does not interact with estradiol (Greene *et al.*, 1977). Although the antibody was raised against purified calf nuclear estrophilin, it nonetheless recognizes and strongly interacts with estrophilin from calf cytosol (Fig. 5). Under the high salt conditions used for the experiment illustrated in Fig. 5, the cytosol estrophilin-estradiol complex itself sediments in the 4S region whereas, after incubation with specific antibody, the complex moves beyond the 7S region. Under low salt conditions, where the cytosol estrophilin-estradiol complex appears in the 8S region, the interaction with antibody leads to a 10 to 12S moiety.

The antiestrophilin antibody does not interact with any other steroid receptors studied thus far, specifically androgen or progestin receptors. However, it does detect and react with estrophilin from a variety of species and tissues (Green *et al.*, 1977). In particular the antibody to the calf uterine nuclear estrophilin interacts with cytosol estrophilin from calf, rat, mouse, rabbit, sheep and guinea pig uterus, the transplantable rat endometrial tumor line, U15, and the pituitary tumor line $C_2$9RAP, both tumors obtained from the laboratory of Dr. Carlos Sonnenshein. The antibody does not interact with estradiol associated with nonspecific binding components such as bovine serum albumin and rat α-fetoprotein. It therefore appears to be specific for estrogen receptors whatever source or type.

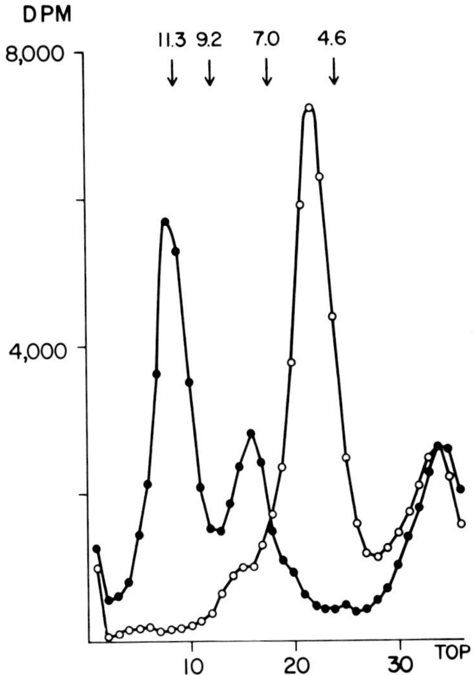

FIGURE 4. Sedimentation pattern of calf nuclear estrophilin complex incubated with estrophilin antibody. Nuclear estrophilin tritiated estradiol complex, extracted with 400 mM KCl from washed nuclear sediment which had been incubated with tritiated estradiol and calf uterine cytosol at 25°C, was incubated with immunoglobulin from normal rabbit serum (o) or from estrophilin-immunized rabbit serum (●) and analyzed by sedimentation analysis on high salt (400 mM KCl) sucrose gradients. Arrows indicate sedimentation positions of the protein markers, bovine serum albumin (4.6S), bovine immunoglobulin (7.0S), β-amylase (9.2S), and catalase (11.3S) run in a separate gradient tube. For experimental details see Greene et al., *1977.*

C. Interaction with Breast Cancer Estrophilin

It was of considerable interest to us to determine whether the estrophilin antibody also interacts with estrophilin of mammary cancers. As shown in Fig. 6, the antibody completely reacts with the cytosol estrophilin complex of the DMBA-induced rat mammary tumor. It is of interest that, in this tumor from an estrogen-treated adult female rat, the cytosol estrophilin sedimented largely as the 4S form that did not change to 8S in

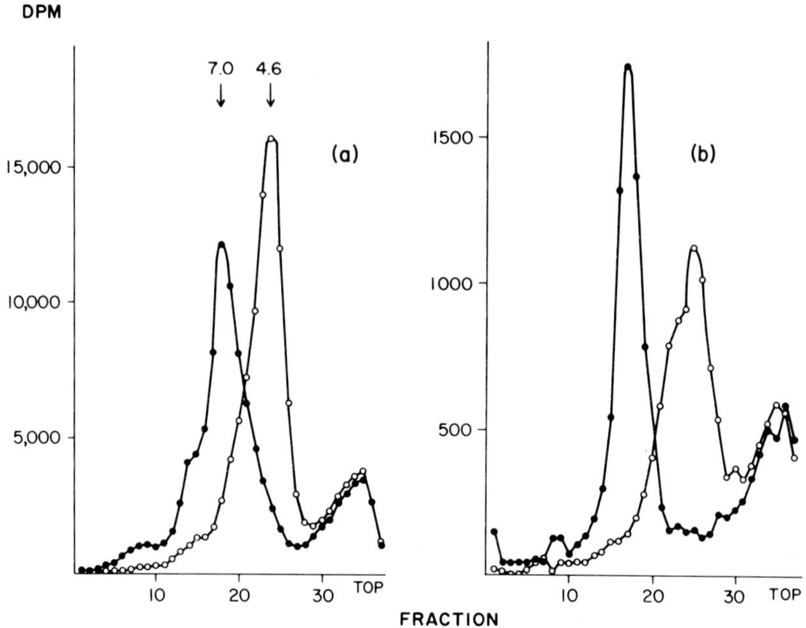

FIGURE 5. Sedimentation patterns of cytosol estrophilin from calf uterus and human breast cancer incubated with estrophilin antibody. Cytosols prepared from 250 mg/ml homogenates of (a) minced calf uterus in 10 mM Tris pH 7.4 and (b) frozen powder of a human breast cancer in the same buffer but including also 0.5 mM dithiothreitol, were incubated with tritiated estradiol followed by incubation with immunoglobulin from normal rabbit serum (o) or from estrophilin-immunized rabbit serum (•) and sedimentation analysis in 10-30% sucrose gradients containing 400 mM KCl (high salt). For details see Greene et al., *1977.*

low salt gradients. Nonetheless, under both high and low salt conditions this rat mammary tumor estrophilin appeared to interact completely with the antibody.

The estrophilin antibody also reacts with human breast cancer estrophilin. As shown in Fig. 5, using high salt sedimentation analysis, the cytosol, tritiated estradiol-estrophilin complex of the human breast cancer, sedimenting in the 4S region in the presence of IgG from a nonimmune rabbit, is converted to a faster sedimenting complex after incubation with IgG from the immunized rabbit. As is evident in Fig. 5, antiestrophilin antibody interacts very similarly with cytosol estrophilin from calf uterus and human breast cancer.

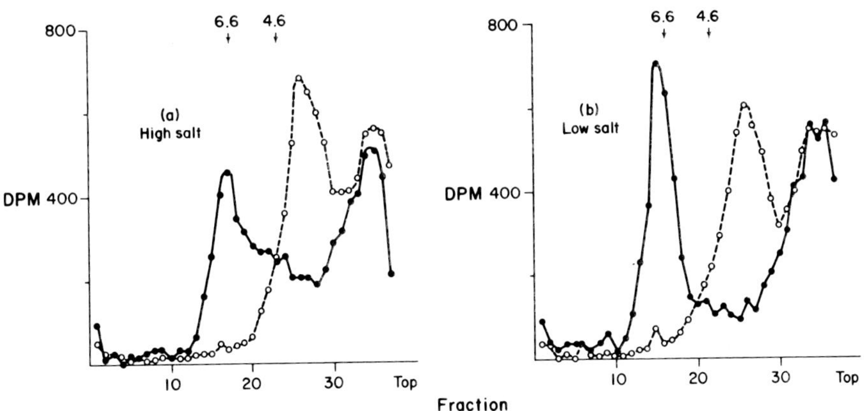

FIGURE 6. Sedimentation analysis of rat mammary tumor cytosol estradiol-estrophilin complex incubated with estrophilin antibody. An intact female rat bearing a DMBA-induced mammary tumor was given 2 μg unlabeled estradiol at 68, 44, and 20 hr prior to sacrifice. The tumor was removed, frozen, thawed, minced, homogenized in 10 mM Tris pH 7.4 buffer and centrifuged at 253,000 x g to obtain the cytosol fraction. The cytosol was incubated with 2.5 nM tritiated estradiol followed by treatment with dextran-coated charcoal to remove unbound steroid, and then incubated with immunoglobulin from normal rabbit serum (o) or estrophilin-immunized rabbit serum (o). The mixtures were layered on 10-30% sucrose gradients in 10 nM Tris, pH 7.4 buffer with 1.5 mM EDTA containing (a) high salt, 400 mM KCl, or (b) low salt, 10 mM KCl, centrifuged 16 hr at 253,000 x g, fractionated and tritium determined by scintillation counting. Cytosol incubated with excess diethylstilbestrol (not shown) was also analyzed to demonstrate that the sedimentation peaks shown represented specific estrophilin binding. The sedimentation markers, bovine serum albumin (4.6S) and rabbit immunoglobulin (6.6S), were run in a separate gradient tube.

Considerable interest has been generated by the availability of certain well-characterized human breast cancer cell lines. In particular the MCF-7 cell line is being actively investigated in a number of laboratories, especially with regard to hormone action in breast cancer. Since this human breast cancer cell line has for some time been recognized as having estrogen receptor (Brooks *et al.*, 1973), we were interested to see if our estrophilin antibody would show a similar interaction with it. Fig. 7 illustrates that the antibody completely shifts the sedimentation of the MCF-7 estrophilin-estradiol complex from the 3.6S region to the 7S region under high salt conditions. Similar sedimentation profiles have been obtained with the nuclear estrophilin complex extracted from the nuclei of cells incubated with tritiated estradiol (DeSombre *et al.*, 1978), as well as by addition of tritiated estradiol to the "free" nuclear estrophilin. Thus the estrophilin antibody interacts with all characterized forms of the MCF-7 cell line estrogen receptor, human breast cancer estrophilin as well as the rat mammary tumor estrogen receptors. This antibody would therefore appear to be well suited to use for the development of various new technologies for breast cancer estrophilin detection and quantitation based on immunochemistry.

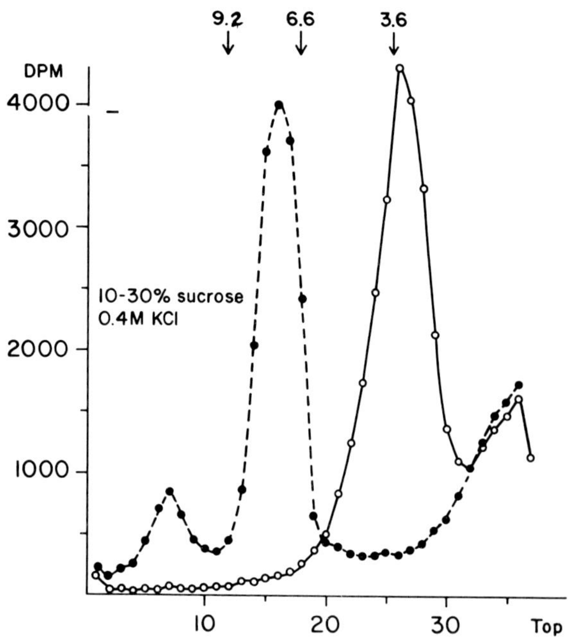

FIGURE 7. Interaction of MCF-7 cytosol estrogen-receptor complex with estrophilin antibody. MCF-7 cytosol, saturated with tritiated estradiol by 2°C incubation with excess steroid followed by treatment with dextran-coated charcoal to remove unbound estradiol, was incubated in the cold with immunoglobulin from normal rabbit serum (o) or from estrophilin-immunized rabbit serum (●) prior to sedimentation analysis on high salt (400 mM KCl) sucrose gradients as described by DeSombre et al., *1978. Arrows indicate sedimentation position of ^{14}C-labeled ovalbumin (3.6S), rabbit immunoglobulin (6.6S), and amylase (9.2S) run in a separate gradient tube.*

SUMMARY

Estrogen target tissues in general are characterized by their significant concentration of estrogen receptor, called estrophilin, which appears to be intimately involved in the tissue response to the hormone. Knowledge of the content of estrophilin in breast cancer specimens has proved to be of considerable clinical value. Although most breast cancer specimens contain at least some estrophilin, only those patients whose cancer contains moderate to high concentrations of cytosol estrophilin appear to respond to endocrine therapy. Prediction of patient response to such therapy based on the critical level of estrophilin appears to be over 80% correct in our series of 170 metastatic patients.

Estrophilin assay of the mastectomy specimen in our smaller series of 34 patients shows a similar prediction success rate for response to endocrine therapy at time of recurrence, despite the often extended time between mastectomy and treatment of disseminated disease. These data also provide additional support for the suggestion that patients with estrophilin-poor cancers may have a shorter disease-free interval than patients with estrophilin-rich tumors.

Rabbit antibody to purified calf uterine nuclear estrogen receptor has been found to react not only with both cytosol and nuclear estrophilin from uteri of a number of species but has been found to interact with rat mammary tumor and human breast cancer cytosol estrophilin. All forms of estrophilin of the human breast cancer cell line, MCF-7, also react with this estrophilin antibody.

ACKNOWLEDGMENTS

These investigations were supported by the National Cancer Institute, grants PO1 CA 14599 and CA 09183 as well as contract CB-43969 from the Breast Cancer Task Force.

REFERENCES

Arbogast, L. Y., and DeSombre, E. R. (1975). *J. Natl. Cancer Inst. 54,* 483-485.

Beatson, G. T. (1896). *Lancet 2,* 104-107.

Boylan, E. S., and Wittliff, J. L. (1975). *Cancer Res. 35,* 506-511.

Brooks, S. C., Locke, E. R., and Soule, H. D. (1973). *J. Biol. Chem. 248,* 6251-6253.

DeSombre, E. R., and Gorell, T. A. (1975). *In* "Methods in Enzymology" (B. W. O'Malley and J. G. Hardman, eds.), Vol. 36, Part A, pp. 349-365. Academic Press, New York.

DeSombre, E. R., and Jensen, E. V. (1979). *Rev. Endocrine Related Cancer,* in press.

DeSombre, E. R., Smith, S., Block, G. E., Ferguson, D. J., and Jensen, E. V. (1974). *Cancer Chemother. Rep. 58,* 513-519.

DeSombre, E. R., Greene, G. L., and Jensen, E. V. (1978). *In* "Hormones, Receptors, and Breast Cancer" (W. L. McGuire, ed.), pp. 1-14. Raven Press, New York.

Engelsman, E., Persijn, J. P., Korsten, C. B., and Cleton, F. J. (1973). *Brit. Med. J. 2,* 750-752.

Folca, P. J., Glascock, R. F., and Irvine, W. T. (1961). *Lancet 2,* 796-798.

Gorski, J., and Gannon, F. (1976). *Annu. Rev. Physiol. 38,* 425-450.

Greene, G. L., Closs, L. E., Fleming, H., DeSombre, E. R., and Jensen, E. V. (1977). *Proc. Natl. Acad. Sci. 74,* 3681-3685.

Horwitz, K. B., McGuire, W. L., Pearson, O. H., and Segaloff, A. (1975). *Science 89,* 726-727.

Huggins, C., and Bergenstal, D. M. (1952). *Cancer Res. 12,* 134-141.

Jensen, E. V., and DeSombre, E. R. (1972). *Annu. Rev. Biochem. 41,* 203-230.

Jensen, E. V., and DeSombre, E. R. (1973). *Science 182,* 126-134.

Jensen, E. V., Suzuki, T., Kawashima, T., Stumpf, W. E., Jungblut, P. W., and DeSombre, E. R. (1968). *Proc. Natl. Acad. Sci. 59,* 632-638.

Jensen, E. V., Block, G. E., Smith, S., Kyser, K. A., and DeSombre, E. R. (1971). *Natl. Cancer Inst. Monograph 34,* 55-70.

Jensen, E. V., Block, G. E., Smith, S., and DeSombre, E. R. (1972). *In* "Estrogen Target Tissues and Neoplasia" (T. L. Dao, ed.), pp. 23-57, University of Chicago Press, Chicago.

Jensen, E. V., Block, G. E., Smith, S., and DeSombre, E. R. (1973). *In* "Breast Cancer: A Challenging Problem" (M. L. Griem, E. V. Jensen, J. E. Ultmann, and R. W. Wissler, eds.), pp. 55-62. Springer-Verlag, Heidelberg.

Jensen, E. V., Mohla, S., Gorell, T. A., and DeSombre, E. R. (1974). *Vit. Hormones 32,* 89-127.

Jensen, E. V., Polley, T. Z., Smith, S., Block, G. E., Ferguson, D. J., and DeSombre, E. R. (1975). *In* "Estrogen Receptors in Human Breast Cancer" (W. L. McGuire, P. P. Carbone, and E. P. Vollmer, eds.), pp. 37-55. Raven Press, New York.

Knight, W. A., Livingston, R. B., Gregory, E. J., and McGuire, W. L. (1977). *Cancer Res. 37*, 4669-4671.

Leung, B. S., Fletcher, W. S., Lindell, T. D., Wood, D. C., and Krippaehne, W. W. (1973). *Arch. Surg. 106*, 515-519.

Luft, R., Olivecrona, H., Ikkos, D., Nilsson, L. B., and Mossberg, H. (1958). *In* "Endocrine Aspects of Breast Cancer" (A. R. Currie, ed.), pp. 27-35. E and S Livingston, Edinburgh.

Maass, H., Engel, B., Hohmeister, H., Lehmann, F., and Trams, G. (1972). *Am. J. Obstet. Gynecol. 113*, 377-382.

McGuire, W. L., Carbone, P. P., and Vollmer, E. P., editors (1975). "Estrogen Receptors in Human Breast Cancer." Raven Press, New York.

McGuire, W. L., Horwitz, K. B., Pearson, O. H., and Segaloff, A. (1977). *Cancer 39*, 2934-2947.

O'Malley, B. W., and Means, A. R. (1974). *Science 183*, 610-620.

Ray, B. S., and Pearson, O. H. (1958). *In* "Endocrine Aspects of Breast Cancer" (A. R. Currie, ed.), pp. 36-45. E and S Livingston, Edinburgh.

Sluyser, M., Evers, S. G., and DeGoeij, C. C. (1976). *Nature 263*, 386-389.

Toft, D., and Gorski, J. (1966). *Proc. Natl. Acad. Sci. 55*, 1574-1581.

Vaitukaitis, J., Robbins, J. B., Nieschlag, E., and Ross, G. T. (1971). *J. Clin. Endocrinol. Metab. 33*, 988-991.

Wittliff, J. L., and Savlov, E. D. (1975). *In* "Estrogen Receptors in Human Breast Cancer" (W. L. McGuire, P. P. Carbone, and E. P. Vollmer, eds.), pp. 73-86. Raven Press, New York.

Zava, D. T., and McGuire, W. L. (1977). *J. Biol. Chem. 252*, 3703-3708.

ESTROGEN AND ANTIESTROGEN ACTION IN HUMAN BREAST CANCER: ROLE OF NUCLEAR ESTROGEN RECEPTOR PROCESSING

*K. B. Horwitz**
and
W. L. McGuire

Department of Medicine
The University of Texas Health Science Center
San Antonio, Texas

I. INTRODUCTION

Since the original identification of cytoplasmic estrogen receptors (ER) in human breast cancer (Jensen *et al.*, 1971; Jensen and DeSombre, 1972), rapid progress has been made towards linking the presence of the receptor with endocrine responsiveness of the tumor. It is now known that the likelihood of a successful response to endocrine therapy is increased at least 10-fold in patients whose tumors are positive for ER (McGuire *et al.*, 1975). However, not all ER-containing tumors respond, and this has led to the concept that ER are necessary but not sufficient markers of hormone dependence.

We have demonstrated progesterone receptors (PgR) in human breast tumors (Horwitz *et al.*, 1975a) and have proposed that this receptor, whose synthesis is known to be controlled by estrogen in the uterus, might serve as a marker of estrogen action in breast cancer (Horwitz *et al.*, 1975b). Thus, the presence of PgR in a tumor would indicate that the entire sequence involving estrogen binding to cytoplasmic receptor, movement of the receptor complex into the nucleus, and stimulation of a specific end product can be achieved in the tumor cell, and would rule out the existence of a defect beyond the binding step.

**Present address: University of Colorado Medical Center, Department of Medicine, Denver, Colorado.*

ISBN 0-12-131150-3

Though this proposal assumes that PgR are under control of estrogen acting through ER, this priming effect has not been demonstrated in human breast cancer. We have used the MCF-7 human breast cancer cell line to study the response of PgR to estrogens and antiestrogens. The MCF-7 cell line derived from a patient with metastatic breast cancer (Soule *et al.*, 1973) is ideally suited to study the mechanism of PgR induction. These cells are in permanent tissue culture, contain estrogen receptors (Brooks *et al.*, 1973; Horwitz *et al.*, 1975a) and are estrogen responsive (Lippman *et al.*, 1976). Cells grown without estradiol have low PgR levels (Horwitz *et al.*, 1975a). MCF-7 cells have an unusual estrogen receptor distribution; unfilled receptor sites can be demonstrated in the cytoplasm (Rc) and are also associated with nuclei (Rn) (Zava and McGuire, 1977; Zava *et al.*, 1977). This chapter summarizes our recent work in this model system, which shows that PgR are under estrogen control and that PgR synthesis involves the estrogen receptor. We have also studied the effects of antiestrogens and find that tamoxifen is a potent inducer of progesterone receptor (PgR) in these cells. This estrogenic property (Leavitt *et al.*, 1977) of tamoxifen is masked at very high doses (1 nM), which also inhibit cell growth. Another antiestrogen, nafoxidine, has by contrast, little if any effect on PgR when tested over a wide dose range. The fact that growth inhibitory effects of both antiestrogens can be reversed by estradiol (Zava *et al.*, 1977; Lippman *et al.*, 1976) suggests that the effects of these compounds are mediated through the estrogen receptor system.

Furthermore, we describe (Horwitz and McGuire, 1978a,b) a complex response system in these cells in which estrogen receptor binding, translocation, and turnover of nuclear receptors or their "processing" mediate induction of PgR by estradiol. Though antiestrogens can bind and translocate Rc and bind Rn, the subsequent nuclear receptor processing step is partially (tamoxifen) or completely (nafoxidine) impaired. This may explain the differential effect of these two antiestrogens on PgR induction.

II. ESTRADIOL: EFFECTS ON PgR MEDIATED THROUGH THE ESTROGEN RECEPTOR

A. *Binding, Translocation, and Processing of ER*

Fig. 1 shows, in general outline, the reactions we have studied in estrogen treated cells. Estradiol enters the cell and binds to unfilled receptor sites that are found both in cytosol (Rc) or more or less firmly associated with nuclear

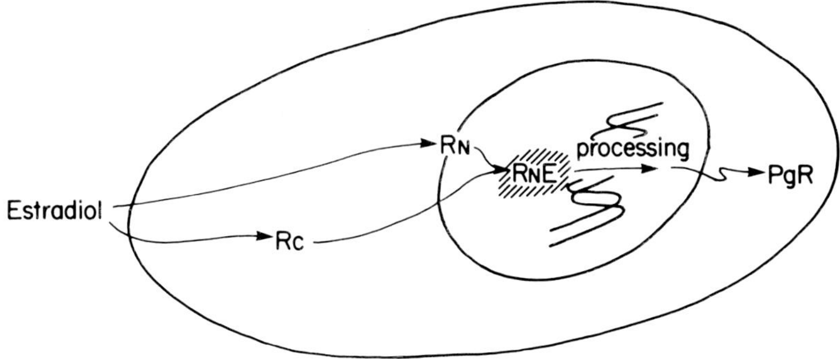

FIGURE 1. Model of estradiol effect on ER in human breast cancer cells.

components (Rn). The newly formed hormone receptor complex is rapidly translocated to sites in the nucleus from which it can only be extracted with buffers of high ionic strength (RnE). Bound nuclear receptors then undergo rapid turnover or "processing"; within 3 to 5 hr, 70% or more of RnE sites are lost from the cells without reappearance of unfilled sites. Much later (a period of several days for progesterone receptor induction) we see formation of specific products or effects on growth or DNA synthesis.

The data from an experiment in which we follow these movements and changes in estrogen receptor levels are shown in Fig. 2. The untreated cells (C) have approximately half their unfilled sites associated with the nucleus (Rn) and half in the cytoplasm (Rc). There are no filled nuclear sites (RnE). Within 5 min of 10^{-8} M estradiol addition, Rc and Rn are no longer measurable and all cellular receptors appear in the nucleus bound to estradiol. Starting at about 30 min and continuing for 3 to 5 hr, we see a progressive loss of RnE. Processing is essentially complete by 5 hr; thereafter RnE levels stabilize at the new steady state level as long as the cells are kept on estradiol. If the hormone is removed (Horwitz and McGuire, 1978) there are several effects: The binding of estradiol as RnE is remarkably prolonged. At least some estrogen always remains bound to nuclear receptors even eight days after the hormone has been removed. However, in addition unfilled cytoplasmic and nuclear sites are restored. Restoration of cell ER cannot be explained by loss of E from the nuclear receptor followed by redistribution of the newly emptied sites. Instead, both cytoplasmic receptors (Rc) and nuclear receptors (Rn) are clearly being synthesized *de novo,* and this synthesis is reflected in the restoration of total cellular ER.

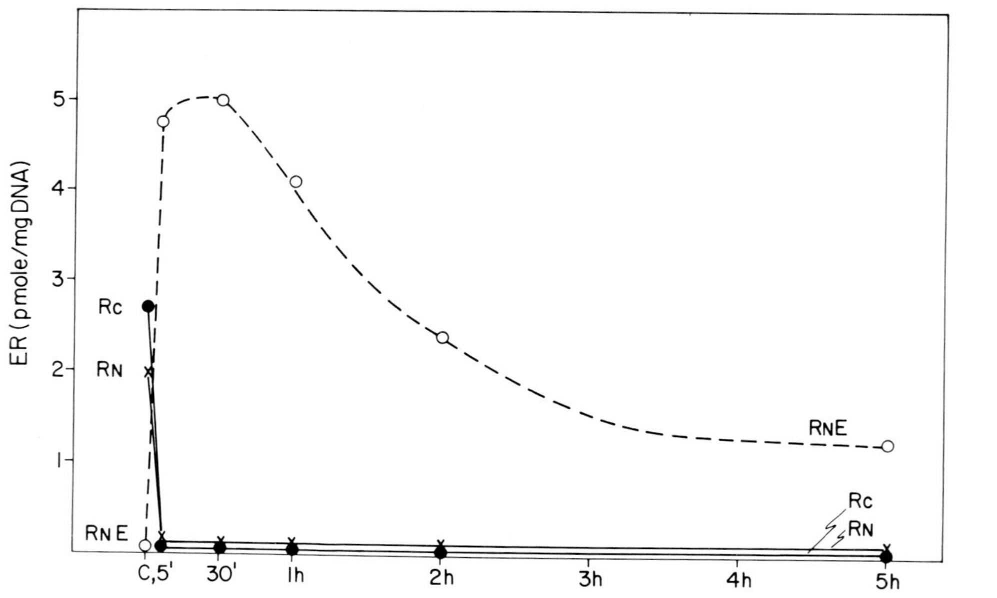

FIGURE 2. Effect of estradiol on estrogen receptor distribution in MCF-7 cells. Cells were treated for the times indicated with 10 nM estradiol added to MEM containing stripped calf serum, insulin, hydrocortisone and prolactin. Control flasks received the same medium without estradiol. Cytoplasmic and nuclear estrogen receptors were measured by the single saturating dose protamine assay (Zava and McGuire, 1977). Values have been corrected for nonspecific binding. Unoccupied cytoplasmic receptors (●, Rc, 4°C incubation), unoccupied nuclear receptors (x, Rn, 4°C incubation), occupied nuclear receptors (o, RnE, 30°C–4°C incubations). (Adapted from Horwitz and McGuire, 1978, submitted.)

B. ER Processing and Estradiol Dose

The extent of receptor loss during processing depends on the dose of estradiol, as shown in Fig. 3. The cells grown on estrogen-free medium have approximately equal levels of Rc and Rn. With increasing doses of estradiol there is progressive depletion of these unfilled sites. At 0.1 nM only 15% of sites

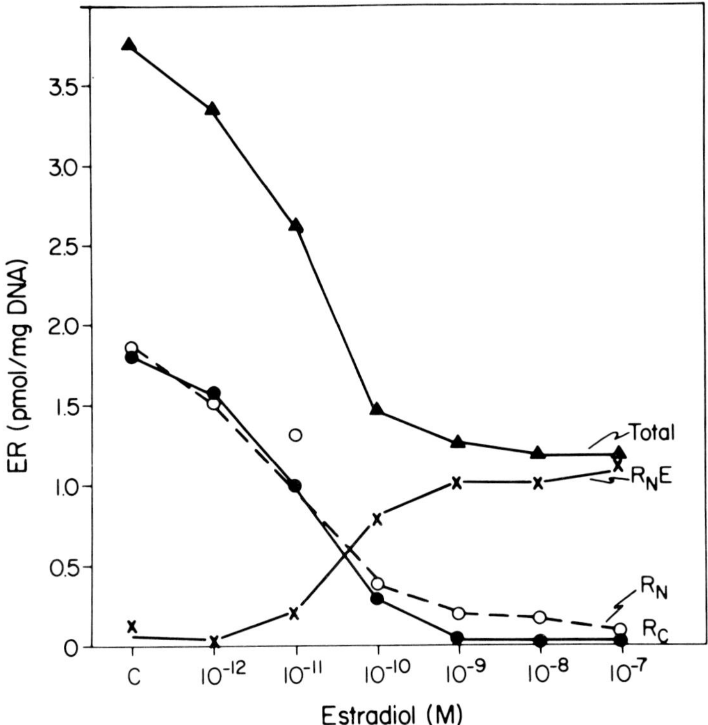

FIGURE 3. Effect of estradiol on estrogen receptor distribution in MCF-7 cells. Cells (four T-75 flasks per treatment group) were treated four days with increasing estradiol concentrations (0.001 to 100 nM) added to MEM containing stripped calf serum, insulin, hydrocortisone and prolactin. Control flasks received the same medium without estradiol. Cytoplasmic and nuclear estrogen receptors were measured by the single saturating dose protamine assay described in Fig. 2. Values have been corrected for nonspecific binding. Unoccupied cytoplasmic receptors (●, Rc, 4°C incubation), unoccupied nuclear receptors (o, Rn, 4°C incubation), occupied nuclear receptor (x, RnE, 30°C - 4°C incubations), total cell receptors (▲, Rc + Rn + RnE). (From Horwitz and McGuire, 1978.)

remain unfilled and virtually complete depletion occurs at higher doses. Rc does not remain in the cytoplasm in bound form (RcE, 30°C incubation; not shown) or in cytoplasmic organelles (0.6*M* KCl extract of high speed pellet). We conclude that Rc is translocated to the nucleus while Rn sites are filled so that all receptor is in the nucleus in bound form (RnE).

However, the quantity of RnE measured at different doses varies. After four-day treatment at the lower doses, though Rc and Rn decrease, there is little accumulation of occupied nuclear receptors (RnE). Instead total cellular receptors (Rc + Rn + RnE) are progressively lower. At the higher estradiol doses, free cytoplasmic and nuclear receptors are entirely depleted but total receptor levels (as RnE) are only 30% of total cell receptor present in controls. There appears to be a limit to amount of receptor loss, however, so that at higher doses RnE accumulation occurs.

C. ER Processing and PgR Induction

Figure 4 compares the amount of ER that is processed at different estradiol doses with the amount of progesterone receptor induced. The extent of free receptor binding and processing parallels PgR induction. Induction is incomplete at low doses if receptor binding and processing is incomplete, reaches a maximum at 0.1 nM when RnE processing is maximal, and is not increased further by accumulation of unprocessed RnE. This suggests that processing may be an essential step in induction of a specific protein by estradiol. These studies with cells of human breast cancer origin show that one response to estradiol treatment is an increase in levels of PgR, as would be predicted from studies of chick oviduct (Sherman *et al.*, 1970), rat uterine PgR priming (Faber *et al.*, 1972), and cyclic changes in PgR levels observed in the human endometrium (Bayard *et al.*, 1975). Our results clearly show that human breast cells that have undergone malignant transformation can continue to synthesize a specific protein under hormone control. Furthermore, these results lend credence to our hypothesis (Horwitz *et al.*, 1975b) that presence of PgR in biopsies of human breast tumors indicates that *in situ* the tumor was exposed to, and was capable of responding to circulating estrogens. Since the tumor, in one instance, has remained hormone responsive, one might suspect that other estrogen sensitive effects have also been retained.

We must emphasize, however, that PgR induction is only one product of estrogen action. The data cannot be construed to mean that other estrogen responses will necessarily be present. We find, for instance, that growth of MCF-7 cells is estrogen

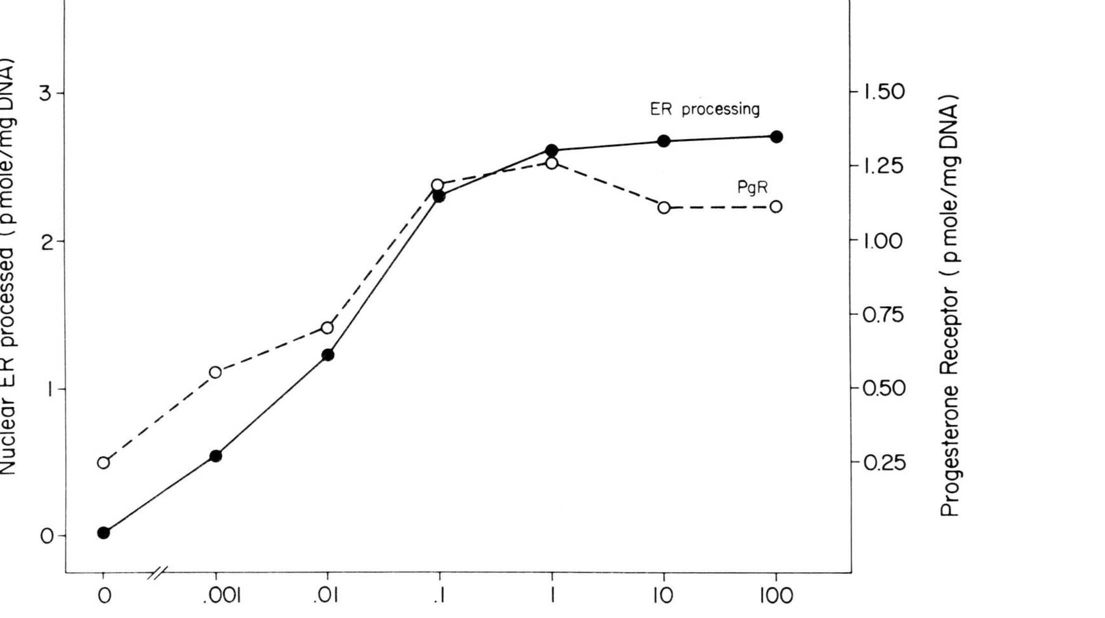

FIGURE 4. Comparison of ER processing and PgR induction. Cells were incubated as described in Fig. 3. ER was measured and the amount of ER lost at each dose (control - total) is plotted. PgR measured by single saturating dose assay: 200 µl cytosol incubated 4 hr at 4°C, in triplicate, with 20 nM [^{3}H]R5020 alone or with 100-fold excess R5020. After 15 min incubation with dextran-coated charcoal suspension, cytosols were centrifuged, and aliquots of the supernatant counted to determine bound radioactivity. Data shown are corrected for nonspecific binding. (Adapted from Horwitz and McGuire, 1978.)

sensitive, but unlike PgR, growth is not estrogen-dependent. Thus, effects of estrogens on growth and PgR induction might well be dissociated. We find this to be true in some DMBA tumors as well. Occasional tumors grow in castrate rats so that growth can be considered estrogen autonomous, while tumor PgR levels decline and could therefore be considered estrogen dependent (Horwitz and McGuire, 1977). Conversely, we would predict that tumors regressing while on high dose estradiol would have elevated PgR levels.

Our studies strongly suggest that estrogen stimulation of PgR involves ER. First, the extent of PgR induction parallels closely both the binding and translocation of Rc and the binding of Rn. Second, PgR induction is correlated with ER processing during estradiol stimulation; when processing ceases PgR levels fall.

The nature of processing is unclear. It may be an active state in which a new equilibrium between receptor degradation and synthesis is achieved (Sarff and Gorski, 1971; Williams and Gorski, 1972), or a redistribution of receptor within nuclear binding sites of differing affinities (DeHertogh *et al.*, 1973), or specificities (Schrader *et al.*, 1972), or sequestration of receptor to sites inaccessible to salt extraction (Clark and Peck, 1976; Ruh and Baudendistel, 1977). We will return to these questions later. Regardless, our data would suggest that the processing step is saturable, that peak activation occurs when RnE processing is maximal, and that the RnE accumulated in excess of that which is processed may be superfluous. That is, a dose of 0.1 nM estradiol is equal to 10 nM estradiol despite the fact that for the former some Rc remains, while for the latter, some unprocessed RnE remains.

In attempts to understand further the role of nuclear processing in ER action, we have studied the effects of antiestrogens.

III. ANTIESTROGENS: EFFECTS ON PgR AND ER PROCESSING

A. *ER Compartmentalization and Processing*

Tamoxifen (Tam) and nafoxidine (Naf), two nonsteroidal antiestrogens, are potent growth inhibitors of MCF-7 cells when present in high doses (Lippman *et al.*, 1976; Horwitz *et al.*, 1978; Zava *et al.*, 1977). Doses above 50 nM are inhibitory for nafoxidine, above 100 nM are inhibitory for tamoxifen. These effects are probably mediated through the ER system and are not simply toxic effects of the compounds, since they can be reversed by addition of estradiol at concentrations 100- to 1000-fold lower than the antiestrogen.

Estradiol, tamoxifen and nafoxidine have distinctly different effects on ER in MCF-7 cells. Fig. 5 shows the levels of total cytoplasmic and total nuclear receptors in cells during 5 hr of hormone or antagonist treatment. Untreated control cells have only unfilled ER. When estradiol (10 nM) is added, Rc binds the hormone and the receptor-hormone complex is rapidly translocated as shown by the reciprocal increase of receptor in the nucleus (RnE) and decrease in the cytoplasm by 5 min. Rn also binds the hormone rapidly so that in 5 min all cell receptors are in the nucleus in bound form (RnE); they then fall rapidly to processed levels. In the presence of tamoxifen or nafoxidine Rc also translocates, and receptor accumulates in the nucleus. This recompartmentalization is slower with antiestrogens than with estradiol. The subsequent processing step is quite different for the antiestrogens. With tamoxifen processing also results in decreased nuclear receptor levels; however, whereas the decrease represents 30 to 50% loss from control levels, it is never as extensive as that seen with estradiol. This processed level is also maintained as long as cells are exposed to tamoxifen. In cells treated with nafoxidine, all cell receptors also accumulate in the nucleus, but no subsequent processing of receptor occurs.

B. Effect of Dose on ER Processing and PgR Induction

As we have shown above, the steady state level of ER achieved when cells are incubated with estradiol in excess of 5 hr depends on the estradiol dose used.

With increasing doses of tamoxifen, Rc are also progressively depleted. At 100 nM more than 95% of Rc are translocated. However, total receptor levels fall to only 70% of control values even at the highest doses (Fig. 6). No processing at all is seen with nafoxidine despite complete Rc depletion.

Again, with antiestrogens, as with estradiol, processing parallels PgR induction. Fig. 6 shows that tamoxifen is a potent inducer of PgR. While low doses have only minimal effects at intermediate doses, PgR induction equals or exceeds that obtained with estradiol (not shown). When doses are raised further, PgR levels are suppressed even below control levels. This high (1 μM) tamoxifen dose is markedly antiestrogenic: At this dose but not at lower doses we see inhibition of cell growth and eventual cell death. Nafoxidine, in contrast to tamoxifen, has little or no effect on PgR at any dose studied. The slight increase at high doses may represent an effect on another receptor (D. T. Zava, unpublished).

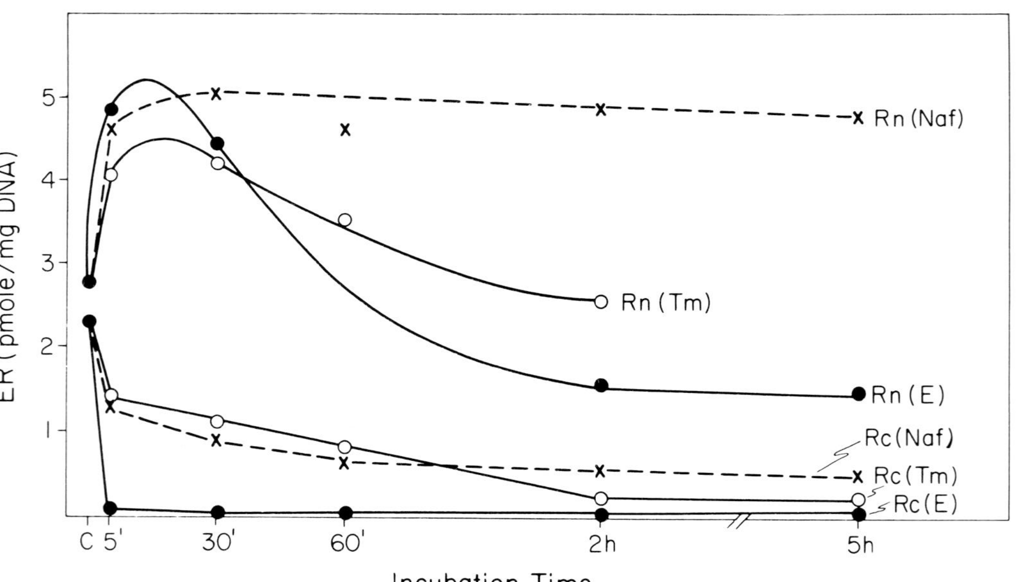

FIGURE 5. Kinetics of ER distribution after estradiol or antiestrogen treatment. Cells were treated as in Fig. 2 with estradiol (●, 10 nM), tamoxifen (o, 0.1 μM), or nafoxidine (x, 1 μM). ER measured by protamine sulfate precipitation as described in Fig. 2. (From Horwitz and McGuire, 1978b).

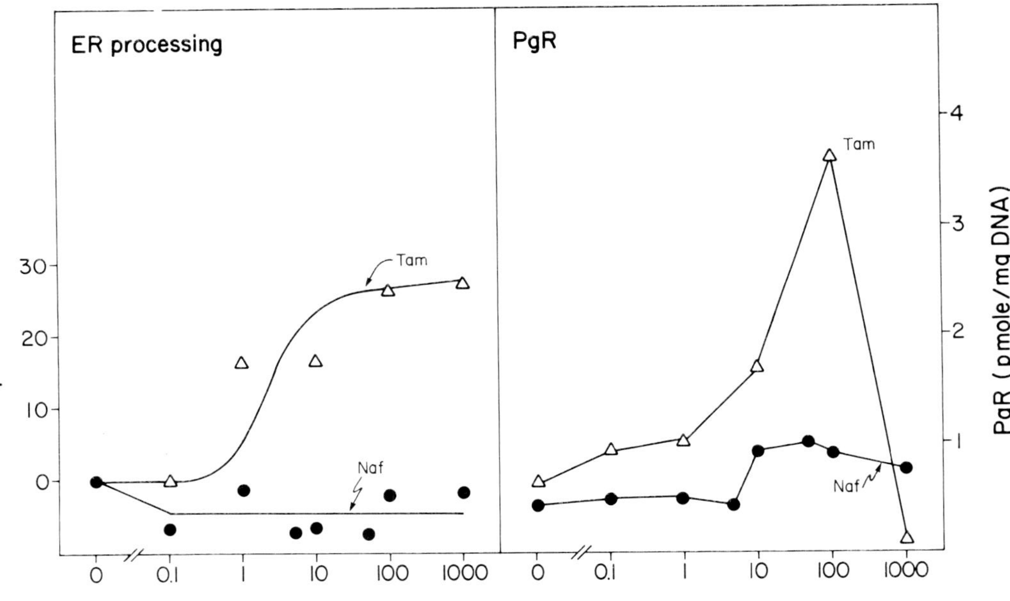

FIGURE 6. ER processing compared to PgR induction with varying doses of the antiestrogens tamoxifen (Tam) and nafoxidine (Naf). Cells were treated four days with increasing concentrations (0.1 to 1000 nM) of the antagonists as described in Fig. 3, and assayed for ER by protamine sulfate precipitation and for PgR by dextran-coated charcoal. ER processed describes the % of sites lost (compared to untreated controls) at each dose. Adapted from Horwitz and McGuire, 1978; Horwitz et al., *1978.)*

These results show that in breast cancer cells of human origin, the ER system mediates antiestrogen action. Antiestrogens bind and translocate cytoplasmic ER; they also bind the free nuclear receptor present in the cells. In these respects estrogen antagonists resemble estradiol. However, the subsequent nuclear processing reactions of estrogen and antiestrogen-bound receptors are dissimilar. After estradiol, nuclear hormone-receptor complexes fall rapidly to less than one third of control values. This pathway of receptor processing is either impaired (tamoxifen) or fails entirely (nafoxidine) for the antiestrogen-receptor complex. Our data would further suggest that processing is an active step in ER function at least in the special case of PgR induction and does not simply serve to return receptor to the cytoplasm. This step appears to be defective when antiestrogens bind the receptor.

With estradiol and tamoxifen, processing of receptor occurs despite the continuous presence of the hormones. This differs from the loss of nuclear ER described in the rat uterus by Giannopoulos and Gorski (1971) and Anderson *et al.* (1975) following a single pulse of estradiol. The latter have shown that if estradiol is administered to the rat so as to maintain elevated blood levels of the hormone, nuclear receptors rise to very high levels. Thus, significant differences are found in the early nuclear reactions of the estrogen receptor-hormone complex of human tumor cells compared to the rat uterus, the usual model of estrogen action. Other tissue differences in mechanisms of ER action have also been reported (Lazier and Alford, 1977; Cidlowski and Muldoon, 1976), suggesting perhaps that studies of estrogen action in uteri may not be extrapolated to other tissues.

Estrogenic and antiestrogenic responses in the rat uterus are characterized as early (<6 hr) or late (24 hr) (Hardin *et al.*, 1976; Lan and Katzenellenbogen, 1976; Stormshak *et al.*, 1976) and different control mechanisms may be required for each. Upon initial injection both responses are evoked by antiestrogens (Clark *et al.*, 1974; Katzenellenbogen and Ferguson, 1975; Capony and Rochefort, 1975); however, late responses cannot be elicited either by estradiol or by antiestrogens if preceded 24 hr by a primary antiestrogen injection (Katzenellenbogen *et al.*, 1977; Ferguson and Katzenellenbogen, 1977). This has led to models of estrogen action having at least two nuclear binding sites for the ER-complex, one of which is accessible to antiestrogen-receptor complexes. These models are further supported by evidence of differential salt extractability of estrogen and antiestrogen bound nuclear receptors (Clark and Peck, 1976; Meites and Baulieu, 1975; Juliano and Stancel, 1976; Ruh and Baudendistel, 1977) and by their differential nuclear retention time (Clark *et al.*, 1973). Our data lend support to the concept of dual nuclear sites of action of estrogen-receptor complexes; they suggest moreover that processing of ER occurs at only one of these. These sites may be temporally as well as structurally distinct since, as we show below, binding to the processing site can be prevented without affecting initial nuclear binding.

IV. ACTINOMYCIN D: EFFECTS ON ER COMPARTMENTALIZATION AND PROCESSING

A. *Inhibition of ER Processing*

Actinomycin D (AcD) has been a powerful tool in investigations into the biochemistry of nucleic acids and their involvement in replication and transcription (Goldberg and Friedman, 1971). The antibiotic intercalates into double-stranded DNA with its chromophore between successive G-C base pairs; two pentapeptides lie in the minor groove of the double helix (Sobel and Jain, 1972). Two binding sites distinguished by different affinities for DNA have been described; both are partially blocked by the presence of chromosomal proteins (Kleiman and Huang, 1971).

The nature of the inhibitory action of AcD is complex and partially concentration dependent. AcD suppresses the synthesis of all cellular RNA fractions by preferentially blocking chain elongation catalyzed by DNA-directed RNA polymerase. However, at low concentrations there is differential inhibition of various RNA classes with ribosomal RNA being most sensitive (Goldberg and Friedman, 1971). DNA synthesis in intact cells or by isolated DNA polymerases is also sensitive to AcD but requires the presence of much higher inhibitor concentrations (Hyman and Davidson, 1970).

More recently it has been further suggested that AcD may inhibit protein synthesis through direct effects on mRNA movement or translation (Leinwald and Ruddle, 1977; Bastos and Aviv, 1977).

Fig. 7 shows the effect of addition of AcD (2 μM) to estradiol-treated cells. In this study cells were treated simultaneously with the hormone and inhibitor and receptor levels were measured at the indicated times. AcD completely inhibits the normal processing of estrogen-charged nuclear receptor. The result is analogous to the effects of nafoxidine. Interestingly, neither the initial binding of estradiol to unfilled sites, nor the translocation of the hormone receptor complex to the nucleus is affected by actinomycin.

These measurements were made with an exchange assay on protamine-precipitated receptor extracted from nuclei with high salt. However, actinomycin is not simply enhancing salt ex-

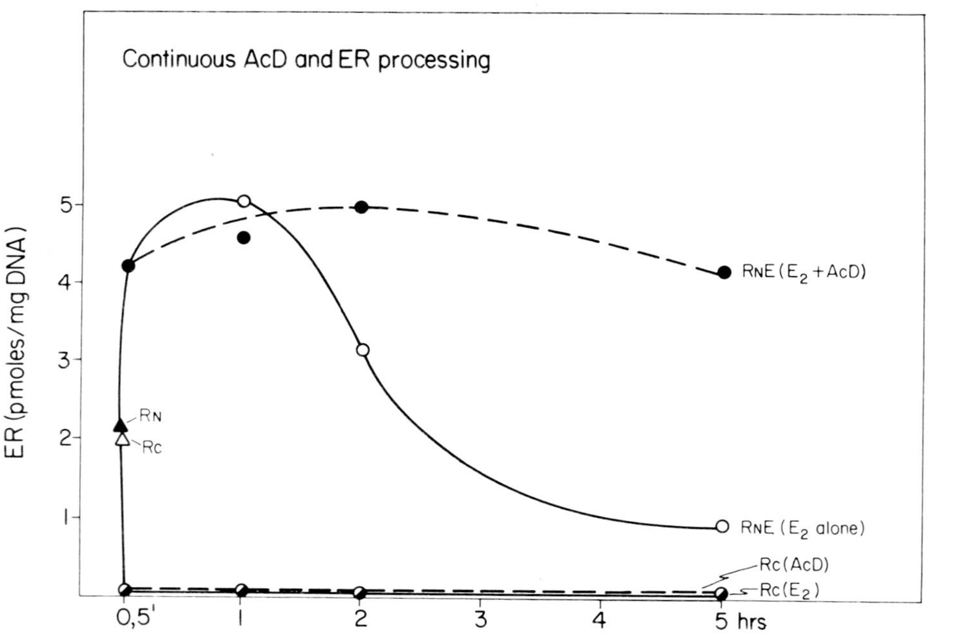

FIGURE 7. Effect of continuous actinomycin treatment on processing of MCF-7 estrogen receptor. Cells were treated at time 0 with 10 nM estradiol alone (o,Δ) or together with 2 μM actinomycin D(●,▲). At the indicated times cells were harvested and assayed for ER by protamine sulfate precipitation. Rn, Rc, RnE as described in Fig. 2.

tractability of RnE since a similar loss of ER and its inhibition by AcD can be demonstrated when nuclear receptors are labeled directly with [^{3}H]estradiol, thereby obviating the need to extract receptors (not shown) (Horwitz and McGuire, 1978.)

B. Dose of AcD and ER Processing

The inhibitory effects of AcD on ER processing are only achieved when it is present in high concentrations (Fig. 8). In this study cells were treated with estradiol alone or with estradiol plus increasing doses of actinomycin. With estradiol only, or with estradiol plus low AcD levels, normal receptor loss is seen (0% inhibition). As AcD doses are increased we see progressive inhibition of ER processing.

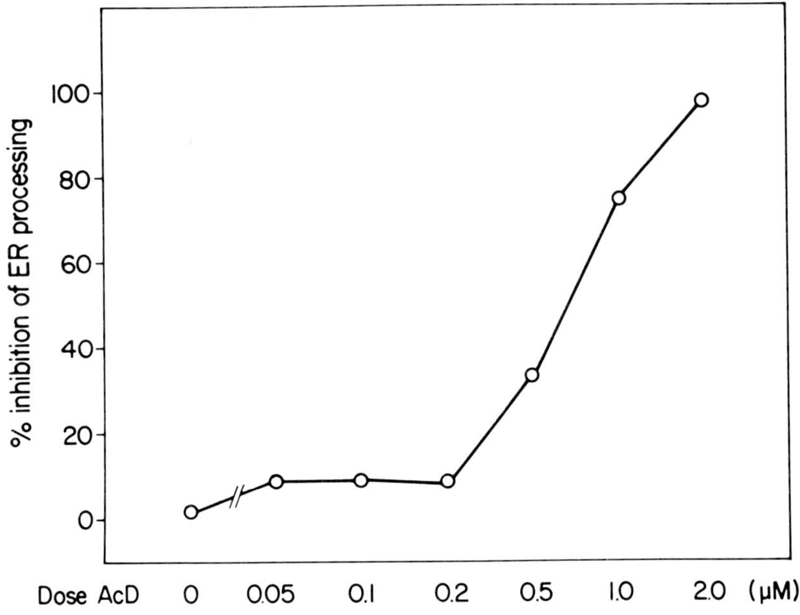

FIGURE 8. Dose of actinomycin D required to inhibit processing of estrogen receptor. Cells were incubated for 5 hr with 10 nM estradiol alone (o AcD) or together with increasing doses of AcD as shown. Cells were harvested and assayed for ER as described in Fig. 2. Maximum processed levels seen in the absence of AcD represent 0% inhibition. Total receptor in untreated cells (not shown) equals 100%. (Adapted from Horwitz and McGuire, J. Biol. Chem. 253, 6319-6322, 1978).

Actinomycin could be working in at least two ways: Its effect could be direct, physically blocking ER access to a specific DNA binding site. Alternatively its effect may be indirect, by inhibiting RNA and protein synthesis. We have several indirect lines of evidence based on the rate of inhibition and the effects of other inhibitors that suggest that AcD acts directly to block processing.

C. *Rate of AcD Block and Effect of Other Inhibitors*

First, the inhibitory effect of actinomycin is rapid as shown in Fig. 9. In this study cells were treated with estradiol, while addition of actinomycin was delayed from 5 min to

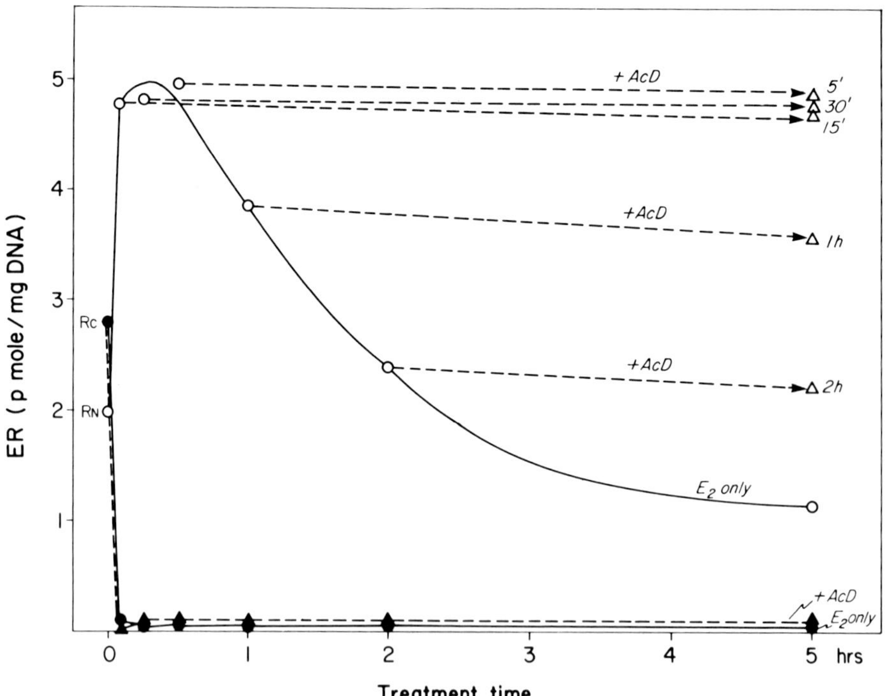

FIGURE 9. Effect of delayed AcD treatment on ER levels. MCF-7 cells were treated with 10 nM estradiol alone (o,•) or with estradiol, followed by AcD given 5 min to 2 hr later (Δ). Cells were harvested at the end of 5 hr of estradiol treatment and assayed for ER as described in Fig. 2. Dashed lines represent the changes in ER levels from the time of AcD addition to the end of the experiment. (From Horwitz and McGuire, J. Biol. Chem. 253, 6319-6322, 1978).

2 hr. The effect of AcD is to immediately fix ER at the levels they had reached before addition of the inhibitor. If estradiol and AcD are added together at the start of treatment (not shown), estrogen binding and translocation of Rc and binding to Rn and the initial accumulation of total receptor in the nucleus are not inhibitable. However, all subsequent processing stops. The slight downward slopes of the dotted lines show that the effect on ER processing occurs within 15 min of AcD addition, so that entry of AcD into nuclei must be quite rapid, and an intermediate effect of AcD on protein synthesis is unlikely.

We have also tested several other inhibitors of cell function for their effect on ER binding, translocation, and processing during estradiol treatment. At 1 μM all other intercalators and inhibitors tested were ineffective; the list includes other inhibitors of transcription (daunomycin, adriamycin, distamycin A, α-amanatin), inhibitors of replication (chloroquine, nalidixic acid, mitomycin C, novobiocin, ethidium bromide), a translation inhibitor (cycloheximide), and inhibitors of other cell processes (colchicine, cytochalasin B). The sole exception was chromomycin A_3. This compound behaves identically to AcD, and like AcD is the only inhibitor that shows specificity for G-C base pairs (Goldberg and Friedman, 1971).

The failure of other intercalators and translation inhibitors to prevent ER processing suggests that the AcD effect is not indirect, resulting from its property of inhibiting RNA and protein synthesis. Instead, AcD (and chromomycin) may directly block ER action at DNA. AcD may distinguish between two RnE binding sites in nuclei. Newly translocated receptor binds to a site on chromatin or DNA insensitive to inhibition. AcD or chromomycin A_3 stop subsequent processing by preventing RnE insertion at a second base specific region on DNA or by preventing its release from those sites (Fig. 10). The existence of two receptor binding sites in nuclei, one for chromatin, another for DNA, have been postulated in the chick oviduct for progesterone receptor (Schrader *et al.*, 1972). Palmiter *et al.*(1976) have also proposed a two-step nuclear receptor translocation mechanism involving a rate-limiting movement of steroid receptors from initial nonproductive chromatin binding sites to productive sites. As described above, the actions of actinomycin are complex and there are several alternative models that can be invoked to explain our data. A model involving only one binding site requires that nuclear ER binding is immediately to DNA; AcD may then mechanically prevent ER release from this site. It is also possible that actinomycin is somehow preventing ER egress from the nucleus (Bastos and Aviv, 1977) or altering its turnover at some extranuclear site.

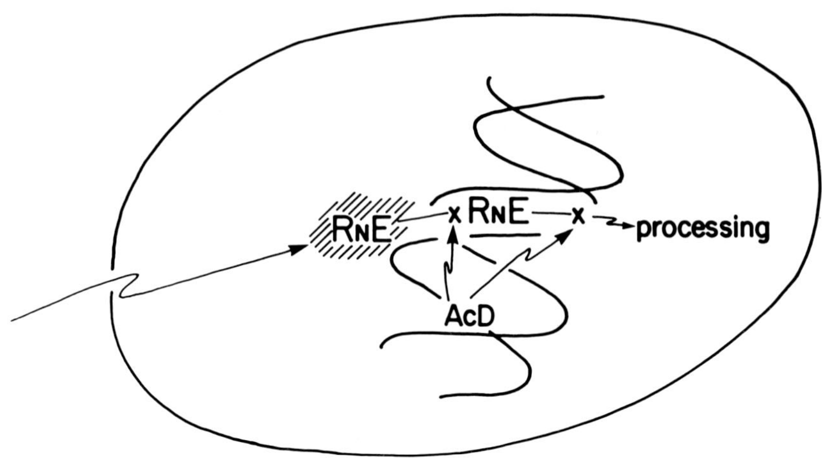

FIGURE 10. A model of the nuclear sites of action of actinomycin D. Though the initial accumulation of RnE in the nucleus is not prevented, AcD may act to prevent insertion of RnE on DNA, or to prevent its release from DNA. Other mechanisms of AcD action are discussed in the text.

In summary, we have provocative data that suggest that the nuclear estrogen-receptor complex interacts with DNA, that this interaction is required for appropriate receptor turnover or processing, and that processing may be essential for induction of a specific protein by estrogen. If the receptor is improperly inserted into DNA, as for instance when it is bound by nafoxidine, processing fails and the biological effect is blunted.

ACKNOWLEDGMENTS

This work is presently supported by the National Institutes of Health (CA11378, CB23862) and the American Cancer Society.

REFERENCES

Anderson, J. N., Peck, E. J., Jr., and Clark, J. H. (1975). *Endocrinology 96*, 160-167.
Bastos, R. N., and Aviv, H. (1977). *Cell 11*, 641-650.
Bayard, F., Damilano, S., Robel, P., and Baulieu, E. E. (1975). *C. R. Acad. Sci.* (Paris) *281*, 1341-1344.

Brooks, S. C., Locke, E. R., and Soule, H. D. (1973). *J. Biol. Chem. 248,* 6251-6253.
Capony, F., and Rochefort, H. (1975). *Molec. Cell. Endocrinol. 3,* 233-251.
Cidlowski, J. A., and Muldoon, T. G. (1976). *Biol. Reprod. 15,* 381-398.
Clark, J. H., and Peck, E. J., Jr. (1976). *Nature 260,* 635-637.
Clark, J. H., Anderson, J. N., and Peck, E. J., Jr. (1973). *Steroids 22,* 707-718.
Clark, J. H., Peck, E. J., Jr., and Anderson, J. N. (1974). *Nature 251,* 446-448.
DeHertogh, R., Ekka, E., Vanderheyden, I., and Hoet, J. J. (1973). *J. Steroid Biochem. 4,* 313-320.
Faber, L. E., Sandman, M. L., and Stavely, H. E. (1972). *J. Biol. Chem. 247,* 5648-5649.
Ferguson, E. R., and Katzenellenbogen, B. S. (1977). *Endocrinology 100,* 1242-1251.
Giannopoulos, G., and Gorski, J. (1971). *J. Biol. Chem. 246,* 2524-2529.
Goldberg, I. H., and Friedman, P. A. (1971). *Annu. Rev. Biochem. 40,* 775-810.
Hardin, J. W., Clark, J. H., Glasser, S. R., and Peck, E. J., Jr. (1976). *Biochemistry 15,* 1370-1374.
Horwitz, K. B., and McGuire, W. L. (1977). *Cancer Res. 37,* 1733-1738.
Horwitz, K. B., and McGuire, W. L. (1978a). *J. Biol. Chem. 253,* 2223-2228.
Horwitz, K. B., Costlow, M. E., and McGuire, W. L. (1975a). *Steroids 26,* 785-795.
Horwitz, K. B., McGuire, W. L., Pearson, O. H., and Segaloff, A. (1975b). *Science 189,* 726-727.
Horwitz, K. B., and McGuire, W. L. (1978b). *J. Biol. Chem. 253,* 8185-8191.
Horwitz, K. B., Koseki, Y., and McGuire, W. L. (1978). *Endocrinology, 103,* 1742-1751.
Hyman, R. W., and Davidson, N. (1970). *J. Mol. Biol. 50,* 421-438.
Jensen, E. V., and DeSombre, E. R. (1972). *Annu. Rev. Biochem. 41,* 203-230.
Jensen, E. V., Block, G. E., Smith, S., Kyser, K., and DeSombre, E. R. (1971). *Natl. Cancer Inst. Monographs 34,* 55-79.
Juliano, J. V., and Stancel, G. H. (1976). *Biochemistry 15,* 916-920.
Katzenellenbogen, B. S., and Ferguson, E. R. (1975). *Endocrinology 97,* 1-12.
Katzenellenbogen, B. S., Ferguson, E. R., and Lan, N. C. (1977). *Endocrinology 100,* 1252-1259.

Kleiman, L., and Huang, R. C. C. (1971). *J. Mol. Biol. 55*, 503-521.

Lan, N. C., and Katzenellenbogen, B. S. (1976). *Endocrinology 98*, 220-227.

Lazier, C. B., and Alford, W. S. (1977). *Biochem. J. 164*, 659-667.

Leavitt, W. W., Chen, T. J., and Allen, T. C. (1977). *Ann. N.Y. Acad. Sci. 286*, 210-225.

Leinwald, L., and Ruddle, F. H. (1977). *Science 197*, 381-383.

Lippman, M., Bolan, G., and Huff, K. (1976). *Cancer Res. 36*, 4595-4601.

McGuire, W. L., Carbone, P. P., Sears. M. E., and Escher, G. C. (1975). *In* "Estrogen Receptors in Human Breast Cancer" (W. L. McGuire, P. P. Carbone, and E. P. Vollmer, eds.), pp. 1-7. Raven Press, New York.

Meites, J., and Baulieu, E. E. (1975). *Biochem. J. 146*, 617-623.

Palmiter, R. D., Moore, P. B., Mulvihill, E. R., and Emtage, S. (1976). *Cell 8*, 557-572.

Ruh, T. S., and Baudendistel, L. J. (1977). *Endocrinology 100*, 420-426.

Sarff, M., and Gorski, J. (1971). *Biochemistry 10*, 2557-2563.

Schrader, W. T., Toft, D. O., and O'Malley, B. W. (1972). *J. Biol. Chem. 247*, 2401-2407.

Sherman, M. R., Corval, P. I., and O'Malley, B. W. (1970). *J. Biol. Chem. 245*, 6085-6096.

Sobel, H. M., and Jain, S. C. (1972). *J. Mol. Biol. 68*, 21-34.

Sonnenschein, C., Soto, A. M., Cologiore, J., and Farookhi, R. (1976). *Exp. Cell Res. 101*, 15-22.

Soule, H. D., Vasquez, J., Long, A., Albert, S., and Brennan, M. J. (1973). *J. Natl. Can. Inst. 51*, 1409-1416.

Stormshak, F., Leake, R., Wertz, N., and Gorski, J. (1976). *Endocrinology 99*, 1501-1511.

Williams, D., and Gorski, J. (1972). *Proc. Natl. Acad. Sci. 69*, 3464-3468.

Zava, D. T., and McGuire, W. L. (1977). *J. Biol. Chem. 252*, 3703-3708.

Zava, D. T., Chamness, G. C., Horwitz, K. B., and McGuire, W. L. (1977). *Science 197*, 663-664.

THE REGRESSION PROCESS IN HORMONE-DEPENDENT MAMMARY CARCINOMAS[1]

Pietro M. Gullino

Laboratory of Pathophysiology,
National Cancer Institute,
Bethesda, Maryland

This is a summary of work carried out in our laboratory and aimed at the understanding of the mechanism of cell destruction in mammary carcinomas after alteration of the host hormonal balance.[2] Rat mammary carcinomas used as models were: primary, 7,12-dimethylbenz(α)anthracene (DMBA)- and *N*-nitrosomethylurea (NMU)-induced and transplantable MTW9 and Walker 256 (W256). Regression of DMBA and NMU tumors was obtained by castration or injection of dibutyryl cyclic adenosine 3',5'-monophosphate (DBcAMP). MTW9 was transplanted into the inguinal fat pads of Wistar/Furth inbred females and grew only in the presence of strong mammotropin stimulation that was obtained by the transplantation of a pituitary tumor into the interscapular subcutaneous tissue. W256 was transplanted s.c. into the lumbar region of Sprague-Dawley random-bred females and regression was obtained by s.c. injections of DBcAMP (10 mg/day/200 g rat). The rapidity of regression varied according to treatment and tumor type. A reduction in tumor volume from 2 to 1 g required 3-4 days for MTW9, 7-10 days for DMBA or NMU, and about 1 week for W256.

[1]*Presented at the 11th Meeting on Mammary Cancer in Experimental Animals and Man, Detroit, Michigan, June 25-28, 1978.*

[2]*The experiments were carried on in collaboration with Drs. J. Bodwin, Y. S. Cho-Chung, R. H. Lanzerotti, and M. Rouleau. The help of T. Clair, F. H. Grantham, I. Losonczy, and U. Walz is gratefully acknowledged.*

ISBN 0-12-131150-3

MORPHOLOGY

The overall morphology of the regressing tumor does not show any peculiarity that permits a diagnosis until the process of tissue destruction is well advanced. Moreover, none of the structural changes recognizable in the regressing tumor can be considered as a specific consequence of hormonal deprivation or imbalance. Pathological events that can take place during cell destruction include: cytoplasmic "loosening" as a result of an altered connection between the cell and its neighbor, disruption of the endoplasmic reticulum, disappearance of ribosomes, mitochondrial swelling with loss of membranous structures, clumping of nuclear chromatin with increased electron opacity in both nuclei and cytoplasm, extensive indentation of the plasma membrane, and fragmentation of the cytoplasm. One or more of these events can also be seen in cells of growing tumors and the increase in frequency is usually the only difference of the regressing tissue. However, it is deceiving to believe that the number of regressing cells visible on a histologic section reflects the extent of cell destruction and turnover.

At the tissue level, the morphology of tumor regression requires a distinction between coagulative necrosis and apoptosis (Arstila and Trump, 1968; Kerr, Wyllie, and Currie, 1972). Coagulative necrosis is the consequence of deficiencies in blood supply, involving complete sections of a tissue and common to every tumor, but there is no evidence that coagulative necrosis plays a role of any consequence in determining hormone-related mammary tumor regression. On the contrary, apoptosis, which is characterized by cell-limited digestion and suggests a programmed phenomenon, appears to be the prevalent and possibly the determining process. Three morphological aspects of hormone-dependent regression must be stressed: The relative abundance of phagocytic cells, the absence of lymphocytic "infiltrates," and the persistence of an evident cell membrane, even when the cell is fragmented. Phagocytic activity is acquired very rapidly by neoplastic cells, and MTW9 carcinoma is a good example to highlight the difficulty of discerning bona fide macrophages from phagocytizing neoplastic epithelium. On the fourth to fifth day of regression the majority of MTW9 cells have numerous phagosomes engulfing fragments of cytoplasm. If mammotropin stimulation is restored, the phagosomes are rapidly cleared and the tumor volume starts to increase again at about the same rate as before hormonal alteration. Thus, the majority of cells containing phagosomes must be neoplastic, otherwise the restoration of hormonal stimulation should first cause tumor shrinkage due to the disappearance of macrophages followed by growth of the remaining neoplastic cell population. Phagocytic activity is less evident in DMBA, NMU, and W256 carcinomas than in MTW9. It is surprising what little morphological evidence is found on histological examination of the vast turnover of tissue occurring during regression.

PATHOPHYSIOLOGY

Any tissue, neoplastic or not, may be viewed in a simplistic way as a three-compartment system constituted by vessels, cells, and interstitial spaces. We measured the sizes of these compartments in growing and regressing tumors with the objective of establishing whether shrinkage of the mass occurred in a coordinated fashion (Gullino *et al.*, 1972a). The vascular space was measured with high molecular weight dextran (Gullino and Grantham, 1964), the extracellular space by ^{24}Na (Gullino, Grantham, and Smith, 1965), and the cellular component was calculated from the difference. MTW9 had a vascular space of about 4.5%, an extracellular space of approximately 45%, and a cellular volume about 50% of the total mass. When tumor volume shrank to about one-half, the relative proportion of the compartment sizes remained about the same. Primary DMBA tumors followed the same pattern. We concluded that shrinkage of the tumor mass was a coordinated event and that the gross physiological structure of the tumor was preserved during regression.

Next we compared the gross composition of the growing and regressing tumors in search of any conspicuous differences (Gullino *et al.*, 1972a). In both DMBA and MTW9 carcinomas that had regressed to about one-half their original size of 3 g, collagen and DNA contents were higher than in their growing counterparts, the water content remained unchanged, and all other components were reduced by varying degrees, whether the data were referred to DNA or to tissue weight. In particular, when referred to the DNA content, the RNA concentrations were about 30% lower in both tumors but the loss of proteins was more pronounced in MTW9 than in DMBA: 40% of total proteins and 53% of phosphoproteins in the former as compared with 19% and 35%, respectively, in the latter. Loss of triglycerides and phospholipids was about 30% in regressing MTW9, whereas regressing DMBA accumulated triglycerides to about twice the content measured in the growing counterpart, but phospholipids did not change significantly. An explanation of the DMBA behavior is not available at this time. Nuclear and cytoplasmic fractions were also separated from growing and regressing tumors and the ratios of DNA, RNA, and proteins were compared. The percent difference of these ratios was within 20% for MTW9 and 25% for DMBA. On the whole, the observed changes in compartment size and gross composition of growing and regressing DMBA and MTW9 carcinomas suggested that tissue destruction followed the pattern of a programmed or coordinated event.

In a subsequent set of experiments (Gullino *et al.*, 1972a), we compared the physiological regulation of blood supply and the metabolic activity of regressing vs. growing tumors. The determinations were made *in vivo* and we utilized as a model MTW9 carcinoma transplanted at the extremity of the ovarian pedicle, according to a procedure developed in our laboratory (Gullino, 1970). The principal feature of this approach is the possibility of studying *in vivo* a tumor completely isolated from the surrounding tissues and connected to the host by a single artery and vein. By cannulating the tumor vein, one can measure the amount of blood passing through the tumor and by sampling the aortic blood as it flows into the tumor artery, one can measure differences in metabolites between arterial and venous tumor blood, and thus evaluate metabolite consumption *in vivo*. It was observed (Gullino *et al.*, 1972a) that the blood supply to both growing and regressing tumors was equally high and that regulation of blood flow under conditions of altered volemia or epinephrine action was as efficient in regressing as in growing tumors. On a weight basis, the regressing tumor, *in vivo*, utilized as much oxygen and glucose as the growing tumor. Pulse labeling with [2-^{14}C]-glycine, [5-^{3}H]uridine, or [U-^{16}C]glucose indicated that incorporation of the label into DNA, RNA, proteins, and lipids was increased during the first 6 to 8 hr of regression and decreased thereafter (Gullino *et al.*, 1972a,b). When the labeled precursor was continuously infused for a 20-hr period, regressing MTW9 incorporated less of the label in all fractions than growing MTW9, but DMBA tumors incorporated equal or larger amounts of the label in each fraction measured than the growing counterparts, whether the results were expressed per gram of wet tissue or as specific activity. At 72 hr after hormone removal, MTW9 tumors were unable to incorporate the label into DNA, and at 24 and 48 hr the incorporation was reduced to levels one-third to one-fifth those of the growing tumors. DMBA behaved as MTW9 except that arrest of incorporation into DNA ceased at 96 hr. Label incorporation into RNA and proteins of nuclear and cytoplasmic fractions was still present when incorporation into DNA had ceased. A sharp difference, however, was observed between MTW9 and DMBA tumors. During 20 hr of continuous infusion, regressing MTW9 incorporated from two- to fivefold less label than growing tumor within a 96-hr period after hormone removal. During the same period, however, regressing DMBA continued to incorporate at least as much label as the growing tumor.

Moreover, in both MTW9 and DMBA the ratios of specific activities for RNA and proteins, in nuclear and cytoplasmic fractions, were different when the label was incorporated during regression.

The overall impression derived from the *in vivo* measurements of blood flow, oxygen and glucose consumption, and incorporation of labeled precursors was that regression resulted in a complex modification of the cell turnover within the tumor, with prevalence of lysis over reproduction, not a simple arrest of cell proliferation.

TISSUE LYSIS

An indication of the extent of the lytic process was given by the observation (Gullino *et al.*, 1972a; Gullino and Lanzerotti, 1972) that the levels of free amino acid nitrogen in the serum of blood leaving the regressing tumor was 40 to 60% higher than that of the afferent serum. When this elevation was related to blood flow and changes in tumor volumes, one could roughly estimate that 60 to 90% of protein loss by the regressing tumors could be accounted for by the loss of amino acids. Thus, an almost complete digestion was occurring within the regressing tumors.

The involvement of lysosomes in tissue digestion is a well-known event (Dingle, 1969). We analyzed whether lysosomal enzyme activity was enhanced during hormonally induced regression, as expected, and whether the enzymatic activities *in vivo* were predominant within or outside of the neoplastic cells. The approach we followed was to compare the enzymatic activity of the interstitial fluid collected *in vivo* with that of the total homogenate. The tumor interstitial fluid was sampled with a micropore chamber following a procedure developed in our laboratory (Gullino, 1970). The enzymes studied were β-glucuronidase, β-galactosidase, acid phosphatase, arylsulfatase, acid RNase, and cathepsin. An increase of activity was observed during regression for all enzymes studied. The increment varied from 50 to 70% and was found in the tumor homogenate. There was no enzymatic activity in the tumor interstitial fluid, whether the tumor was growing or regressing (Lanzerotti and Gullino, 1972). This observation was carefully controlled and it should be kept in mind when "leakage" of lysosomal enzymes is assumed to occur *in vivo* just because it may be observed *in vitro*. An increase in the number of enzyme molecules per gram of tumor was also observed when the increment of enzymatic activity appeared. Moreover, the half-life of acid ribonuclease decreased from 7.8 to 2.6 days; thus, synthesis and turnover of lytic enzymes were sharply enhanced during regression (Cho-Chung and Gullino, 1973; Lanzerotti and Gullino, 1972). However, the peak enzymatic activity, as measured in whole homogenates, was reached after varying periods of time, about 6 hr for acid ribonuclease but 48 hr or more for the other enzymes (Lanzerotti and Gullino, 1972).

This elevation of activity can be interpreted in at least two ways: either as an indication that during regression lysosomes are actively destroying the neoplastic cells or that turnover of cells and molecules is being sharply increased by the removal of hormones, which implies that lysosomes do not cause regression but simply expand their physiological activity during regression. If the second hypothesis is correct, one would expect that hormonal deprivation has the ultimate effect of increasing the substrate available to the lytic enzymes for lysis. Rouleau and Gullino (1977) examined this possibility and demonstrated that: (a) the rate of labeled amino acid incorporation into proteins did not change during the first 24 hr after hormonal deprivation; (b) within 24 hr of hormone withdrawal cytosol fractions of MTW9 became more easily degraded by trypsin, α-chymotrypsin or subtilisin BPN; (c) labilization of cytosol proteins occurred much earlier than any change in either protein synthesis or lysosomal enzyme activity; and (d) the data showing increased susceptibility to proteolysis could not be explained by the presence of endogenous proteases, by the destruction of the exogenous proteins used in the assay, or by the existence of protease inhibitors. Moreover, the increased susceptibility to proteolysis of regressing cytosol persisted after preincubation with dithiothreitol, prolactin, 17β-estradiol, progesterone, or hydrocortisone (0.5 μg/ml concentration for each) but it disappeared after heat denaturation. The presence of hormones was not sufficient to stabilize the cytosol proteins, suggesting that the increased susceptibility to lysis was probably a precondition of the increment of protein turnover (Goldberg and Dice, 1974; Goldberg and St. John, 1976) observed during regression, although the relationship between change in protein turnover and hormonal deprivation has yet to be defined.

As a contribution to this objective, Rouleau, Losonczy, and Gullino studied the pattern of leucine incorporation into cytosol proteins of growing and regressing MTW9 carcinomas and observed that the electrophoretic pattern differed in three bands and this change occurred within 6 hr after hormonal deprivation of the host, or about 4 hr after prolactin levels in the blood were lower than the concentration needed by MTW9 to grow. None of these changes were observed in the nuclear proteins. These observations on the cytosol proteins coupled with the finding of their increased susceptibility to digestion within a few hours after hormonal deprivation support but do not prove the hypothesis that the augmented activity of lysosomol enzymes observed during tumor regression may be triggered by a change in the protein profile of the cell, followed by a sharp increment in the amount of substrate to be lysed, which, in turn, requires an elevation in the number and activity of the lysosomes.

INDUCTION OF REGRESSION

As the work following this approach progressed, it became clear that the possibility of understanding the mechanism of regression would be enhanced if a hormone-unresponsive tumor could be induced to regress and we could study the related events under the same conditions as pertained to hormone removal. Cho-Chung and Gullino (1974) found that s.c. injections of DBcAMP induced growth arrest in about 30% of W256 and several of these regressed completely. When regressing tumors were retransplanted into the untreated host, they resumed growth, thus a line of regressing W256 could be maintained by injecting DBcAMP into the rat bearing the susceptible W256 and retransplanting it as soon as regression was measurable. DBcAMP was also able to induce growth arrest in MTW9 and DMBA carcinomas while growth of NMU tumors was only slowed to about one-half the original doubling time (Cho-Chung, 1974; Cho-Chung and Gullino, 1974 a,b,). One of the first differences observed between responsive and unresponsive W256 carcinomas following DBcAMP treatment, was in the binding affinity of the cytosol to cAMP. Cyclic AMP-binding proteins and protein kinase were present in both DBcAMP-responsive and -unresponsive W256 but showed both qualitative and quantitative differences. In the responsive W256 (a) maximum binding was higher under all conditions tested, (b) the binding equilibrium was reached faster and the peak binding lasted longer, (c) the electrophoretic mobility of the major cAMP binding component of the cytosol was distinct from that of unresponsive W256, (d) preincubation at 50°C for 15 min had no effect on the binding whereas it decreased the binding of unresponsive W256 by 50%, (d) cAMP stimulated the protein kinase activity of the cytosol fivefold compared to a twofold stimulation of unresponsive W256, and (e) cAMP caused a decrease in the Km of protein kinase for ATP but had no effect on the affinity of the enzyme in unresponsive W256 (Cho-Chung *et al.*, 1977). A comparison between cytoplasmic cAMP and nuclear cAMP binding revealed that within 24 hr after DBcAMP treatment, the nuclear cAMP binding increased threefold while cAMP binding to the cytosol decreased by 50%. No change was observed in

W256 unresponsive to DBcAMP treatment. Scatchard analysis showed that the increment of nuclear binding after DBcAMP treatment depended on the transfer into the nuclei of 3.6 S binding proteins found in the cytosol. This predominant species showed kinase activity with a substrate specificity similar to that of cAMP-dependent protein kinase but distinct from that of the kinase present in control nuclei. DBcAMP treatment of the host produced a shifting of the heavier binding and kinase components toward the lighter components in the cytosol of responsive but not in unresponsive W256.

The interaction of cAMP with cytoplasmic and nuclear binding molecules was also studied using tumor slices incubated at 30°C with labeled nucleotide. As incubation progressed the level of cytoplasmic binding decreased and that of nuclear binding increased in responsive but not in unresponsive W256. The same shifting was observed when protein kinase activity was measured. The lack of transfer of cAMP + receptor complex from the cytoplasm into the nuclei of DMcAMP-unresponsive W256 could be due to a defect of the complex in the cytoplasm or of the acceptor site in the nuclei. To clarify this point, cAMP + receptor complexes as well as nuclear pellets were prepared from DBcAMP-responsive and -unresponsive W256. Incubation of isolated nuclei with [^{3}H]cAMP + receptor complexes revealed that translocation occurred only if the latter derived from a DBcAMP-responsive W256, regardless of the origin of the nuclei. Lack of translocation was evidently due to a "defect" of the cAMP + receptor complex in the cytosol of DBcAMP-unresponsive W256 (Cho-Chung and Clair, 1977; Cho-Chung, Clair, and Huffman, (1977).

The consequences of the nuclear penetration of the cAMP + receptor complex were studied in the following experiments (Cho-Chung and Redler, 1977). The nuclear pellet of a DBcAMP-responsive W256 was incubated with [γ-^{33}P]ATP and the nuclear proteins phosphorylated by the nuclear kinases were then shown by acrylamide gel electrophoresis to be concentrated within a relatively narrow and high peak. When W256 was treated with DBcAMP for a few days until regression was measurable, the nuclear proteins phosphorylated by the same assay constituted two large peaks; one peak was in the same position as shown for untreated nuclei, although almost 40% smaller; the second peak was much less mobile, clearly distinct on the gel and almost as large as the first one. When nuclei from an untreated tumor were first isolated from the cytoplasm, then incubated with DBcAMP, the second peak of phosphorylation did not appear, suggesting that the presence of the cytoplasm was necessary at the time of DBcAMP treatment. In order to assess whether this endogenous phosphorylation of nuclear proteins was related to the regression process, the experiment was repeated using DMBA-induced primary tumors regressing after ovariectomy. The nuclear pellet isolated from a tumor that had regressed to about 70% of the original size was also able to phosphorylate proteins moving as two major peaks, as shown by DBcAMP-treated W256. Moreover, when the DMBA tumor was induced to regrow by injections of 17β-estradiol, the slow moving peak of phosphorylated proteins disappeared as it did with W256 when DBcAMP treatment was interrupted.

The interdependence between the regression induced by DBcAMP in W256 and by castration in DMBA tumors was further clarified by comparing cAMP- and estrogen-binding activities. After ovariectomy the cAMP content of DMBA tumors doubled within 24 hr, while the cAMP binding doubled in the cytosol and tripled in the nuclei. The total protein content was not appreciably changed during the first 24 hr following castration. Six days after ovariectomy the cAMP content was fourfold the original level, the binding activity in the nuclei was increased fivefold over the growing counterpart, while the cytosol cAMP binding was decreased. The estrogen receptor pattern changed in the opposite direction. In sucrose gradients the growing tumor showed, as expected, two major fractions in the cytosol, sedimenting at 4 S and 8 S, whereas the nuclear fraction contained an estrogen binding component of a 5 S species. As regression progressed after ovariectomy the estrogen binding activity decreased both in the nuclei and cytosol by 80% and 50%, respectively, while cAMP binding increased. Growth of the tumor induced by injections of 17β-estradiol reversed the trend, i.e., estrogen receptor levels increased and cAMP binding decreased. In a few DMBA tumors that were hormone-independent, ovariectomy failed to modify cAMP- and estrogen-binding activities.

CONCLUSIONS

The study of the regression process in hormone-dependent mammary carcinomas has been carried out in our laboratory with the major objective of understanding the control of cell death and cell turnover. It has been shown that during regression:

The size of tissue compartments maintained the same relative proportion as during growth;

Regressing tumors used as much energy *in vivo* as growing tumors and the physiological regulation of blood supply and oxygen, and glucose comsumption was equally efficient in both tumors;

The incorporation of precursors continued during regression, especially in the RNA and protein fractions, but the degree and duration of incorporation varied depending on the tumor type;

Free amino acid nitrogen increased in the efferent blood of

regressing tumors at levels that suggested almost complete digestion of proteins within the tumor;

Activities and turnover rates of lysosomal enzymes increased within the cells but active lysosomal enzymes were not found within the interstitial compartment *in vivo*, suggesting that the regression process is an intracellular event;

Cytosol proteins of regressing tumors were more rapidly lysed by trypsin than those of growing tumors and some changes in the leucine incorporation pattern were observed, suggesting that a protein "labilization" may be involved during regression;

The cAMP system is involved during regression and the concentration of cAMP- and estrogen receptors changed in opposite directions;

Hormone-unresponsive mammary carcinomas, like W256, could be induced to regress by DBcAMP treatment if they had high affinity receptors for cAMP;

The cAMP + receptor complex migrated to the nucleus and thereafter phosphorylated proteins appeared.

The role, if any, of these processes in regression is being investigated further.

REFERENCES

Arstila, A. U., and Trump, B. F. (1968). Studies on autophagocytosis. The autophagic vacuoles in the liver after glucagon administration. *Am. J. Pathol. 53;* 687-733.

Cho-Chung, Y. S. (1974). *in vivo* inhibition of tumor growth by cyclic adenosine 3',5'-monophosphate derivatives. *Cancer Res. 34;* 3492-3496.

Cho-Chung, Y. S., and Clair, T. (1977). Altered cyclic AMP-binding and db cyclic AMP-unresponsiveness *in vivo*. *Nature (London) 265;* 452-454.

Cho-Chung, Y. S., Clair, T., and Huffman, P. (1977). Loss of nuclear cyclic AMP binding in cyclic AMP-unresponsive Walker 256 mammary carcinoma. *J. Biol. Chem. 252;* 6349-6355.

Cho-Chung, Y. S., Clair, T., Yi, P. N., and Parkison, C. (1977). Comparative studies on cyclic AMP-responsive and -unresponsive Walker 256 mammary carcinomas. *J. Biol. Chem. 252;* 6335-6341.

Cho-Chung, Y. S., and Gullino, P. M. (1973). Mammary tumor regression. V. Role of acid ribonuclease and cathepsin. *J. Biol. Chem. 248;* 4743-4749.

Cho-Chung, Y. S., and Gullino, P. M. (1974a). Effect of dibutyryl cyclic adenosine 3',5'-monophosphate on *in vivo* growth of Walker 256 carcinoma: Isolation of responsive and unresponsive cell populations. *J. Natl. Cancer Inst. 52;* 995-996.

Cho-Chung, Y. S., and Gullino, P. M. (1974b). *In vivo* inhibition of two hormone-dependent mammary tumors by dibutyryl cyclic AMP. *Science 183*; 87-88.

Cho-Chung, Y. S., and Redler, B. H. (1977). Dibutyryl cyclic AMP mimics ovariectomy: Nuclear protein phosphorylation in mammary tumor regression. *Science 197*; 272-275.

Dingle, J. T., (1969). The extracellular secretion of lysosomal enzymes. *In* "Lysosomes in Biology and Pathology" (J. T. Dingle and H. B. Fell eds.) Vol. 2, pp. 421-436. American Elsevier Publishing Co., New York.

Goldberg, A. L., and Dice, J. F., (1974). Intracellular protein degradation in mammalian and bacterial cells. *Annu. Rev. Biochem. 43*; 835-869.

Goldberg, A. L., and St. John, A. C., (1976). Intracellular protein degradation in mammalian and bacterial cells: Part 2. *Annu. Rev. Biochem. 45*; 747-803.

Gullino, P. M. (1970). Techniques for the study of tumor physiopathology. *In* "Methods in Cancer Research" (H. Busch, ed.) Vol. 5, pp. 45-91. Academic Press, New York.

Gullino, P. M., and Grantham, F. H., (1964). The vascular space of growing tumors. *Cancer Res. 24*; 1727-1732.

Gullino, P. M., Grantham, F. H., and Smith, S. H., (1965). The interstitial water space of tumors. *Cancer Res. 25*; 727-731.

Gullino, P. M., Grantham, F. H., Losonczy, I., and Berghoffer, B. (1972a). Mammary tumor regression. I. Physiopathologic characteristics of hormone-dependent tissue. *J. Natl. Cancer Inst. 49*; 1333-1348.

Gullino, P. M., Grantham, F. H., Losonczy, I., and Berghoffer, B. (1972b). Mammary tumor regression. III. Uptake and loss of substrates by regressing tumors. *J. Natl. Cancer Inst. 49*; 1675-1684.

Gullino, P. M., and Lanzerotti, R. H., (1972). Mammary tumor regression. II. Autophagy of neoplastic cells. *J. Natl. Cancer Inst. 49*; 1349-1356.

Kerr, J. F. R., Wyllie, A. H., and Currie, A. R., (1972). Apoptosis: A basic biological phenomenon with wide-ranging implications in tissue kinetics. *Brit. J. Cancer 26*; 239-257.

Lanzerotti, R. H., and Gullino, P. M., (1972). Activities and quantities of lysosomal enzymes during mammary tumor regression. *Cancer Res. 32*; 2679-2685.

Rouleau, M., and Gullino, P. M., (1977). Increased susceptibility of cytosol proteins to proteolytic digestion during regression of a hormone-dependent mammary tumor. *Cancer Res. 37*; 670-677.

Rouleau, M., Losonczy, I., and Gullino, P. M., (1978). Arrest of synthesis of specific proteins at the onset of mammary tumor regression. *Cancer Res. 38*; 926-931.

PROLACTIN REGULATION OF CASEIN GENE EXPRESSION: A MODEL SYSTEM FOR STUDYING PEPTIDE HORMONE ACTION

Jeffrey M. Rosen
Robert J. Matusik
William A. Guyette
and
Scott C. Supowit

Department of Cell Biology
Baylor College of Medicine
Houston, Texas

I. INTRODUCTION

In order to elucidate the mechanism by which peptide hormones regulate gene expression, a system is required in which the rapid induction of a specific mRNA can be accurately measured following the addition of the hormone. An ideal model system should permit pulse-labeling studies of the specific mRNA, so that the rates of mRNA synthesis and degradation can be analyzed independently. Such experiments are necessary because mRNA accumulation has been shown to be a function not only of the rate of synthesis, but also of the rate of turnover of the specific mRNA (Kafatos, 1972). For example, differential mRNA turnover has been suggested to be an important factor regulating the accumulation of histone mRNA during the cell cycle (Melli *et al.*, 1977), of globin mRNA during erythroid development (Aviv *et al.*, 1976), and ovalbumin mRNA following estrogen treatment in the chick oviduct (Cox, 1977).

In addition, quantitative measurements of mRNA levels require the availability of a specific cDNA hybridization probe synthesized from a well-characterized, purified mRNA. This cDNA probe can also be used for the synthesis and amplification of the structural gene sequence, and eventually for the identification and cloning of a larger genomic DNA fragment. Using cDNA probes synthesized from these steroid-inducible mRNAs, it has been possible to demonstrate that the primary effect of

ISBN 0-12-131150-3

steroid hormones is to rapidly increase the rate of specific gene transcription (Ringold *et al.*, 1977). These hormones appear to regulate gene expression through a mechanism involving translocation of the steroid-cytoplasmic receptor complex to the cell nucleus, followed by an interaction of the receptor complex with specific chromosomal proteins and DNA sequences (O'Malley and Means, 1974). However, because of the enormous complexity of eucaryotic DNA, it has not been possible to elucidate the precise mechanism of steroid hormone action using total genomic DNA and nuclear protein fractions.

In contrast to steroid hormones, the mechanism by which peptide hormones regulate gene expression remains a complete enigma. In the following section, some of our recent studies on prolactin regulation of casein gene expression in the mammary gland are reported. The mammary gland fulfills the above criteria as an excellent model system in which to study peptide hormone action. Casein mRNA comprises between 50 to 60% of the total mRNA activity and is therefore readily purified in large quantities (Rosen, 1976). Furthermore, a full-length complementary DNA probe has been synthesized using purified casein mRNA as a template, and well characterized (Rosen and Barker, 1976). Utilizing this cDNA probe, the rapid induction of casein mRNA accumulation by prolactin in organ culture of mid-pregnant rat mammary tissue has been demonstrated (Matusik and Rosen, 1978). Finally, mammary gland organ culture is performed in a serum-free, chemically defined medium, thereby allowing a detailed examination of the mechanism by which prolactin regulates the synthesis of casein mRNA. In addition to these studies of peptide hormone regulation of differentiated function in the normal mammary gland, a brief discussion of gene expression in hormone-dependent mammary cancer is also included in the following section.

II. PEPTIDE HORMONE ACTION ON GENE EXPRESSION

A. *Indirect Second Messenger Pathway*

Prolactin does not appear to act through the classical peptide hormone pathway, involving the initial binding of the hormone to a membrane receptor followed by the activation of adenylate cyclase and a subsequent activation of protein kinase (Fig. 1A). The binding of prolactin to a membrane receptor has been shown by the elegant studies of Friesen and his colleagues (Shiu and Friesen, 1976) to be a necessary prerequisite for the induction of casein synthesis. This was demonstrated by blocking the induction of casein synthesis with an antibody prepared against the solubilized prolactin receptor. However, prolactin

A. CLASSICAL PATHWAY: SECOND MESSENGER

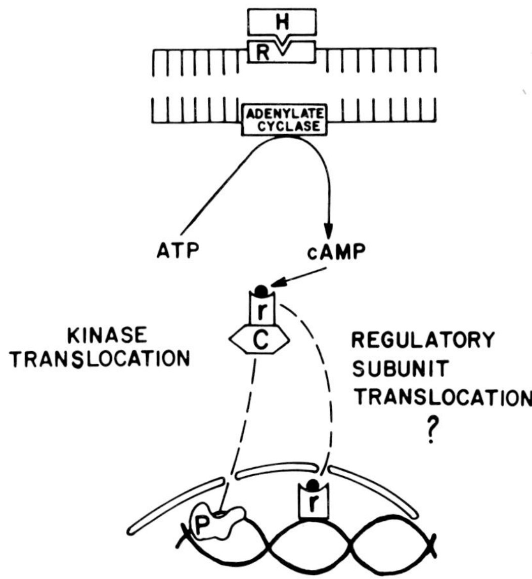

B. INTERNALIZATION: DIRECT ACTION

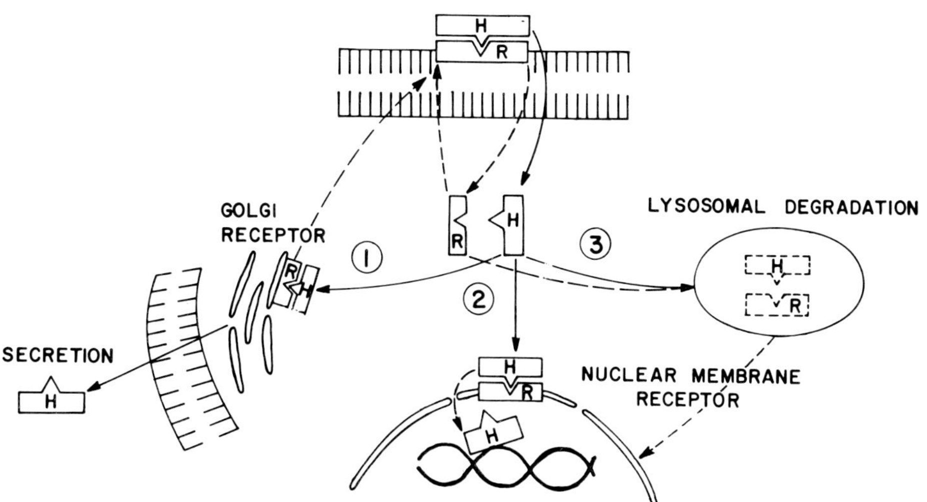

FIGURE 1. (A) Peptide hormone action. Classical pathway: second messengers. (B) Internalization and direct action. H = peptide hormone; R = receptor; r = regulatory subunit of protein kinase; C = catalytic subunit of protein kinase; P = nuclear phosphoprotein; 1, 2, and 3 are described in the text. Dashed lines refer to speculative pathways.

activation of adenylate cyclase and an increased net accumulation of intracellular cyclic AMP has not been demonstrated in the mammary gland (Majumder and Turkington, 1971; Oka and Perry, 1976). A similar failure to demonstrate prolactin activation of adenylate cyclase has been reported in the corpus luteum, which contains prolactin receptors and a peptide hormone (LH)-sensitive adenylate cyclase system (Birnbaumer *et al.*, 1976). Finally, dibutryryl cyclic AMP when added to mammary explants is unable to either induce or inhibit casein synthesis (Matusik and Rosen, 1980).

Following the binding of prolactin to specific membrane receptors, a rapid induction of cyclic AMP-stimulated protein kinase and cyclic AMP binding protein has been reported with half-maximal levels observed within 30 min and maximal levels observed by 4 hr (Majumder and Turkington, 1971). These early effects of prolactin were, however, prevented by both actinomycin D and cycloheximide, suggesting that the concomitant synthesis of RNA and protein was required for induction. Thus, the induction of cyclic AMP-dependent protein kinase probably did not result from the usual mechanisms operable during kinase activation, although conclusions drawn from these inhibitor experiments must be viewed with caution. Furthermore, it was not clear whether increased kinase activity was a cause or an effect of prolactin-regulated gene expression. Presumably, translocation of the catalytic subunit of protein kinase to the nucleus may result in nuclear protein phosphorylation and gene activation (Fig. 1A). Alternatively, translocation of cyclic AMP bound to the regulatory subunit of protein kinase might result in positive regulation of casein gene transcription in an analogous fashion to the action of the CAP protein in bacteria (Anderson *et al.*, 1974). However, there is no proof that either of these mechanisms are operable in regulating gene expression in the mammary gland or, in fact, in any other peptide hormone responsive system.

A comparable system appears to exist for the formation of cGMP by guanylate cyclase and the subsequent activation of cGMP-dependent protein kinase. However, in contrast to the activation of protein kinase by cAMP, dissociation of the catalytic and regulatory subunits of cGMP-dependent protein kinase apparently does not occur upon cGMP binding (Gill *et al.*, 1977). In addition, both soluble and particulate guanylate cyclase activities have been identified (Garbers, 1978). Furthermore, alterations in the intracellular distribution of both cGMP and guanylate cyclase activity have been reported to occur during rat liver regeneration in the absence of net changes in total tissue cGMP (Koide *et al.*,1978). Thus, it may be important to study intracellular compartmentalization of cyclic nucleotides rather than whole tissue levels. As with cAMP, the role of cGMP in the mammary gland is not well defined. While it has been suggested that cGMP may act as a direct mediator of prolactin action on casein synthesis in the mammary gland (Rillema *et al.*, 1977), recent studies in our laboratory using casein mRNA levels as a specific marker of prolactin action have been unable to confirm this hypothesis (Matusik and Rosen, 1980).

B. *Direct Action of Internalized Hormone on Receptor*

In addition to the "second messenger" models, recent studies have also indicated that certain peptide hormones, including prolactin (Nolin, 1978; Nolin and Witorsch, 1976), insulin (Goldfine *et al.*, 1977; Schlessinger *et al.*, 1978), and epidermal growth factor (Schlessinger *et al.*, 1978; Carpenter and Cohen, 1976) may enter the cell (Fig. 1B). Furthermore, the recovery of intact internalized prolactin from rat hepatocytes has been reported (Posner *et al.*, 1977). Uptake of a fragment or a specific subunit of peptides such as diphtheria and cholera toxins has also been demonstrated (Boquet and Pappenheimer, 1976). Furthermore, internalization and processing of the hormone-receptor complex has been suggested recently for epidermal growth factor and its putative membrane receptor (Das and Fox, 1978). Three possible pathways may exist following the entry of peptide hormones and their receptors into cells (Fig. 1B):

(1) Intracellular polypeptide hormone receptors have been demonstrated in rat liver Golgi fractions (Bergeron *et al.*, 1978). While it is conceivable that these receptors are precursors for those receptors in the plasmalemma, they might also function intracellularly or participate in the secretion of the intact hormone. Thus, the presence of prolactin in milk might result from such a process. Alternatively, it may result from the normal process of exocrine secretion.

(2) Direct interaction of the peptide hormone with unique nuclear envelope receptors may provide a mechanism for specific nuclear localization. It has been suggested that such distinct receptors for insulin exist on the rat liver nuclear envelope and that these binding sites have characteristics different from plasma membrane receptors (Vigneri *et al.*, 1978).

(3) If uptake is mediated by endocytosis and subsequent fusion with lysosomes, the internalized hormone and receptor may be ultimately degraded as a means of desensitization. Alternatively, specific processing may occur in lysosomes and a fragment or fragments of the hormone or receptor may act directly or indirectly to activate specific genes. Lysosomal transport of the hormone-receptor complex to the nucleus is also a possibility. Following internalization, some receptors may also be reutilized in the absence of new receptor biosynthesis.

Possible support for a direct role of internalized prolactin comes from the studies of Chomczynski and Topper (1974). They have reported that prolactin and placental lactogen can directly stimulate the rate of UTP incorporation into RNA in nuclei isolated from mammary epithelial cells. However, the significance of these results is difficult to assess in the absence of experiments to analyze the newly synthesized RNA or to delineate effects of these hormones at the level of initiation or elongation of RNA synthesis. Furthermore, prolactin unexpectedly stimulated UTP incorporation in nuclei isolated from both pregnant and lactating tissue, and in the latter case the rates of RNA synthesis should already have been maximal in the presence of high levels of endogenous prolactin. Because of the multiplicity of artifacts that are known to occur in these *in vitro* transcriptional assays, it is necessary to reassess these results using specific cDNA probes and more sophisticated techniques to determine the fidelity of transcription.

Recent synthesis of an artificial hybrid protein-containing diptheria toxin fragment A conjugated to human placental lactogen has also provided investigators with a probe to study the biological effect of the internalization process (Chang *et al.*, 1977). In this hybrid probe, both the toxin A enzymatic activity and the placental lactogen receptor binding activity were partially conserved. However, binding of the probe during mammary gland organ culture did not permit the subsequent entry of the toxin A fragment as assessed by its failure to inhibit protein synthesis. Whether this indicates that the placental lactogen-receptor complex is not specifically internalized or that the toxin A-placental lactogen hybrid is a nonfunctional analog requires further investigation, especially since the ability of the toxin-placental lactogen complex to induce casein synthesis was not determined. Other studies have suggested that it may be possible to uncouple peptide hormone activation of steroidogenesis from its lysosomal uptake and degradation (Ascoli and Puett, 1978). Thus, the role of internalized peptide hormones and their receptors in the regulation of gene expression remains to be established.

Although the "second messenger" system and internalization provide us with two alternative models by which peptide hormones may regulate gene expression, it has not yet been possible to delineate the precise mechanism for their regulation of specific mRNA accumulation. In order to elucidate such a mechanism, we have directed our attention toward studying prolactin induction of casein mRNA im mammary gland organ culture.

III. PROLACTIN INDUCTION OF CASEIN mRNA IN MAMMARY GLAND ORGAN CULTURE

A. *Kinetics of Induction*

Some progress has recently been made in obtaining hormonally responsive primary epithelial cell cultures from pregnant mammary tissue in which the maintenance and induction of differentiated function has been possible (Emerman *et al.*, 1977). However, since no cloned, prolactin-responsive mammary epithelial cell line is presently available for study, we have chosen mammary gland organ culture as a well-characterized and operable system in which to study peptide hormone regulation of a specific mRNA. One advantage of mammary gland organ culture is that it is performed in a serum-free, chemically defined medium, in which the effective concentration of both peptide and steroid hormones can be carefully controlled.

In the experiments to be described, mid-pregnant mammary gland explants were employed rather than explants derived from virgin tissue in order to study the early effects of prolactin in preexisting, differentiated alveolar cells. Because of the high levels of casein mRNA (Rosen *et al.*, 1975; Rosen *et al.*, 1978), which existed in the mid-pregnant rat, explants were initially exposed for 48 hr to a medium containing only insulin and hydrocortisone. Following the first 24 hr in culture, only 10% of the original amount of casein mRNA remained and after the next 24 hr, a further decrease to 4% of the original level was observed (Fig. 2). In the continued presence of insulin and hydrocortisone for 72 hr, the casein mRNA level decreased to *near* steady-state conditions. Routinely, ovine prolactin was added after the initial 48 hr insulin and hydrocortisone time period. In agreement with our previous results (Matusik and Rosen, 1978), a rapid induction of casein mRNA was observed following the addition of prolactin. The rate of accumulation appeared to be linear resulting in 1.6-fold increase by 4 hr and a 7-fold increase from the insulin-hydrocortisone baseline within 24 hr. A small effect of prolactin on casein mRNA levels, i.e., 1.3-fold, was also usually observed within one hour (Matusik and Rosen, 1978). Similar kinetics of induction have been observed following prolactin addition when the level of casein mRNA sequences were determined by either RNA excess or cDNA excess hybridization. The latter technique was especially useful when only small quantities of RNA were available for hybridization. These results suggested that prolactin had a rapid effect on either the transcription or turnover of casein mRNA.

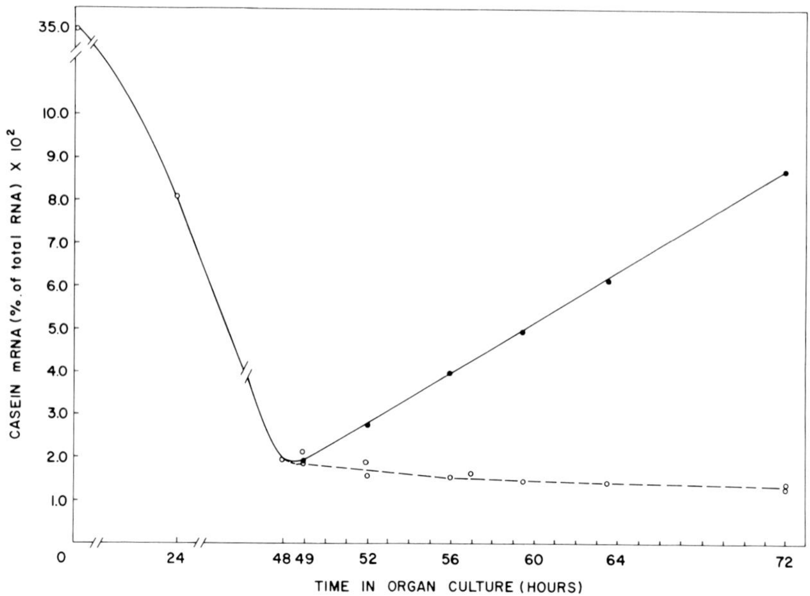

FIG. 2. Prolactin induction of casein mRNA in organ culture. Casein mRNA levels were determined by cDNA excess hybridization as described by Pauley et al. (1978). The conditions of organ culture were essentially the same as those described by Matusik and Rosen (1978). The open circles represent casein mRNA levels in cultures of 15 day pregnant rat mammary explants in the presence of insulin and hydrocortisone (IF). The closed circles show the effect of adding prolactin (M) after 48 hr in culture with IF alone. Fresh media were added after 48 hr to both groups. The data are expressed as the percentage casein mRNA of the total cellular RNA, e.g., the zero time value = 0.35%.

B. *Calculation of the Transcriptional Rate and Half-Life of Casein mRNA*

Using the above data for the prolactin induction of casein mRNA, it is possible to estimate the rate of transcription and the half-life of casein mRNA. In order to perform these calculations, the following assumptions were made: First, the RNA/DNA ratio of the alveolar cell is 1.5. This is the average ratio observed in 13-day pregnant tissue (Matusik, unpublished observations; Richards and Hilf, 1972). Second, at this stage in organ culture the alveolar cells comprise 35% of the total population (Munford, 1963). Third, during the early time periods, i.e., less than 24 hr, no significant increase occurs in alveolar cell number. Finally, a total complexity of 850,000 daltons for the two casein mRNAs was used (Rosen, 1976). This value has been confirmed recently by electron microscopic measurement (Rosen and Robberson, unpublished observations). A comparison of the initial slope of the hybridization of highly purified casein mRNA and total explant RNA under the conditions of cDNA excess was employed to determine the percentage of casein mRNA in a total RNA extract as follows: 100 x slope total extracted RNA ÷ slope pure back hybrid. The RNA/DNA ratio was then used to calculate the picogram of casein mRNA per picogram DNA. Then assuming 35% alveolar cells with 6.5 pg DNA/cell (Sober, 1970), the number of picograms of casein mRNA per cell was determined. The final calculation using the complexity of casein mRNA yielded the number of molecules of mRNA per cell.

It was now possible to calculate the number of molecules of mRNA synthesized per minute per cell and to analyze the rate of synthesis of casein mRNA in the presence and absence of prolactin. Converting the number of molecules of casein mRNA per cell to the rate of accumulation (molecules mRNA per min per cell, dC/dt) allows the determination of the rate of transcription (T) by plotting the rate of accumulation of casein mRNA versus the concentrations of casein mRNA at any given time (C_t). Using the expression $\frac{dC}{dt} = T - DC_t$, the value of T can, therefore, be estimated by extrapolation back to the Y axis. The slope of each line yields the value of D, the rate of degradation, where D is related to the half-life of the mRNA by the first-order decay expression, $D = \ln 2/t_{1/2}$ (Fig. 3). Using this method of analysis, the transcription rates for casein mRNA were estimated to be 11 and 5.2 molecules/min/cell in the presence and absence of prolactin, respectively. Thus, the addition of prolactin increased the rate of casein mRNA transcription approximately 2-fold above control. This increase in transcription was not, however, sufficient to account for the experimental accumulation of casein mRNA (7-fold above control). Thus, these data suggested that in addition to increasing the rate of transcription prolactin might also increase the half-life of casein mRNA. The values estimated for the half-life of casein mRNA in the presence and absence of prolactin were 92 and 5.4 hr, respectively, as shown in Fig. 3. This represents a 17-fold change in the half-life of casein mRNA and, coupled with the 2-fold change in its rate of synthesis, accounts for the observed accumulation of casein mRNA following prolactin addition.

The effect of varying the mRNA half-life on the accumulation of casein mRNA is illustrated in Fig. 4. The actual accumulation of casein mRNA is compared to theoretical mRNA accumulation curves in the presence of prolactin as predicted for several different casein mRNA half-lives (Fig. 4) using the following equation (Kafatos, 1972; Harris *et al.*, 1975):

$$C_t = \frac{T}{D} - \left(\frac{T}{D} - C_o\right)e^{-Dt}$$

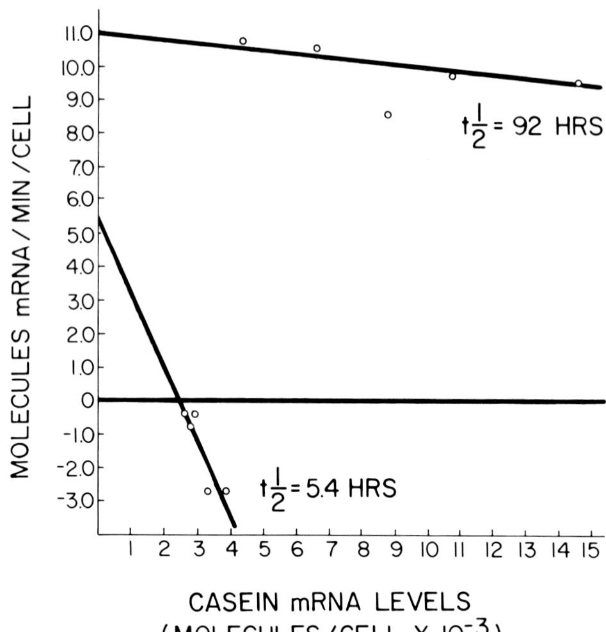

FIGURE 3. Transcription rate and half-life of casein mRNA in the presence (●) and absence (o) of prolactin. The data shown in Fig. 2 were analyzed as described in the text and replotted as the number of molecules of casein mRNA synthesized per minute per cell vs. the concentration of mRNA at a given time. Extrapolation back to the Y axis yields as estimate of the initial rate of transcription, and the slope yielded a value for D, the rate of degradation.

This equation is derived from the previous equation for analyzing mRNA accumulation (see above). C_o is the initial concentration of casein mRNA and a value of 11 molecules/min/cell was used for T as shown above. In the presence of prolactin, the observed accumulation of casein mRNA is best approximated from theoretical mRNA accumulation curves using a half-life of greater than 48 hr (Fig. 4). However, this analysis may be complicated by the fact that prolactin in addition to regulating casein mRNA may be acting mitogenicly. Thus a slight increase in the epithelial cell number at the later times possibly due to prolactin, which was not evident by measuring total DNA content, would influence the number of molecules per cell and the shape of the curve. Therefore, at present these results are best interpreted conservatively, and in the presence of prolactin a long half-life of casein mRNA between 48 and 92 hr is a valid approximation. Similar computer analysis for the fall-off of casein mRNA that occurs in the absence of prolactin has been

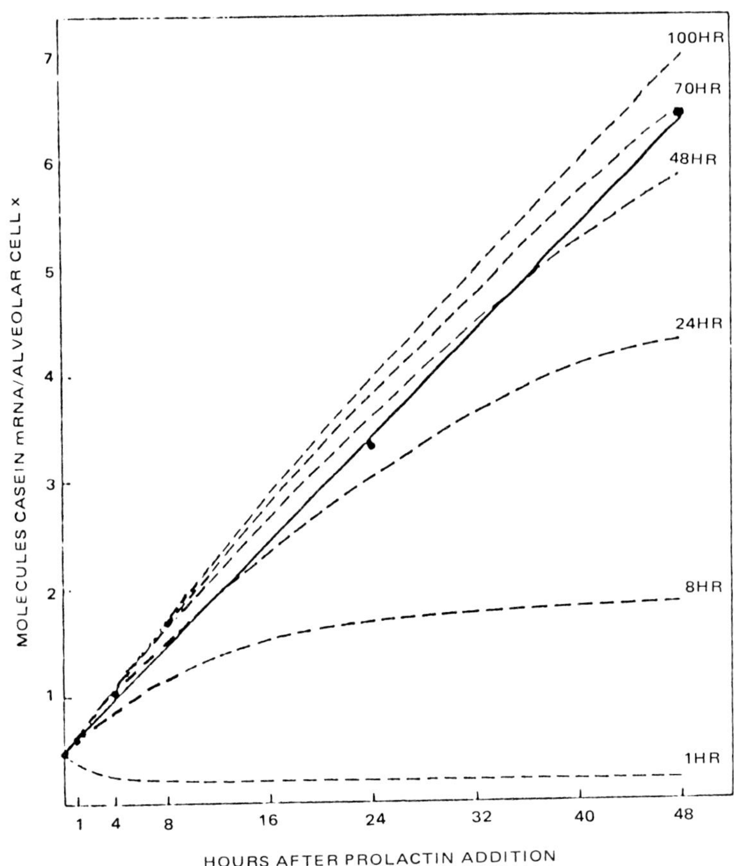

FIGURE 4. Estimation of the half-life of casein mRNA in the presence of prolactin. The data shown by the solid line were taken from Matusik and Rosen (1978). The dashed lines represent theoretical accumulation curves using the different mRNA half-lives shown calculated as described in the text and by Kafatos (1972).

performed. Thus, the addition of prolactin to the mammary gland organ culture increased the rate of casein mRNA transcription by approximately 2-fold and increased the mRNA half-life from 5.4 hr to a value greater than 48 hr. This dual effect of prolactin on both the rates of transcription and degradation of casein mRNA could account for observed accumulation of casein mRNA seen during organ culture. These results also suggest that prolactin regulation of casein gene expression may be a complex process requiring multiple signals that may control transcription as well as the processing and degradation of casein mRNA.

The half-life and transcription rate estimates obtained for casein mRNA appear to be reasonable approximations. They are similar to the reported half-lives and transcription rates of several other abundant mRNAs in specialized cells including ovalbumin mRNA (Harris *et al.*, 1975; Palmiter, 1973), globin mRNA (Aviv *et al.*, 1976), and vitellogenin mRNA (Burns *et al.*, 1978). Although the relative differences between these parameters in the presence and absence of prolactin are valid approximations, their absolute values should be interpreted conservatively since they are based upon a number of assumptions: (1) notably, that transcription rates can be assessed accurately by extrapolation to the *Y* axis; (2) that no marked increase in epithelial cell content occurs during the time in culture. Previous results have suggested that a slight increase in the content of epithelial cell DNA occurs in midpregnant mouse explants after 48 hr in culture with prolactin, insulin, and hydrocortisone (Owens *et al.*, 1973). These half-life and transcription rate values should, therefore, be confirmed by a more direct method that measures the rate of transcription and turnover of pulse-labeled casein mRNA sequences. Such studies using a specific cDNA-cellulose affinity matrix are reported in the following section.

IV. cDNA-CELLULOSE AFFINITY CHROMATOGRAPHY

A. *Selectivity and Fidelity*

The study of specific mRNA transcription is complicated by the fact that each messenger represents only a small fraction of the initial RNA transcripts. Thus, hybridization in solution to a specific cDNA will result in a high-background level of radioactivity due to both nuclease-resistant secondary structure in the radioactive RNA and due to trapping during Cl_3COOH-precipitation. This level may reach 1% of the input radioactivity, making it impossible to detect specific transcripts of unique gene sequences, which may represent only 0.1% of the rapidly labeled RNA. To overcome this problem, cDNA can be covalently attached to an inert matrix and several cycles of hybridization performed or, alternatively, RNase may be used to digest any RNA not present as a true hybrid with the immobilized cDNA.

Several chemical methods are available for coupling DNA to cellulose (Noyes and Stark, 1975), phosphocellulose (Shih and Martin, 1974), and agarose (Robberson and Davidson, 1972). A poly(dC)-tail can also be enzymatically attached to the cDNA and following hybridization in solution, the cDNA-mRNA hybrid is isolated on a poly(I)-sephadex column (Curtis and Weissman, 1976). We have utilized another enzymatic method, originally described by Venetianer and Leder (1974), which allows the cDNA to be reutilized. A purified 15S-casein-mRNA fraction was used as the template to direct the synthesis of casein cDNA by avian myeloblastosis virus, RNA-directed DNA polymerase, with oligo-dT cellulose serving as the DNA-primer. Following synthesis, the 15S casein mRNA was hydrolyzed with 0.1*N* NaOH, leaving casein cDNA attached to the cellulose via the deoxythymidylate residues.

To test the selectivity of this casein-cDNA cellulose, 1 mg of RNA, extracted from an 8-day lactating rat mammary gland, was allowed to hybridize with the cDNA cellulose (Guyette *et al.*, 1979). The nonbinding RNA was saved and following extensive washing the bound mRNA was eluted by "melting" the cDNA-mRNA hybrid. This bound fraction was then rehybridized to generate a second bound fraction. The initial bound RNA was purified 18-fold as assessed by hybridization in solution to casein-specific cDNA. The resultant second bound fraction was purified 340-fold with respect to the total RNA and reacted with the same kinetics as those observed with purified 15S-casein mRNA. The nonbinding RNA from the first hybridization was rehybridized and the resultant nonbinding RNA contained no casein mRNA sequences detectable by hybridization to labeled cDNA. Thus, two passages were sufficient to purify casein-specific sequences from a large amount of total RNA.

This procedure was then used to analyze RNA radio-labeled in mammary gland organ culture. Following 48 hr in the presence of insulin and hydrocortisone, the media was changed and labeling performed for an additional 8 hr in the presence of insulin, hydrocortisone, and prolactin, or only insulin and hydrocortisone. Under these conditions prolactin resulted in a 6-fold increase in the incorporation of ^{3}H-uridine into casein mRNA, in close agreement with the previously determined effect of prolactin on the accumulation of casein mRNA in organ cultures of 15-day pregnant mammary tissue.

To facilitate the handling of more samples, the RNA from pulse-labeling experiments was not subjected to two cycles of hybridization, rather RNase treatment was used to reduce the background level of radioactivity resulting from RNAs other than casein mRNA adsorbing to the cellulose or interacting with the cDNA-mRNA hybrid in a nonspecific manner (Levy and Aviv, 1976). Briefly this procedure involved hybridization in 50% formamide for 24 hr, elution of the nonbound RNA, RNase treatment, and elution of the RNase-sensitive material, and finally elution of the remaining RNA with 0.1*N* NaOH. A further correction for background binding was also made by hybridizing a duplicate labeled sample to ovalbumin cDNA cellulose and subtracting the small percentage of counts released by 0.1*N* NaOH from the percentage released from casein cDNA cellulose. The kinetics and efficiency of hybridization under these conditions was tested using ^{125}I-labeled 15S casein mRNA. In the presence and absence of mammary gland explant RNA, 32% of the input iodinated casein mRNA was hybridized to the cDNA cellulose after 24 hr (Fig. 5A). This number represents the efficiency of hy-

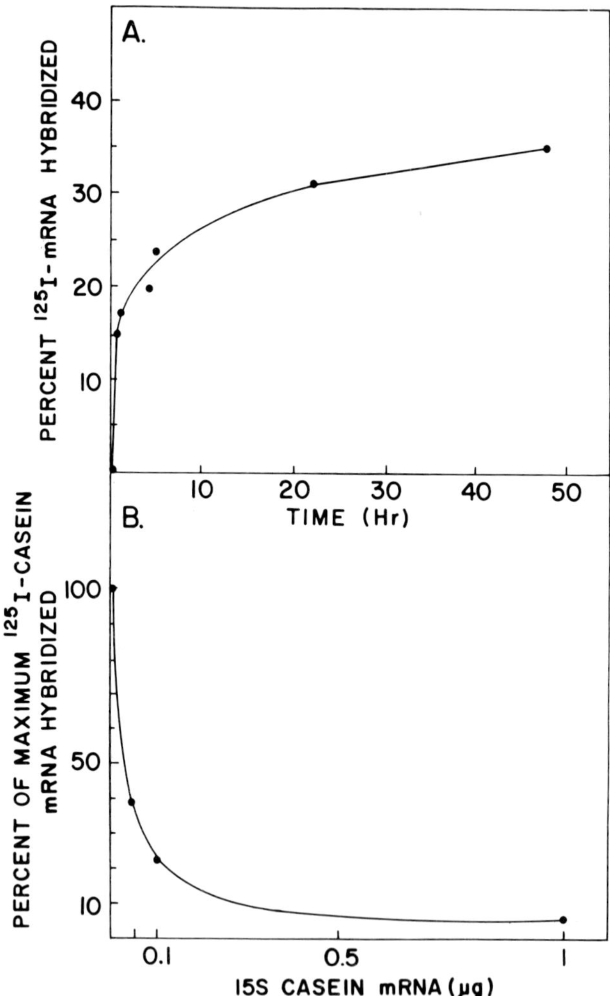

FIGURE 5. Selectivity of cDNA-cellulose affinity chromatography. (A) Kinetics of hybridization of ^{125}I-labeled 15S casein mRNA to casein mRNA. (B) Competition of ^{125}I-casein mRNA hybridization with unlabeled 15S casein mRNA. The conditions of hybridization and elution were essentially the same as those described in the text and by Levy and Aviv (1976) and Guyette et al., *1979).*

bridization under the above conditions and thus can be used to calculate the percent of casein sequences present from the percent of the radioactivity that binds to casein-cDNA cellulose. Unlabeled casein mRNA competed greater than 90% of the ^{125}I-mRNA binding while excess amounts of both poly (A) and oviduct RNA were unable to compete with the binding of iodinated casein mRNA (Fig. 5B). Thus, under these "RNase elution conditions" the cDNA-cellulose affinity matrix was able to bind selectively casein mRNA. This procedure was then used to analyze RNA, extracted from rat mammary gland after a 30-min pulse-label with ^{3}H-uridine in organ culture.

B. Analysis of Casein-Specific Transcripts

The accumulation of labeled RNA, following a long labeling period, as in the previous experiment, reflects the combined effects of synthesis and degradation. To make an accurate judgment concerning the effects of hormones on the rate of transcription, it is necessary to label for a time much shorter than the half-life of the RNA in question. The half-life of casein mRNA in the presence of prolactin has been estimated to be greater than 50 hr and approximately 5 hr in the absence of prolactin. (Section III,B). Thus, a labeling pulse of 30 min was considered sufficiently short to accurately indicate alterations in the rate of transcription.

Approximately 1 x 10^6 cpm of labeled RNA (50 μg) extracted after different times of exposure to hormone was hybridized to casein cDNA cellulose and to ovalbumin cDNA cellulose, and the percent of specific casein transcripts was calculated from the specifically hybridized radioactivity as described above. The results from many such experiments are shown in Fig. 6. In the absence of prolactin, a low percentage of casein transcripts was observed, the mean (from 11 experiments) = 0.09%. During the first 30 min of exposure to prolactin (when ^{3}H-uridine was added simultaneously with the hormone), there was no measurable effect on the transcription of casein mRNA. However, if the pulse was delayed by as little as 30 min following prolactin addition, a large increase in casein specific transcripts was detectable by the end of 30 min. This increased level of transcription appears to remain constant for at least 24 hr. The percent casein transcripts (mean value from nine experiments) in the presence of prolactin was 0.38%. The determination in the presence and absence of prolactin were significantly different at a p value of less than 0.01. Thus, a 4.2-fold increase in casein transcription occurred within 30 min after the

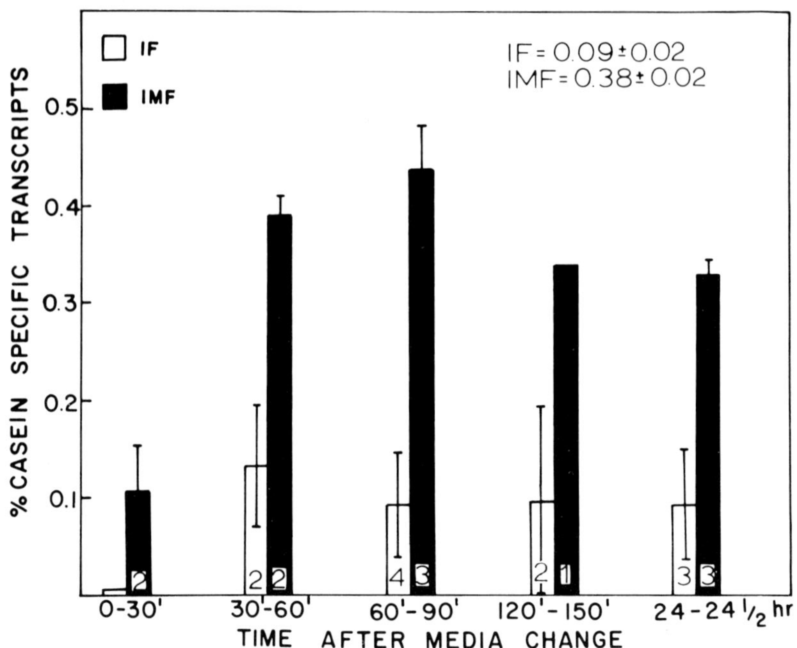

FIGURE 6. Prolactin-induced casein mRNA transcription. The conditions of organ culture are essentially the same as those described in the legend to Fig. 2. After the initial 48 hr in culture with IF alone, the medium was changed and 30-min pulse-labeling performed with ^{3}H-uridine (3 mCi/ml, 50 Ci/mmole) at the times designated. The percentage casein-specific transcripts were calculated as described in the text and the legend to Fig. 5. The error bars indicate the standard errors of the mean and the numbers within each bar represent the number separate experiments. The mean values ±S.E.M. are shown for each group, IF or IMF, in the upper right corner of the figure. Data are taken from Guyette et al., *1979 and reprinted with the permission of Cell.*

addition of prolactin. This is in good agreement with the 2-fold increase in the rate of synthesis determined indirectly by measuring the accumulation of casein mRNA at different times in culture (see Section III,B).

Since a 7- to 13-fold increase in the level of casein mRNA is usually observed following a 24-hr exposure to the hormone, these pulse-labeling studies agree with our hypothesis that prolactin may have a dual mode of action leading to increased casein mRNA levels. To account for the difference in the transcription rate of 2- to 4-fold and the mRNA accumulation of 7- to 13-fold, it is possible that prolactin may also act to increase the half-life of the transcribed RNA either by increasing the efficiency of RNA processing in the nucleus, or perhaps by indirectly stabilizing the mature mRNA. At present, work in our laboratory is aimed at directly testing these hypotheses by measuring the half-life of the mRNA via pulse-chase experiments in organ culture (Footnote 1) and by investigating the possibility of the existence of a higher molecular weight precursor to casein mRNA and the effects of prolactin on its processing.

These studies represent the first demonstration of a rapid effect of a peptide hormone *in vitro* on the transcription and accumulation of a specific mRNA. Studies are also under way to examine the mechanisms by which two steroid hormones, hydrocortisone and progesterone, act to modulate the cells's response to prolactin. Hopefully these studies will increase our understanding of the development and differentiation of the mammary gland and lead to a better understanding of hormonal control of gene transcription and processing in eukaryotic cells.

V. GENE EXPRESSION IN MAMMARY CANCER

A. *Casein-mRNA Levels in DMBA-Induced Mammary Adenocarcinomas*

The expression of differentiated function in hormone-responsive breast cancer has been previously reported in both experimental (Rosen and Socher, 1977) and human breast cancer (Young *et al.*, 1974). Histological examination has revealed the presence of secretory activity in a small proportion of DMBA-induced rat mammary tumors (Archer, 1969) and in a transplantable rat mammary adenocarcinoma (Hilf, 1967). In both cases estradiol treatment caused a lactationlike response in the tumors, and casein was identified in the secretory fluid. Both primary DMBA- and NMU-induced rat mammary carcinomas have recently been reported to contain α-lactalbumin at levels equal to or less than 10% of the amounts found in the 5-day lactating rat mammary gland (Qasba and Guillino, 1977). Transplantation of a pituitary gland under the kidney capsule of the host that leads to elevated serum prolactin levels increased the α-lactalbumin content in the primary DMBA-induced tumors, but unexpectedly reduced the levels observed in the NMU-induced tumors. α-lactalbumin was also detected in the transplantable R3230AC mammary carcinomas, but levels did not increase with pituitary hormone stimulation.

Studies in our laboratory have demonstrated the presence of casein mRNA in approximately 70% of more than 30 DMBA-induced tumors assayed by molecular hybridization (Fig. 7). However,

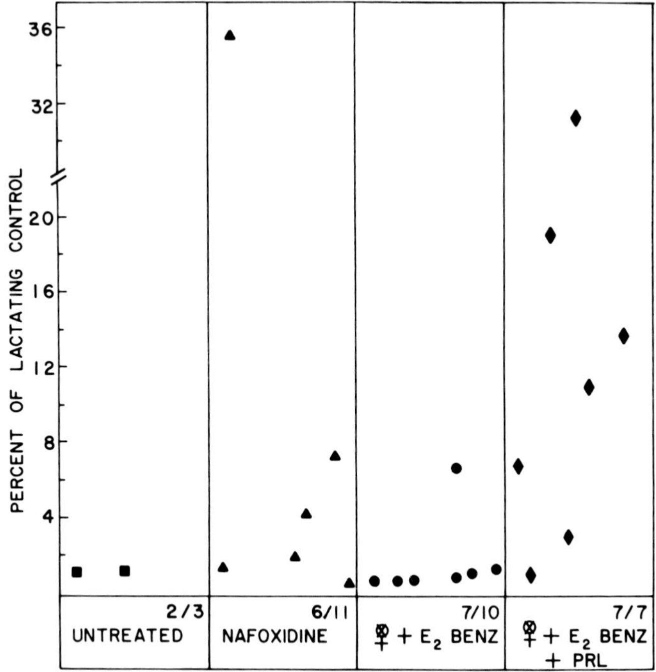

FIGURE 7. Detection of casein mRNA in hormone-dependent mammary cancer by molecular hybridization. The data are taken from Rosen and Socher (1977) and are reprinted with the permission of Nature. *The fractions shown under each group represent the number of tumors in which significant hybridization, i.e., >20% at Rot½ values of 10^3, was observed. The abbreviations used are: ⚥=ovariectomized; E_2BENZ = estradiol benzoate; PRL = prolactin. Experimental details can be found in Rosen and Socher (1977).*

casein mRNA levels were usually only 10% or less of those observed in an 8-day lactating mammary gland. The highest levels of casein mRNA were found in prolactin- and estradiol-treated animals, compared to animals given estradiol treatment alone or in the absence of exogenous hormonal administration. These studies were all performed using the technique of molecular hybridization because the low levels of casein mRNA present in these tumors could not be accurately measured by cell-free translation assays.

At present, it is not possible to determine whether the low

levels of casein mRNA observed in experimental breast cancer are due to a limited proportion of the tumor cell population actively synthesizing casein or a decreased response in the entire cell population (Footnote 2). However, it is clear from both histological examination and autoradiographic localization of prolactin receptors using ^{125}I-prolactin, and casein by immunofluorescence, that heterogeneity of cell types exists within these tumors (Costlow and McGuire, 1977). Thus, in order to correlate the hormonal dependency of tumor growth with hormonally induced differentiated function, it will be necessary to identify theose cell types that produce casein mRNA and casein. This may be accomplished by either *in situ* hybridization using cDNA or immunological localization of casein using fluorescent antibodies.

The absence of casein mRNA in several hormone-independent mammary carcinomas suggested that casein mRNA as detected by cDNA hybridization might be a useful molecular marker for determining hormonal dependence (Rosen and Socher, 1977). Whereas the majority of the DMBA-induced mammary adenocarcinomas in Sprague-Dawley rats are dependent on hormones for growth, those that appear in BALB/c mice are characteristically hormone-independent. Using a homologous mouse 15S casein mRNA-cDNA probe, a number of transplantable mouse mammary tumor lines were also screened for the presence of casein mRNA. In none of these autonomous mouse mammary tumor RNA samples were significant amounts of casein mRNA detected, i.e., levels of casein mRNA of greater than 1 molecule per cell. Thus, casein mRNA may provide a useful marker for prolactin responsiveness in experimental breast cancer.

B. Total mRNA Populations in Normal and Neoplastic Mammary Tissues

In order to study the mechanisms involved in the neoplastic transformation, it will be necessary to identify those molecules responsible for producing altered functions in mammary tumors. One approach is to use molecular hybridization to study the poly(A)-RNA populations in normal and neoplastic tissues. Utilizing molecular hybridization, it is possible to study the transcription of gene products that represent as little as one millionth of the total genomic DNA and to detect specific mRNAs, which may be present in only one copy per cell. Because of the sensitivity and specificity of this technique, it has been used to study gene expression in the developing rat mammary gland and in hormone-dependent mammary tumors.

Total nucleic acids were extracted from DMBA-induced mammary tumors and normal mid-pregnant mammary glands. The poly(A)-RNA populations were then purified by affinity chromatography on oligo dT-cellulose. The poly(A)-RNA was fractionated on 85% formamide, 5-20% sucrose gradients. Hybridization across the gradients with [^{3}H] polyuridine gave average molecular weights of 325,000 and 460,000 for the tumor and mid-pregnant RNAs, respectively. The poly(A) content of both tumor and mid-pregnant RNAs was 5.7% as determined by [^{3}H] polyuridine hybridization. Utilizing the enzyme reverse transcriptase, radio-labeled complementary DNA (cDNA) was synthesized using each of the purified poly(A)-containing RNA populations. Alkaline sucrose gradient centrifugation indicated that the cDNA species were full length copies of the RNA templates.

Molecular hybridization between homologous and heterologous mRNAs and cDNAs was then used to characterize and compare the poly(A)-RNA populations from the neoplastic and the normal tissue (Fig. 8). The extent of both types of hybridizations were greater than 95%. There were no detectable qualitative differences in the poly(A)-RNA sequences found in the tumor and the normal mammary gland. However, differences in the abundancies of various poly(A)-RNA species were observed.

In the normal mammary gland, mRNA sequences for the milk proteins, casein, and α-lactalbumin are specific markers for mammary gland differentiated function. Hybridization of tumor and mid-pregnant cDNAs to a casein and α-lactalbumin-enriched mRNA fraction revealed that these specific gene products comprise 40-50% of the total poly(A)-RNA in the mid-pregnant gland, but were present at a 100-fold lower concentration in the tumor RNA. However, higher levels of casein mRNA might have been induced in these tumors if they were exposed to the same hormonal milieu found in the pregnant rat (Rosen and Socher, 1977).

Thus, the poly(A)-RNA sequences in the tumor are also present in the mid-pregnant mammary gland indicating that large alterations in gene derepresion are not required for the altered function found in neoplastic cells. However, a change in expression of 1% of the mRNA population would probably not be detected by these techniques. These studies also suggest that differences in relative abundancies of specific mRNAs and not the absolute presence or absence of the message are important in determining which mRNAs are expressed. Thus, the regulation of gene expression in neoplastic and normal mammary tissue may not be an "all or none" phenomenon with respect to which mRNAs sequences are transcribed. Differences in cellular phenotype may be brought about by a relatively small number of specific sequences in conjunction with the regulation of the abundancies of sequences that are held in common between the different cell types.

Support for this concept comes from other studies in which molecular hybridization has been used to analyze mRNA populations between different cells and tissues. Molecular hybridization has been used to compare mRNA species in mouse kidney, brain, and

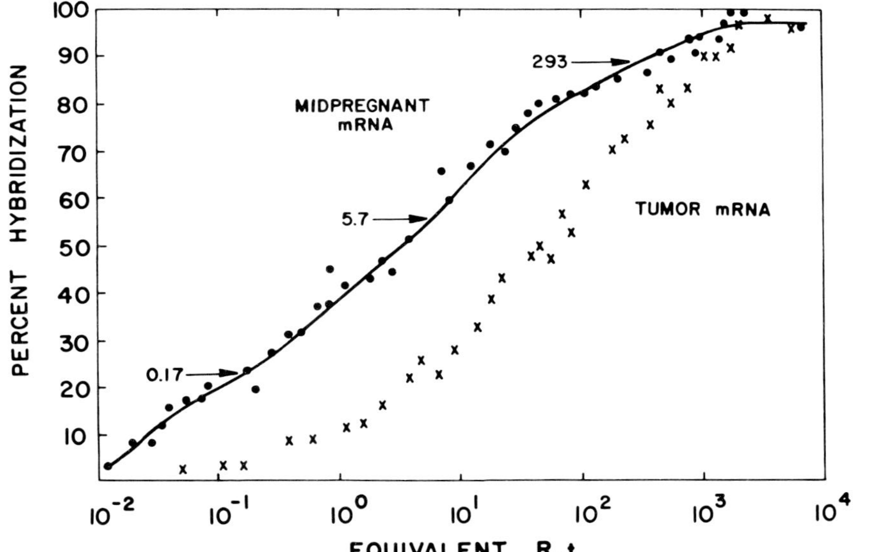

FIGURE 8. Analysis of mid-pregnant and DMBA-induced mammary tumor poly(A)-containing RNA populations. The hybridizations of cDNA synthesized from total cellular poly(A)-containing RNA isolated from a 14-day pregnant rat with its template RNA (⊛) and with total cellular poly(A)-RNA isolated from untreated DMBA-induced mammary carcinomas (x) are shown. The arrows represent the Rot½ values of the three principal abundancy components obtained from a computer-analyzed least-squares fitting program. The conditions of cDNA synthesis and hybridization were essentially the same as those described by Rosen et al. *(1978). The data shown represent RNA pooled from several different DMBA-induced tumors and 14-day pregnant rats and, in some cases, different preparations of cDNA and poly(A)-RNA.*

liver (Hastie and Bishop, 1976). Cross hybridization experiments revealed that a high proportion of the total sequences are held in common among these tissues even though the most abundant class of mRNA is characteristic of a given tissue. For example, the abundant sequences of the liver and kidney were shown to be present also in other tissues, but at a lower frequency. In order to examine nuclear RNA sequences rather than polysomal RNAs that are held in common between various rat tissues, nuclear RNA was hybridized to highly labeled unique sequence DNA (Chikaraishi *et al.*, 1978). These experiments have revealed that the great majority of nuclear RNA sequences homologous to unique sequence DNA are held in common between brain, liver, and kidney.

The poly(A)-RNA in cultured human fibroblasts and SV-40 transformed clones of these cells has also been analyzed using cDNA hybridization (Williams *et al.*, 1977). A class of mRNAs specific for the transformed cells could not be detected by cross hybridization experiments. When the polysomal poly(A)-RNA populations from normal AKR mouse embryo cells and a 3-methylcholanthrene-transformed clone were compared using cDNA hybridization, both mRNA populations were found to be composed of essentially the same sequences (Getz *et al.*, 1977).

These are only a few examples of the qualitative similarities found in mRNA populations in different tissues during different stages of differentiation and in normal and transformed cells. However, it is apparent from these studies that an understanding of gene expression will require an investigation of both the synthesis and processing of specific mRNAs. Differences between normal and transformed mammary cells or between prolactin-stimulated and unstimulated mammary epithelial cells may reflect a coordinated change in both the rates of synthesis and processing of specific transcripts. Regulation of the relative abundancies of certain mRNA sequences may, therefore, provide a mechanism by which the levels of specific proteins and, ultimately, cellular functions are modulated. The search for a unique tumor-specific marker at the molecular level may prove futile if this hypothesis is correct.

ACKNOWLEDMENTS

This work was supported by a grant from the National Institutes of Health CA-16303. J.M.R. is a recipient of a Research Career Development Award CA-00154 and R.J.M. is a recipient of an NIH postdoctoral fellowship CA-05344.

Notes added in proof:

[1]*We have recently demonstrated a selective 20-fold increase in the half-life of casein mRNA by a direct pulse-chase (Guyette* et al., *1979).*

[2]*Recent evidence from our laboratory obtained using a peroxidase-antiperoxidase staining technique and a specific anticasein antibody fraction suggests that only a few cells within the tumor cell population are actively synthesizing casein (Supowit and Rosen, in preparation).*

REFERENCES

Anderson, W. B., Gottesman, M. E., and Pastan, I. (1974). *J. Biol. Chem. 249,* 3592.

Archer, F. L. (1969). *J. Natl. Cancer Inst. 42,* 347.

Ascoli, M., and Puett, D. (1978). *Proc. 60th Annu. Endocrine Soc. Meeting,* Miami, 338a.

Aviv, H., Voloch, Z., Bastos, R., and Levy, S. (1976). *Cell 8,* 495.

Bergeron, J. J. M., Posner, B. I., Josefsberg, Z., and Sikstrom, R. (1978). *J. Biol. Chem. 253,* 4058.

Birnbaumer, L., Yan, P-C., Hunzicker-Dunn, M., Bockaert, J., and Duran, J. M. (1976). *Endocrinology, 99,* 163.

Boquet, P., and Pappenheimer, A. M., Jr. (1976). *J. Biol. Chem. 251,* 5770.

Burns, A. T. H., Deeley, R. G., Gordon, J. I., Udell, D. S., Mullinix, K. P., and Goldberger, R. F. (1978). *Proc. Natl. Acad. Sci. 75,* 1815.

Carpenter, G., and Cohen, S. (1976). *J. Cell Biol. 71,* 159-171.

Chang, Ta-min, Dazord, A., and Neville, D. M., Jr. (1977). *J. Biol. Chem. 252,* 1515.

Chikaraishi, D. M., Deeb, S. S., and Sueoka, N. (1978). *Cell, 13,* 111.

Chomczynski, P., and Topper, Y. J. (1974). *Biochem. Biophys. Res. Commun. 60,* 56.

Costlow, M. E., and McGuire, W. E. (1977). *J. Natl. Cancer Inst. 58,* 1173.

Cox, R. F. (1977). *Biochemistry 16,* 3433.

Curtis, P. J., and Weissman, C. (1976). *J. Mol. Biol. 106,* 1061.

Das, M., and Fox, C. (1978). *Proc. Natl. Acad. Sci. 75,* 2644.

Emerman, J. T., Enami, J., Pitelka, D. R., and Nandi, S. (1977). *Proc. Natl. Acad. Sci. 74,* 4466.

Garbers, D. L. (1978). *J. Biol. Chem. 253,* 1898.

Getz, M. L., Reiman, H. M., Jr., Siegal, G. P., Quinlan, T. J., Prager, J., Elder, P. K., and Moses, H. L. (1977). *Cell 11,* 909.
Gill, G. N., Walton, G. M., and Sperry, P. J. (1977). *J. Biol. Chem 252,* 6443.
Goldfine, I. D., Smith, G. J., Wong, K. Y., and Jones, A. L. (1977). *Proc. Natl. Acad. Sci. 74,* 1368-1372.
Guyette, W. A., Matusik, R. J., and Rosen, J. M. (1979). *Cell 17,* 1013.
Harris, S. E., Rosen, J. M., Means, A. R., and O'Malley, B. W. (1975). *Biochemistry 14,* 2072.
Hastie, N. D., and Bishop, J. O. (1976). *Cell 9,* 761.
Hilf, R. (1967). *Science 155,* 826.
Kafatos, F. C. (1972). *In* "Gene Transcription in Reproductive Tissue" (E. Diczfalusy, ed.) Vol. 5, pp. 319-345. Karolinska Institute, Stockholm, Sweden.
Koide, Y., Earp. H. S., Ong. S. H., and Steiner, A. L. (1978). *J. Biol. Chem. 253,* 4439.
Levy, S., and Aviv, H. (1976). *Biochemistry 15,* 1844.
Majumder, G. C., and Turkington, R. W. (1971). *J. Biol. Chem. 246,* 5545.
Matusik, R. J., and Rosen, J. M. (1978). *J. Biol. Chem. 253,* 2343.
Matusik, R. J., and Rosen, J. M. (1980). *Endocrinology,* in press
Melli, M., Spinelli, G., and Arnold, E. (1977). *Cell 12,* 167.
Munford, R. E. (1963). *J. Endocrinol 28,* 1.
Nolin, J. M. (1978). *Endocrinology 102,* 402-406.
Nolin, J. M., and Witorsch, R. J. (1976). *Endocrinology 99,* 949-958.
Noyes, B. E., and Stark, G. R. (1975). *Cell 5,* 301.
Oka, T., and Perry, J. W. (1976). *J. Biol. Chem. 251,* 1738.
O'Malley, B. W., and Means, A. R. (1974). *Science 183,* 610.
Owens, I. S., Vonderhaar, B. K., and Topper, Y. J. (1973). *J. Biol. Chem. 248,* 472.
Palmiter, R. D. (1973). *J. Biol. Chem. 248,* 8260.
Pauley, R. J., Rosen, J. M., and Socher, S. H. (1978). *Nature 275,* 455.
Posner, B. I., Josefsberg, Z., Patel, B. Z., and Bergeron, J. J. M. (1977). *J. Cell Biol. 75,* 191a.
Qasba, P. K., and Guillino, P. M. (1977). *Cancer Res. 37,* 3792.
Richards, A. H., and Hilf, R. (1972). *Endocrinology 91,* 287.
Rillema, J. A., Linebaugh, B. E., and Mulder, J. A. (1977). *Endocrinology 100,* 529.
Ringold, G. M., Yamamoto, K. R., Bishop, J. M., and Varmus, H. E. (1977). *Proc. Natl. Acad. Sci. 74.* 2879.
Robberson, D. L., and Davidson, N. (1972). *Biochemistry 11,* 533.

Rosen, J. M. (1976). *Biochemistry 15*, 5263.
Rosen, J. M., and Barker, S. W. (1976). *Biochemistry 15*, 5272.
Rosen, J. M., and Socher, S. H. (1977). *Nature 269*, 83.
Rosen, J. M., Woo, S. L. C., and Comstock, J. P. (1975). *Biochemistry 14*, 2895.
Rosen, J. M., O'Neal, D. L., McHugh, J. E., and Comstock, J. P. (1978). *Biochemistry 17*, 290.
Schlessinger, J., Schechter, Y., Willingham, M. C., and Pastan, I. (1978). *Proc. Natl. Acad. Sci. 75*, 2659-2663.
Shih, T. Y., and Martin, M. A. (1974). *Biochemistry 13*, 3411.
Shiu, R. P. C., and Friesen, H. G. (1976). *Science 192*, 259.
Sober, H. A. (1970). "Handbook of Biochemistry, Selected Data for Molecular Biology," 2nd ed., pp. H-112. The Chemical Rubber Publishing Co., Cleveland.
Venetianer, P., and Leder, P. (1974). *Proc. Natl. Acad. Sci. 71*, 3892.
Vigneri, R., Goldfine, I. D., Wong, K. Y., Smith, G. J., and Pezzino, V. (1978). *J. Biol. Chem. 253*, 2098.
Williams, J. G., Hoffman, R., and Penman, S. (1977). *Cell 11*, 901.
Young, S., Pang, L. S. C., and Goldsmith, I. (1974). *J. Clin. Pathol. 27*, 94.

VIRAL ASPECTS OF BREAST CANCER

SYSTEMATICS OF MURINE MAMMARY TUMOR VIRUSES

J. Schlom
D. Colcher
W. Drohan
P. H. Hand
Y. A. Teramoto

National Cancer Institute
National Institutes of Health
Bethesda, Maryland

D. Howard

Life Sciences Division
Meloy Laboratories
Springfield, Virginia

I. INTRODUCTION

The murine model is currently used to study factors involved in the etiology of mammary carcinoma. Over the past four decades, experimental systems have been developed in numerous mouse strains, and in almost every strain studied, a mouse mammary tumor virus (MMTV) has been revealed (Bittner, 1936; Bentvelzen, 1972; Nandi and McGrath, 1973). Various mouse strains differ in incidence of spontaneously occurring mammary tumors, latent period to tumor, types of tumors produced, and whether or not mouse mammary tumor virions are observed in mammary tumors by electron microscopy (Table I). It should be noted that mammary tumors appear "early" (before 1 yr) in the high incidence mouse strains C3H, RIII, and GR, and "late" (after 1 yr) in low and moderate incidence strains C3HfC57BL and BALB/c.

A question that has remained unanswered concerning the origin of mammary oncogenesis in the mouse is: How many mouse mammary tumor viruses are there? There are at least two considerations involved in this question: (a) each mouse strain

ISBN 0-12-131150-3

TABLE I. Mammary Tumor Incidence in Various Mouse Strains

Mouse strain	Virus designation MTV-	Mammary tumor incidence (%)	Latent period (months)	Type of mammary tumor	Virions in tumor
C3H	S	100	7	Fast growing, hormone-independent	++
RIII	SP	96	9	Fast-growing, hormone-independent	++
GR	P	100	3	Hormone-dependent plaques, progress to hormone independent	++
C3HfC57BL	L	35	19	Slow-growing, hormone independent	+
BALB/c	O	10	14	Slow-growing, also acanthomas	-
C57BL	Y	<1	24	Hormone independent	-

may contain its own mouse mammary tumor virus or viruses, which are partially related to or distinct from other viruses of other mouse strains, or (b) there is only one MMTV and each mouse strain exerts its own control over various properties of this virus, such as its expression, or its virulence. The answer to this question is essential to our understanding of the murine model and for a better definition of trans-species reactivities involving MMTV.

MMTVs have been classically characterized on the basis of their host of origin and biological activity (MTV-S, P, O, etc., Table I). Many of the studies conducted as a basis for this classification, however, did not take into account variations in host defense mechanisms from one mouse strain to another. Furthermore, many of these studies employed foster-nursing as a means of virus introduction, thereby making important quantitation of virus inoculum impossible.

A recent achievement has been the ability to productively infect heterologous cells with various MMTV isolates (Lasfargues *et al.*, 1976; Howard *et al.*, 1977). The MMTVs grown in feline cells share nucleic acid and immunologic properties with their mouse-grown counterparts. These reagents have now made possible the delineation between viral-coded vs. host-derived entities.

Recent techniques in nucleic acid chemistry, protein chemistry, and immunochemistry can thus now be used to delineate any differences that may exist among MMTVs. We report here that radioimmunoassays for the major external and internal MMTV proteins, tryptic peptide analyses of MMTV proteins, and nucleic acid hybridization to murine DNAs can all be used to distinguish various MMTVs. These techniques have also been used to detect MMTV-related nucleic acids and proteins in other rodent species and to identify a new virus immunologically related to MMTVs.

In the nucleic acid hybridization and immunologic studies to be presented here, reagents from both murine- and feline-grown MMTVs were employed with identical results, thus demonstrating the viral-coded nature of the nucleic acids and proteins being studied.

II. HETEROGENEITY IN MMTV-CODED GENE PRODUCTS

A. *Type- and Group-Specific Reactivities of the MMTV Envelope Glycoprotein*

The major surface component of the MMTV virion is a 52,000*d* glycoprotein (gp52). The other major protein components of the MMTV virion are a 36,000-38,000*d* glycoprotein (gp36-38), and the 28,000 (p28), 14,000 (p14), and 10,000 (p10) dalton polypeptides. With the development of sensitive radioimmunoassays for the whole MMTV virion (Cardiff *et al.*, 1974), or for purified MMTV polypeptides (Parks *et al.*, 1974; Verstraeten *et al.*, 1975; Ritzi *et al.*, 1976; Sheffield *et al.*, 1977), it has become possible to precisely analyze similarities or differences among MMTVs from different mouse strains. Several investigators have previously shown that the gp52 of MMTVs contains group-specific antigenic determinants (Parks *et al.*, 1974; Verstraeten *et al.*, 1975; Ritzi *et al.*, 1976; Sheffield *et al.*, 1977). Experiments have recently been described (Teramoto *et al.*, 1977a,b) that also demonstrate type-specific antigenic determinants on the gp52 molecule.

MMTVs from RIII and C3H mice, i.e., MMTV(RIII) and MMTV(C3H), were used in a competitive radioimmunoassay (RIA) to compete for the binding of anti-MMTV(C3H) to [^{125}I]-labeled MMTV(C3H) virions. In this system, increasing amounts of MMTV(RIII) competitor gave a shallower slope than that given by the homologous MMTV(C3H) (Fig. 1A). At the highest input of competing MMTV(RIII) protein employed, i.e., 100 μg, only 75% inhibition was obtained while less than 1 μg of MMTV(C3H) resulted in the same competition. In a "group-specific" assay using anti-MMTV(C3H) vs. [^{125}I]-MMTV (RIII), both viruses competed identically, i.e., with comparable inputs and with the same slopes.

The addition of increasing amounts of MMTV(GR) into the anti-MMTV(C3H) vs. [^{125}I]-MMTV(C3H) system did not cause complete inhibition of the precipitation of [^{125}I]-MMTV(C3H) (Fig. 1B). Even at high inputs of protein, MMTV(GR) was incapable of competing for all the antibodies binding to MMTV(C3H). The anti-MMTV(C3H) sera, therefore, appear to contain an antibody population that is directed towards antigenic determinants that are present in MMTV(C3H) but not in MMTV(GR). To further amplify the type specific reactions observed, anti-MMTV(C3H) sera were absorbed with MMTV(GR) and the immune precipitate was removed by centrifugation. The resulting absorbed sera retained their ability to bind [^{125}I]-MMTV(C3H). This binding could be completely inhibited by the addition of MMTV(C3H) or MMTV(C3H) gp52 but was not inhibited by the addition of up to 10,000 ng of MMTV(GR) competitor (Fig. 1C). Additional type-specific reactivities among the various MMTVs also exist. These include differences between MMTV(C3H) and the endogenous MMTV of C3H obtained from C3HfC57BL mice (Teramoto *et al.*, 1977a, b).

The type and group specificities of MMTVs grown in feline cells (Howard *et al.*, 1977) were indistinguishable from the reactivities observed with murine-grown MMTVs, thus providing strong evidence that the MMTV gp52 antigens are viral coded. The analysis of feline grown MMTV further excludes the possibilities that the observed antigenic differences were due to either dif-

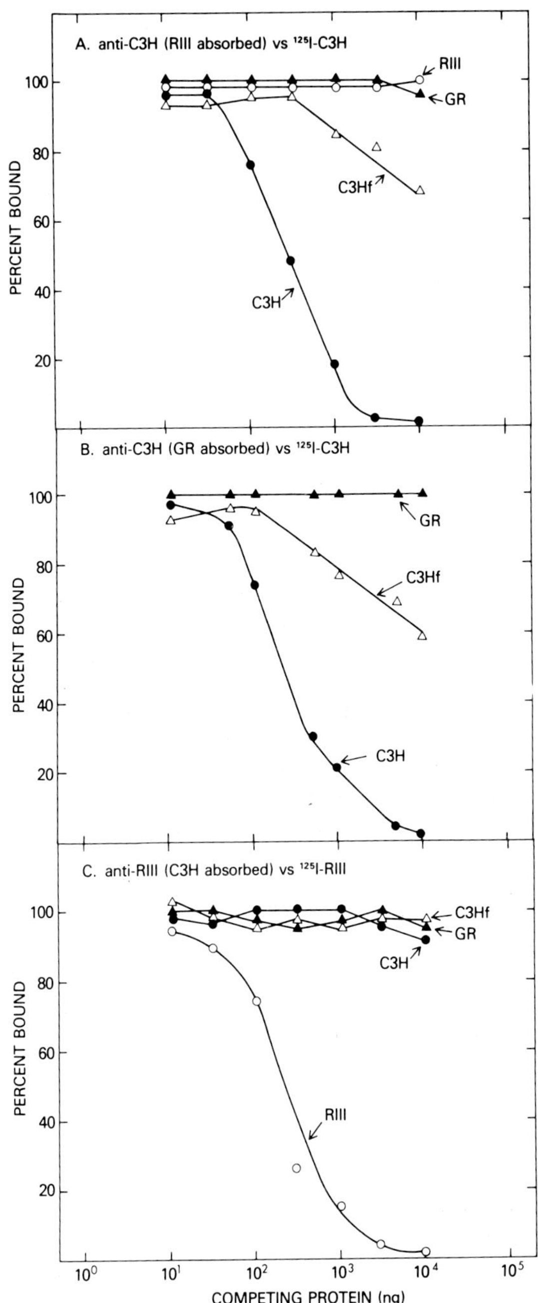

FIGURE 1. Competition radioimmunoassay for MMTV gp52. (A) Anti-MMTV(C3H) serum at a 1:10,000 input dilution was used to precipitate 10,000 cpm of [^{125}I]-MMTV(C3H) intact virions. MMTV(RIII) (O), and MMTV(C3H) (●), were used as

ferences in host antigenic determinants of the different mouse strains producing the virus, or to host-coded differences in glycosylation of virions.

The identification of the type-specific differences for different MMTVs is now being used in several laboratories to monitor the host's immune response to mammary tumorigenesis, as well as in studies seeking trans-species reactivities with MMTVs. These studies further delineate the molecular diversity of viruses that can be involved in the etiology of mammary carcinoma within a given species.

B. *Type- and Group-Specific Reactivities of the MMTV Major Internal Protein*

We have recently developed a competition RIA for the 28,000d major internal protein (p28) of MMTV (Teramoto and Schlom, 1978). When this assay was conducted with high antibody dilutions for maximum sensitivity, no differences were observed among MMTVs from RIII, GR, C3H, or C3HfC57BL mice or with mammary tumor extracts from those mice. To demonstrate type-specific reactivities associated with the MMTV p28 polypeptide, assay conditions of low antibody dilution were used.

The binding of antisera prepared against the p28 of MMTV from RIII mice to [^{125}I]-MMTV(RIII) p28 could be completely inhibited by the addition of 1 μg of purified MMTV(RIII) p28 (Fig. 2A). The addition of increasing amounts of MMTV(C3H) p28 also competed for this binding, but with a shallower slope characteristic of a cross-reacting (Hunter, 1973) but not identical antigen (Fig. 2A). Changing the radioactive antigen from [^{125}I]-MMTV(RIII) p28 to [^{125}I]-MMTV(C3H) p28 and maintaining the same antibody dilution revealed that both MMTV(RIII) p28 and MMTV(C3H) p28 competed identically in the radioimmunoassay (Fig. 2B). Thus, the MMTV p28 appears to contain both indistinguishable, i.e., group-specific, antigenic determinants as well as distinguishable, i.e., type-specific, antigenic determinants (Teramoto and Schlom, 1978).

---

competitors. (B) Anti-MMTV(C3H) serum at a 1:10,000 input dilution was used to precipitate [^{125}I]-MMTV(C3H) whole virions. MMTV(C3H) (●), and MMTV(GR) (▲), were used as competitors. (C) Anti-MMTV(C3H) serum, absorbed with MMTV(GR), was used at a 1:1,000 dilution to precipitate [^{125}I]-MMTVC3H) whole virions. MMTV(C3H) (●), C3H type-C virus (△), MMTV(RIII) (O), and MMTV(GR) (▲) were used as competitors.

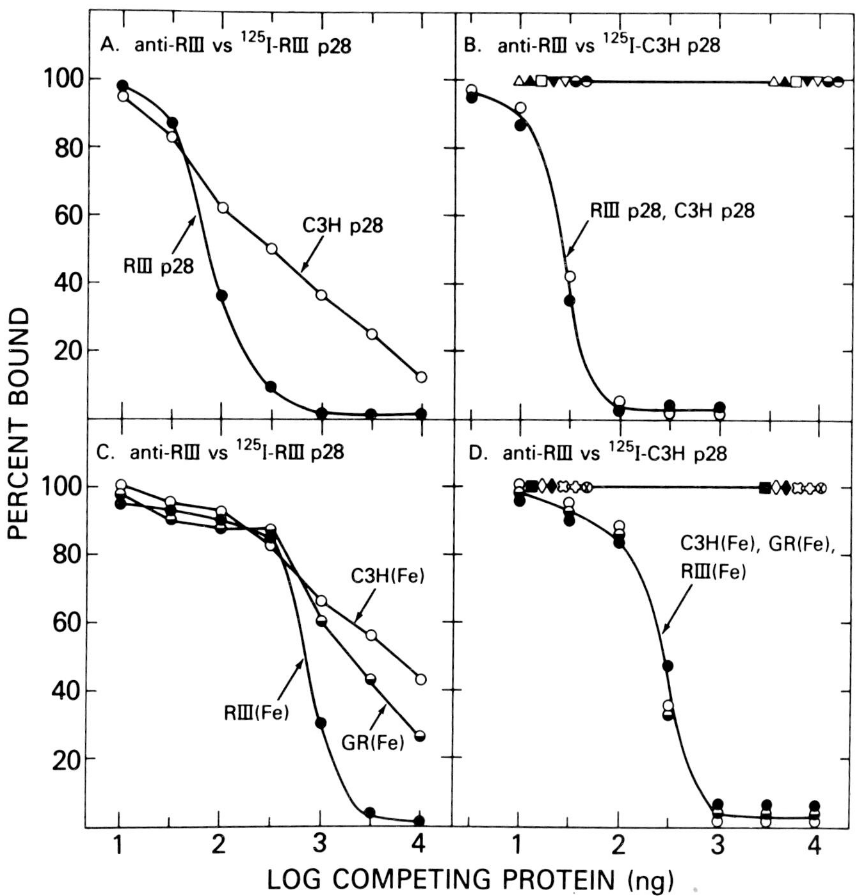

FIGURE 2. Group-specific and type-specific reactivities of MMTV p28. Anti-MMTV(RIII) p28 was used at a final dilution of 1:1000 to precipitate [^{125}I]-MMTV(RIII) p28 in A and C (type-specific assays) and [^{125}I]-MMTV(C3H) p28 in B and D (group-specific assays). Purified MMTV p28s and MMTV virions grown in feline cells (Fe) were used as competitors as indicated. The following were also used as competitors: △, langur type-D retrovirus; ▲, Mason-Pfizer virus: ■, squirrel-monkey retrovirus; ▼, RD-114 virus; ▽, avian myeloblastosis virus; ◐, bovine leukemia virus; ◒, guinea pig virus; ▬, M432 Mus cervicolor *virus; ◊ endogenous MuLV(C3H) virus; ◆, Rauscher murine leukemia virus; X, extract of CrFK feline cells; +, fetal calf serum proteins; ⊗, purified MMTV gp52.*

Both type-specific and group-specific reactivities were retained when MMTVs were used that were grown in the same feline CrFK cell line (Fig. 2C). All three of the MMTVs grown in feline cells, however, competed identically in the anti-MMTV(RIII) p28 vs. [^{125}I] MMTV(C3H) "group specific" p28 radioimmunoassay (Fig. 2D).

Using the combination of gp52 and p28 RIAs, levels of MMTV gene expression can now be analyzed in terms of both viral glycoproteins and nonglycoproteins. This type of comparison is important in light of recent evidence of noncoordinate polypeptide chain initiation of glycosylated vs. nonglycosylated MMTV proteins in infected cells (Schochetman and Schlom, 1976). These combined radioimmunoassays should further elucidate the mechanisms of MMTV replication and gene expression in murine mammary tumors.

C. *Tryptic Peptide Analyses of MMTV Gene Products*

Tryptic peptide analyses (Elder *et al.*, 1977) have been performed on the 52,000 and 36,000-38,000 dalton glycoproteins and the nonglycosylated 28,000, 14,000, and 10,000 dalton proteins of the highly oncogenic MMTVs of C3H, RIII, and GR mice (Gautsch *et al.*, 1978). Each virus was grown in both murine and feline cells to ensure the viral-coded nature of each peptide analyzed. The gp36-38 peptide maps of all three MMTVs were indistinguishable as were the p14 maps for each virus. Both the gp52 (Fig. 3) and the p28 (Fig. 4) of MMTV(C3H), however, could be clearly distinguished from the corresponding proteins of MMTV(RIII) and MMTV(GR), regardless of whether the viruses were grown in feline or murine cells. The p10 of MMTV(RIII), on the other hand, was clearly different from that of MMTV(C3H) and MMTV(GR) (Gautsch *et al.*, 1978). Therefore, tryptic peptide analysis of three MMTV proteins, gp52, p28, and p10 can serve to distinguish these three viruses from one another. These studies represent further strain-specific markers for several MMTV gene products. Thus, as for type-C retroviruses of the mouse (Elder *et al.*, 1977), MMTVs form a multigene family, the final extent of which is not yet known.

III. HETEROGENEITY IN MMTV GENOMES AND MODE OF TRANSMISSION

Studies employing both MMTV radioactive 60-70S RNA and MMTV cDNA probes have demonstrated that MMTV proviral sequences are present in the DNA of all strains of laboratory mice. Copy numbers are in the low repetitive range for normal tissues such

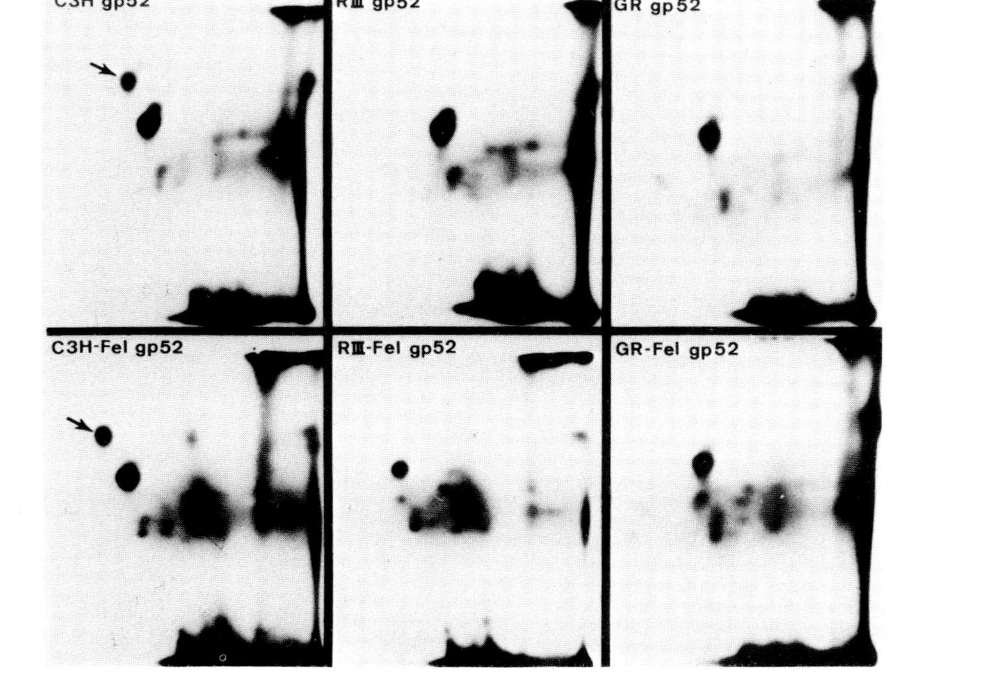

FIGURE 3. Tryptic peptide maps of MMTV gp52s. Two-dimensional fingerprints of the gp52s from the MMTVs were performed as described (Elder et al.*, 1977; Gautsch* et al.*, 1978). The peptide maps of gp52s from mouse- and feline (Fel)-grown viruses are shown in the top and bottom rows, respectively. The arrows in the MMTV(C3H) gp51 maps show an additional peptide which distinguishes this protein from the gp52s of the RIII and GR viruses.*

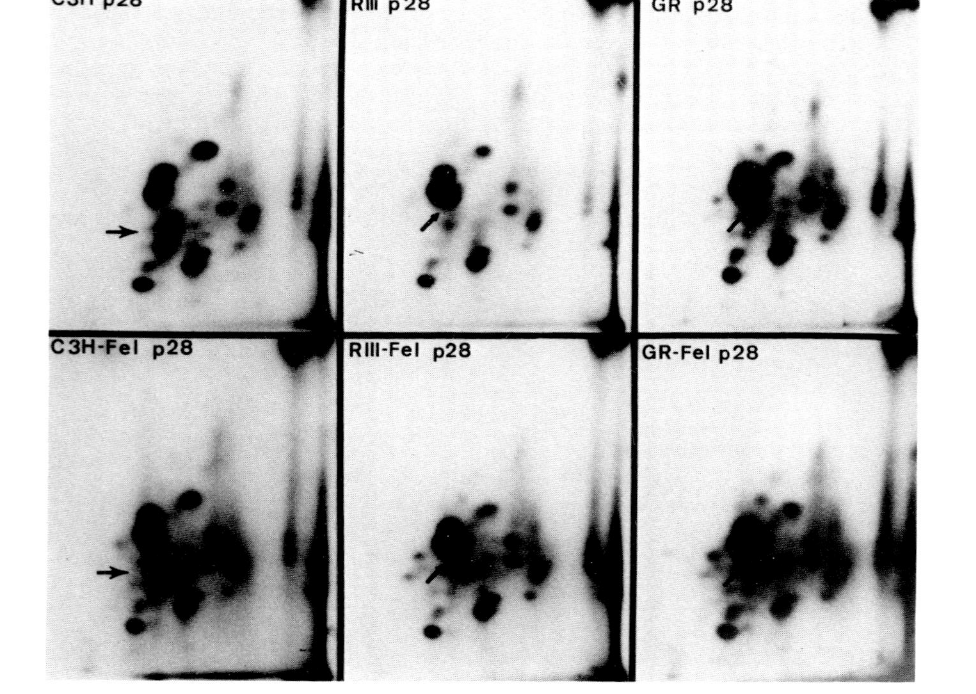

FIGURE 4. Tryptic peptide maps of MMTV p28s. Two-dimensional fingerprints of tyrosine-containing tryptic peptides of the p28s of various MMTVs grown in murine and feline cells. The arrows indicate the difference between the p28 of MMTV(C3H) grown in either murine or feline cells and the MMTVs of RIII and GR mice.

as liver and are higher in mammary tumors (Varmus *et al.*, 1972; Varmus *et al.*, 1975; Drohan *et al.*, 1977; Morris *et al.*, 1977; Schlom *et al.*, 1977; Cardiff, 1978).

Biological studies have shown that MMTVs can be transmitted in different mouse strains either by the milk, or via the germ line (Bittner, 1936; Bentvelzen, 1972; Nandi and McGrath, 1973). Occasionally, MMTV may also be transmitted by male seminal fluids to females, which in turn can transfer the virus to their progeny via the milk (Bentvelzen, 1972; Nandi and McGrath, 1973). Other modes of transmission are, of course, possible. The question that arises is: Can one distinguish if an MMTV has been introduced into a given mouse via the germ line (i.e., as a germinal provirus or virogene) or via some nongerm line mechanism, such as via the placenta, milk, seminal fluid, or as a plasmid? The term "horizontal transmission" is not used here due to the confusion that would arise from such modes of viral transmission as via the placenta or as a plasmid in a germ cell. If an MMTV was introduced into a mouse via the germ line, one would expect to find MMTV proviral sequences equally distributed in the DNA of all tissues of that mouse. On the other hand, if an MMTV was introduced into a mouse by some other mechanism, one would expect to see an uneven distribution of MMTV sequences in the DNA of different tissues of that mouse. To address these points, we used the technique of molecular hybridization.

MMTV(C3H) was isolated from supernatant fluids of a C3H mammary tumor cell line. The 60-70S RNA from these virions was purified and iodinated to a specific activity of approximately 2×10^7cpm/μg as described previously (Drohan *et al.*, 1977). This RNA was then hybridized at various C_0t values to DNA from C3H mammary tumor cells and DNA from an apparently normal C3H liver; hybridization to sheep DNA was used as a control. C_0t is defined as the product of the DNA concentration in moles of deoxyribonucleotide per liter and incubation time in seconds. As assayed by resistance to ribonuclease (RNase A and T_1) digestion, hybridizations to sheep and other nonrodent DNAs remained consistently at less than 6% up to a C_0t of 35,000 and were thus scored as nonspecific background. Hybridization between the iodinated MMTV(C3H) 60-70S RNA and DNA from C3H mammary tumors was approximately 60% (Fig. 5A). This value was consistently higher than the maximum extent of hybridization between this MMTV(C3H) RNA and DNAs from livers or other normal organs of C3H mice (Fig. 5A).

The C_0t 1/2 value was approximately 380 for the hybridization between MMTV(C3H) [^{125}I]-RNA and the C3H mammary tumor DNA, and approximately 440 for C3H liver DNA. For comparison, poly A enriched C3H cellular RNA (selected by poly U Sepharose chromatography), representing messenger RNA, was also iodinated and hybridized to C3H liver DNA. The C_0t 1/2 value obtained using this RNA was approximately 3100, thus representing the value

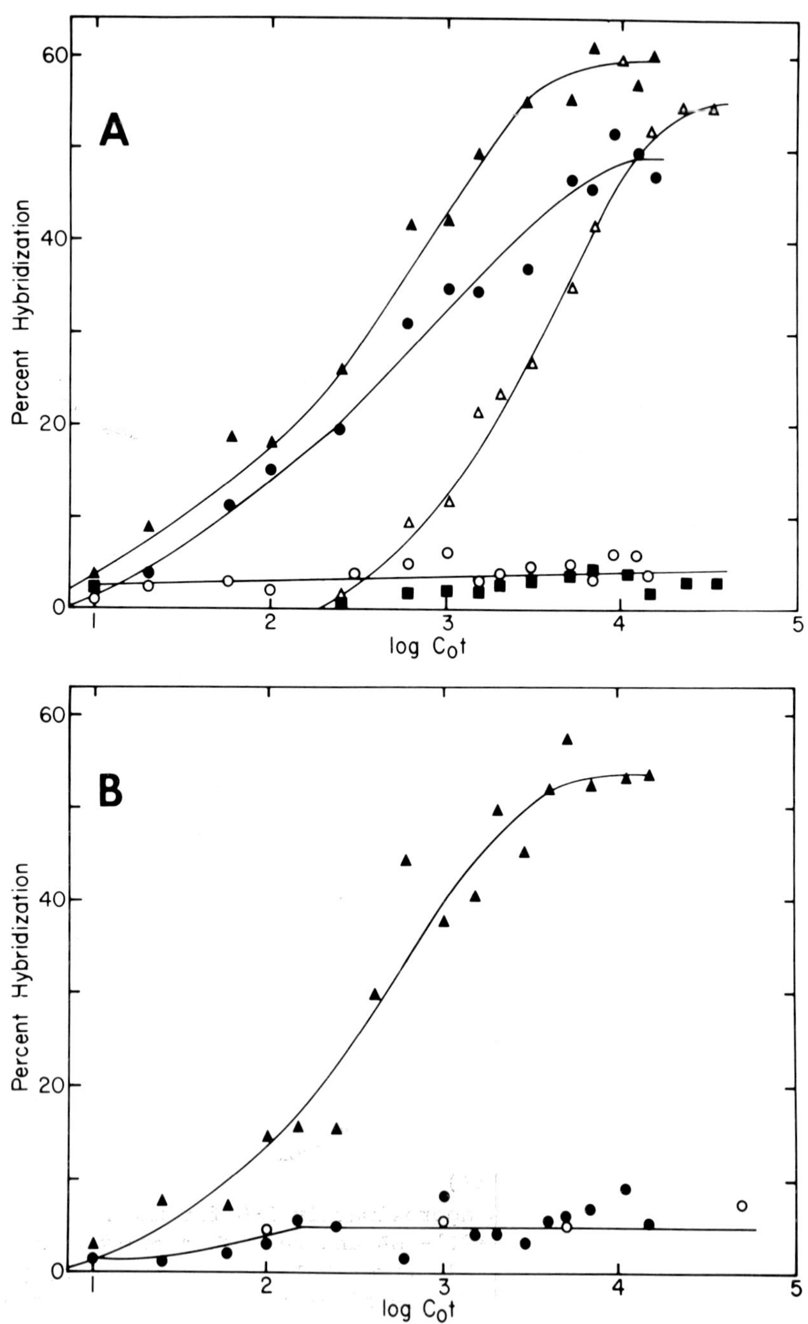

A
Percent Hybridization
0
20
40
60
1
2
3
4
5
log C_0t
B
Percent Hybridization
0
20
40
60
1
2
3
4
5
log C_0t

obtained with "unique" DNA. The results depicted in Fig. 5A demonstrate that both the C3H mammary tumor cell line and C3H liver contain MMTV proviral sequences in the low repetitive range (Drohan *et al.*, 1977). The lower C_0t 1/2 value obtained with the C3H mammary tumor cell line DNA indicates that there are more MMTV proviral sequences in this DNA than in the DNA of the C3H liver. The differences in final percent hybridization, i.e., approximately 60% for the C3H tumor cell line DNA, and approximately 50% for the C3H liver DNA, however, may be indicative of one or a combination of two phenomena: (a) there are quantitatively more MMTV proviral sequences in the mammary tumor DNA than normal cellular DNA; (b) the DNA of the C3H mammary tumor cells contain sequences of the MMTV genome that are not found in the DNA of normal cells of C3H mice. To answer this question, recycling experiments were performed.

A. *Isolation of MMTV(C3H) Tumor-Associated (TA) Sequences*

To determine if there are MMTV proviral sequences present in early C3H mammary tumors that are not present in the DNA of apparently normal C3H tissues, recycling experiments were conducted. Iodinated MMTV(C3H) 60-70S RNA was first hybridized to a vast excess of C3H liver DNA. Liver DNA was chosen because murine livers have been shown to be negative for most MMTV markers (Bentvelzen, 1972; Nandi and McGrath, 1973). 300,000 cpm of [^{125}I]-MMTV(C3H) 60-70S RNA was first annealed to 30 mg of normal C3H liver DNA at 68°C to a C_0t of 20,000 as described previously (Drohan *et al.*, 1977). The unhybridized single-stranded [^{125}I]-RNA eluted from the hydroxylapatite column at 0.14*M* sodium phosphate. This RNA was then concentrated and reannealed to C3H mammary tumor DNA and to C3H liver DNA to a C_0t of 20,000. The recycled MMTV(C3H) RNA failed to

---

FIGURE 5. (A) Cellular hybridization of [^{125}I]-labeled MMTV(C3H) 60-70S RNA to DNAs as described (Drohan et al.*, 1977). DNA from the C3H mammary tumor cell line (▲); normal C3H liver (●); and sheep lung (O). For comparison, hybridizations were performed between [^{125}I]-labeled poly(A)-enriched mouse RNA and C3H liver DNA (△) and calf thymus DNA (■). (B) Hybridization of recycled [^{125}I]-labeled MMTV(C3H) RNA to cellular DNAs. Iodinated MMTV(C3H) 60-70S RNA was extensively hybridized to normal C3H liver, and the unhybridized fraction was recovered by hydroxylapatite column chromatography as described (Drohan* et al.*, 1977). The recycled RNA was then hybridized to the following cellular DNAs: C3H mammary tumor cell line (▲); C3H liver (●); and sheep lung (O).*

hybridize above background levels to the DNA of normal C3H livers (Fig. 5B) or other apparently normal C3H organs (Drohan *et al.*, 1977). This demonstrates that the recycling procedure effectively removed all portions of the MMTV(C3H) [^{125}I]-RNA that are complementary to the DNA of normal C3H tissues. These sequences, however, hybridize extensively with DNA from early occurring C3H mammary tumors (Fig. 5B), thus demonstrating the existence of MMTV(C3H) "tumor associated" sequences.

B. *Natural Distribution of MMTV(C3H) Tumor-Associated Sequences*

Studies were conducted to determine the natural distribution of MMTV(C3H) tumor-associated (TA) sequences in various murine DNAs. The MMTV(C3H) [^{125}I]-RNA representing TA sequences was first hybridized to DNA from RIII livers and RIII mammary tumors that arise early in life. Complementary sequences were found in the DNA of all "early" mammary tumors tested but not in the DNA of livers (Table II).

The GR strain of mice is of great interest as a result of genetic studies that have indicated the possible transmission of MMTV in this strain as a one-gene dominant characteristic (Bentvelzen, 1972). The tumor-associated MMTV(C3H) [^{125}I]-RNA was hybridized to GR mammary tumor and liver DNAs. Complementary sequences are present in the DNAs of both GR mammary tumors and GR livers (Table II) as well as other GR organs tested. These studies demonstrate that MMTV(C3H) tumor-associated sequences may be integrated as a germinal provirus in some mice. We have recently found that certain colonies of C3H mice, designated C3H/Bi (Bittner), also contain MMTV(C3H)-TA sequences integrated in DNA of normal tissues. The possibility exists, therefore, that MMTV(C3H)-TA sequences became integrated into C3H/Bi DNA some time after 1932 when C3H/Bi and C3H/He (Heston) colonies were separated.

DNA of "late" occurring mammary tumors of the low and moderate incidence strains BALB/c and C3HfC57BL (Table I) were also analyzed for the presence of the MMTV(C3H)-TA sequences in their DNA and were consistently found negative. Since the C3HfC57BL strain was originated by foster-nursing C3H mice on C57BL mothers, a strain of mice devoid of overt MMTV in its milk (Bentvelzen, 1972; Nandi and McGrath, 1973), further evidence is provided that the MMTV(C3H)-TA sequences are part of the milk-transmitted MMTV(C3H) and are not germ-line transmitted.

Livers of BALB/c, C57BL/6N, and C57BL/10SCN mice were shown to contain some MMTV proviral information (Varmus *et al.*,

TABLE II. Distribution of MMTV(C3H) Tumor-Associated Sequences[a]

Source of murine DNA		*% Hybridization*
C3H/HeN	*mammary tumor*	*44*
C3H/HeN	*liver*	*7*
RIII	*mammary tumor*	*47*
RIII	*liver*	*7*
DBA/2	*mammary tumor*	*45*
DBA/2	*liver*	*6*
GR	*mammary tumor*	*40*
GR	*liver*	*38*
BALB/c	*mammary tumor*	*7*
BALB/c	*liver*	*7*
C3HfC57BL	*mammary tumor*	*7*
C3HfC57BL	*liver*	*5*
C57BL/6N	*liver*	*4*
C57BL/10SCN	*liver*	*6*
A/He	*liver*	*7*
NIH Swiss	*liver*	*3*
NZB/N	*liver*	*4*
NZW/N	*liver*	*6*
C3H/Bi(Micro. Assoc.)	*liver*	*24*
C3H/Bi(Simonson)	*liver*	*20*

[a]*Six hundred cpm of MMTV recycled [^{125}I]-RNA were hybridized to 500 μg of cellular DNA to a C_0t of 15,000 (in 0.4*M *NaPB, pH 6.8, and 0.05% SDS) and assayed using RNase as previously described (Drohan* et al., *1977).*

1972, 1975; Morris *et al.*, 1977; Schlom *et al.*, 1977; Cardiff, 1978); they do not contain, however, nucleotides homologous to the MMTV(C3H) tumor-associated sequence RNA (Table II).

It thus appears that the virus (or viruses) responsible for causing early mammary tumors in C3H, RIII, and GR mice are easily distinguishable from the virus (or viruses) causing late mammary tumors in C3HfC57BL mice and BALB/c mice by the presence of TA sequences in members of the former group. Furthermore, a virus similar to the highly oncogenic nongerm line-transmitted C3H virus appears to be a germinal provirus in the DNA of the GR strain, the only strain in which genetic evidence has been presented for a one-gene dominant characteristic for MMTV. One possible explanation, therefore, is that a virus similar to the nongerm line-transmitted viruses of C3H and RIII has become integrated as an endogenous virus of GR.

C. *MMTV-Related Genetic Information in the DNAs of Other Rodents*

In view of the varied distribution of MMTV proviral sequences in the mouse, we set out to determine if MMTV-related proviral sequences are present in other rodents. Furthermore, to determine if sequences related to, but not identical to, MMTV could be detected in the DNAs of other rodents, conditions of hybridization were relaxed by lowering the temperature at which hybridizations were carried out from 68° to 54°C. The assay of resulting RNA-DNA duplexes was accomplished by raising the salt concentration from the standard conditions of 2X SSC (1X SSC is 0.15*M* NaCl and 0.15*M* Na citrate) to 8X SSC. Specificity is still maintained using relaxed conditions since no hybridization above 6% background is observed to DNA obtained from bovine and canine tissue or *E. coli*.

Molecular hybridization experiments were carried out to determine the presence of "MMTV-specific" sequences (using standard conditions) and "MMTV-related" sequences (using relaxed conditions of hybridization and RNase assay) (Drohan and Schlom, 1979) in other *Mus* species. Results are given in Table III where values have been normalized by subtracting the 6% background hybridization level and using as 100% the hybridization observed to the homologous C3H mammary tumor cell line DNA. As can be seen in Table III, when standard conditions of hybridization and RNase assay are used, the subspecies of *Mus musculus*, i.e., *M. musculus molossinus* and *M. musculus Peru Atteck*, appear to contain less MMTV sequences as endogenous provirus. When standard conditions of hybridization are used, however, no MMTV-specific sequences are detected in the DNAs of other *Mus* species, i.e., *M. cervicolor* or *M. caroli* (Drohan and Schlom, 1979).

When relaxed conditions of hybridization and RNase assay are used, the degree of hybridization detected using DNAs of C3H or RIII *M. musculus* tissues remains approximately the same as does the degree of hybridization to *M. musculus molossinus* and *M. musculus Peru Atteck* DNAs. Using these relaxed conditions, however, MMTV-related sequences are now detected in the DNAs of *M. cervicolor* and *M. caroli* mice (Table III). Kinetic analysis of this hybridization reveals C_0t 1/2 values of 150

TABLE III. Hybridization of ^{3}H-MMTV(Fel) 60-70S RNA to Rodent DNAs: Normalized Values

Source of DNA	% Hybridization	
	Standard[a]	Relaxed
Mouse		
M. musculus - *mammary tumor (C3H)*	100[b]	100[b]
- *liver (C3H)*	56	56
- *liver (RIII)*	60	56
M. musculus molossinus	22	22
M. musculus Peru Atteck	18	22
M. caroli	0	18
M. cervicolor	0	20
Rat (Rattus norvegicus)		
Wistar	0	20
Lewis	0	17
Osborn-Mendel	0	17
Sprague-Dawley	2	19
AXC	0	22
feral	0	17
Hamster	0	0
Guinea pig	0	0
Mink	0	0
Bovine	0	0
Feline	0	0

[a]*Standard and relaxed conditions of hybridization and RNase treatment are described (Drohan* et al., *1977).*

[b]*Values were normalized as follows: the 6% (average) background hybridization observed to nonrodent DNAs was subtracted from all values. The hybridization value to the DNA of the cell line from which the MMTV RNA was produced was given a value of 100%, and all other values were normalized to that number accordingly.*

and 600 for *M. cervicolor* and *M. caroli* DNAs as compared to 500 for *M. musculus* and 3100 for murine "unique" sequences (Drohan and Schlom, 1979). Thermal analysis studies revealed ΔT_m values 3.2 and 3.4°C lower for hybrids formed between MMTV RNA and DNA from *M. cervicolor* and *M. caroli*, respectively, than observed with *M. musculus* DNAs. These results are in general agreement with a recent report (Morris *et al.*, 1977) using MMTV cDNA probes.

MMTV-related DNA in rats: As seen in Table III, five different laboratory strains of rats, as well as feral rats, all contained approximately the same degree of MMTV-related information in their DNA when using relaxed conditions of hybridization and RNase assay. DNAs from various organs of a feral rat were also tested for the presence of MMTV-related information and they all contained the same degree of MMTV-related information. The sequences detected thus appear to be endogenous, i.e., germ-line transmitted in rats (Drohan and Schlom, 1979).

The MMTV 60-70S ^{3}H-RNA used in these experiments was obtained from virions from the supernatant fluids of MMTV-infected feline and murine cells (Howard *et al.*, 1977). Both RNAs were used to rule out the possibility that normal murine or feline cellular RNA or DNA was contaminating the MMTV 60-70S RNA preparations. No hybridization above background was obtained when this RNA was hybridized to the uninfected feline cells, and thus the hybridization observed to rat DNA is interpreted as the result of the presence of nucleic acid sequences related to the MMTV genome.

Fisher or F344 rats, from several colonies, were also examined and found to contain the same degree of MMTV-related information in their DNA as other rat strains (Table III). However, F344 rats obtained from certain colonies appeared to contain additional MMTV-related information in their DNA, indicating a possible infection and integration by MMTV or an MMTV-related virus. The nature and distribution of these additional sequences is currently being investigated.

To determine at what frequency the MMTV-related sequences are present in rat DNA, MMTV radioactive 60-70S RNA was hybridized to the DNAs of five different laboratory strains of rats as well as C3H mouse liver and mammary tumor DNA. As seen in Fig. 6, the kinetics of hybridization to the DNAs of several strains were extremely similar. The C_0t 1/2 values obtained for all five strains were approximately 800 (Drohan and Schlom, 1979). The hybridization of poly selected radioactive rat RNA to "unique" rat DNA gave a C_0t 1/2 value of approximately 2500, indicating that the endogenous MMTV-related sequences in rat DNAs are present in the "low repetitive" range.

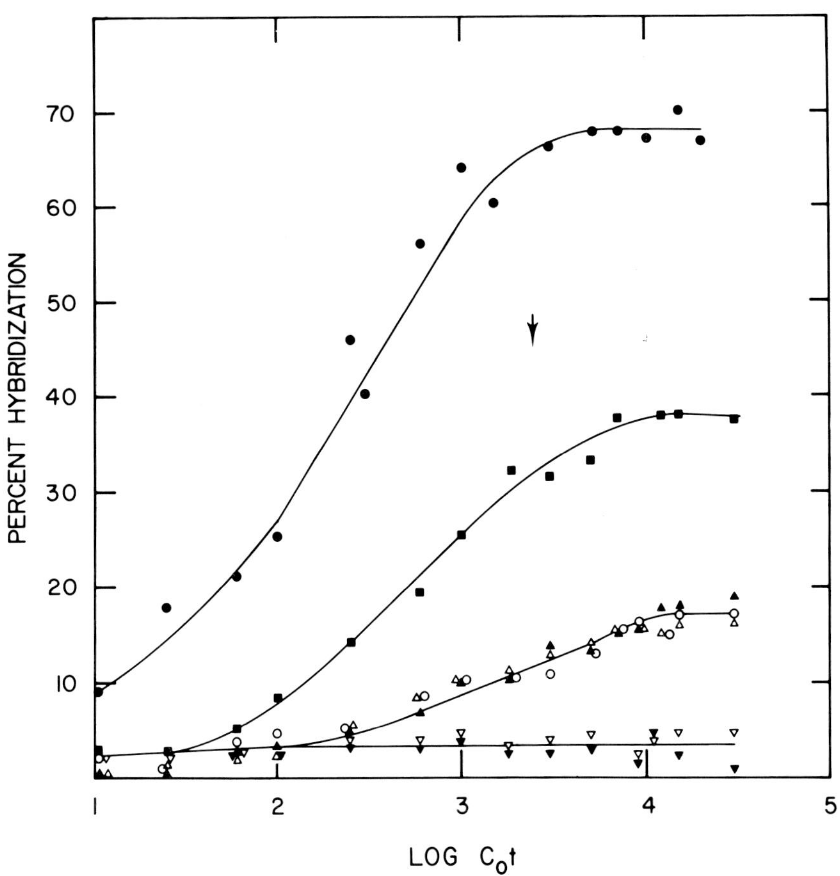

FIGURE 6. Kinetic analysis of hybridization between MMTV 60-70S [^{125}I]-RNA and rat cellular DNAs using relaxed conditions of hybridization and RNase assay (see text). Each point represents the hybridization between 1000 cpm of [^{125}I]-MMTV 60-70S RNA and 500 μg of DNA from the following: C3H mammary tumor cell line (●); C3H liver (■); AXC rat (▲); Lewis rat (O); Wistar rat (Δ); Hamster (▼); and guinea pig (▽). The arrow indicates the C_0t 1/2 for the hybridization between [^{125}I]-labeled polyadenine selected normal rat RNA (selected on Poly U Sepharose 4B [Drohan et al., 1977]), and rat DNA under relaxed conditions of hybridization.

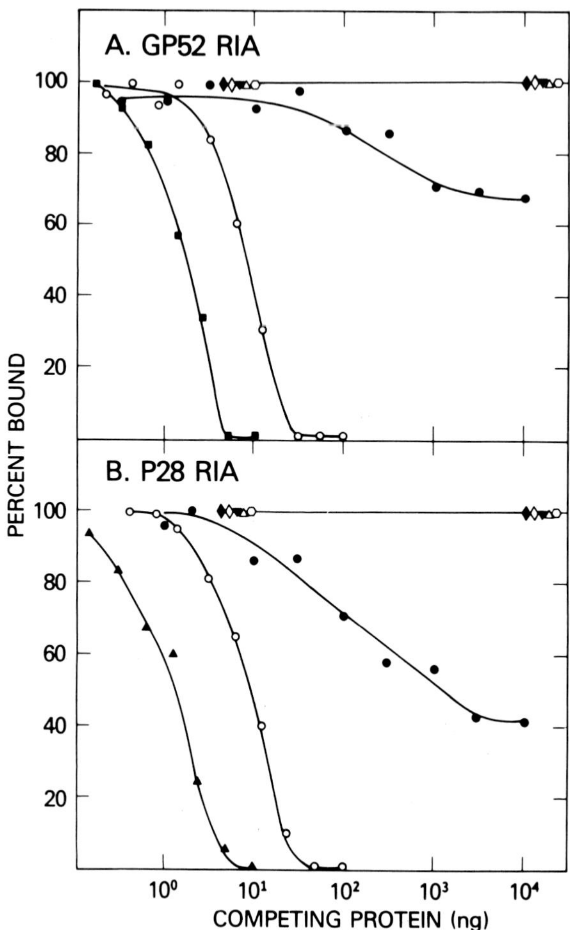

FIGURE 7. Reactivity of M. cervicolor *type-B virus in MMTV gp52 and p28 radioimmunoassays. (A) Anti-MMTV (C3H) gp52 serum was used to precipitate [^{125}I]-labeled MMTV(RIII) gp52. Increasing amounts of the following competitors were used: purified gp52 of MMTV(RIII), (■); MMTV(RIII), (O);* M. cervicolor *type-B virus (●). Other competitors were tested at multiple protein inputs, but only two points are shown for clarity. Symbols: CERV-VI, (◇); CERV-CII, (◆); M432 virus, (▼); C57BL milk, (△); and C3H-T10 MuLV; (⬡). (B) Anti-MMTV(RIII) p28 serum was used to precipitate [^{125}I]-labeled MMTV(C3H) p28. Competitors are as in (A), plus MMTV(C3H) p28 (▲).*

To determine the fidelity of hybrids formed between MMTV radioactive RNA and rat DNA, the thermal stability of the RNA-DNA duplexes formed was analyzed by hydroxylapatite chromatography. The differential T_m values observed were 5°C lower than those obtained with homologous *M. musculus* DNAs.

IV. CHARACTERIZATION OF A NEW VIRUS IMMUNOLOGICALLY RELATED TO MMTVs

A virus, morphologically indistinguishable from the type-B MMTVs of the laboratory mouse *M. musculus,* has been identified in the milk of *M. cervicolor popaeus* mice (Schlom *et al.,* 1978). Group-specific radioimmunoassays for the gp52 (Fig. 7A) and the p28 (Fig. 7B) of MMTV demonstrate that this new virus shares some antigenic determinants with both of these MMTV proteins (Schlom *et al.,* 1978). This reactivity is clearly different, however, from that observed with all MMTVs tested from *M. musculus.* The *M. cervicolor* B-type virus has a density of 1.16 gm/ml in sucrose and virion-associated DNA polymerase with a divalent cation preference for Mg^{2+} over Mn^{2+}. Competitive molecular hybridization experiments showed little if any nucleic acid homology with MMTVs. Radioimmunoassays also clearly differentiate this virus from the other viruses previously identified from *M. cervicolor*: M432, CERV-CI, and CERV-II (Callahan *et al.,* 1977; Callahan and Todaro, 1978). These studies thus identify the first virus from another species that is immunologically related to the MMTVs of *M. musculus.* Similar particles were also observed in a spontaneous *M. cervicolor* mammary tumor (Schlom *et al.,* 1978).

Milk of some feral and various inbred strains of *M. musculus* have previously been shown to be a source of MMTV, regardless of the mode of transmission of the virus (Bittner, 1936; Bentvelzen, 1972; Nandi and McGrath, 1973; Rongey *et al.,* 1973). Similarly, *M. cervicolor* milk appears to be a good source of B-type virus, particularly from mice from the Tak province of Thailand. Experiments are now in progress, involving use of this resource, to develop "interspecies" RIAs for the p28 and gp52 viral proteins to use as probes for the detection of antigen expression related to MTV in other rodent and more distantly related species.

ACKNOWLEDGMENT

These studies were supported, in part, by Contract N01 CP43223 of the National Cancer Institute.

REFERENCES

Bittner, J. J., (1936). *Science 84,* 162.

Bentvelzen, P. (1972). *Int. Rev. Exp. Pathol. 11,* 259-297.

Callahan, R., and Todaro, G. (1978). *In* "Workshop on the Origins of Inbred Mice" (H. C. Morse III, ed.), pp. 689-713. Academic Press, New York.

Callahan, R., Sherr, C. J., and Todaro, G. J. (1977). *Virology 80,* 401-416.

Cardiff, R., (1978). *In* "Workshop on the Origins of Inbred Mice" (H. C. Morse III, ed.), pp. 321-342. Academic Press, New York.

Cardiff, R. D., Puentes, M. J., Termoto, Y. A., and Lund, J. K. (1974). *J. Virol. 14,* 1293-1303.

Drohan, W., and Schlom, J. (1979). *J. Nat. Cancer Inst. 62,* 1279-1286.

Drohan, W., Kettmann, R., Colcher, D., and Schlom, J. (1977). *J. Virology 21,* 986-995.

Elder, J. H., Jensen, F. C., Bryant, M. L., and Lerner, R. A. (1977). *Nature 267,* 23-28.

Gautsch, J. W., Lerner, R., Howard, D., Teramoto, Y. A., and Schlom, J. (1978). *J. Virol. 127,* 688-699.

Howard, D. K., Colcher, D., Teramoto, Y. A., Young, J. M., and Schlom, J. (1977). *Cancer Res. 37,* 2969-2704.

Hunter, W. M. (1978). *In* "Handbook of Experimental Immunology" (D. M. Weir, ed.), pp. 17.1-17.36. Blackwell Scientific Publications, Oxford.

Lasfargues, E. Y., Lasfargues, J. C., Dion, A. S., Greene, A. E., and Moore, D. H. (1976). *Cancer Res. 36,* 67-72.

Morris, V. L., Medeiros, E., Ringold, G. M., Bishop, J. M., and Varmus, H. E. (1977). *J. Mol. Biol. 114,* 73-91.

Nandi, S., and McGrath, C. M. (1973). *Adv. Cancer Res. 17,* 353-414.

Parks, W. P., Howk, R. S., Scolnick, E. M., Oroszlan, S, and Gilden, R. V. (1974). *J. Virol. 13,* 1200-1210.

Ritzi, E., Baldi, A., and Spiegelman, S. (1976). *Virology 75,* 188-197.

Rongey, R. W., Hiavacova, A., Lara, S., Estes, J., and Gardner, M. B. (1973). *J. Natl. Cancer Inst. 50,* 1581-1589.

Schochetman, G., and Schlom, J. (1976). *Virology 73,* 431-441.

Schlom, J., Colcher, D., Drohan, W., and Kettmann, R. *In* "Progress in Experimental Tumor Research" (F. Homburger, ed.) Vol. 21, pp. 140-158. S. Karger, Basel.

Schlom, J., Hand, P., Teramoto, Y. A., Callahan, R., Todaro, G., and Schidlovsky, G. (1978). *J. Natl. Cancer Inst. 61,* 1509-1519.

Sheffield, J. B., Daly, T., Dion, A. S., and Taraschi, N. (1977). *Cancer Res. 37,* 1480-1485.

Teramoto, Y. A., and Schlom, J. (1978). *Cancer Res. 38,* 1990-1995.
Teramoto, Y. A., Kufe, D., Schlom, J. (1977a). *Proc. Natl. Acad. Sci. 74,* 3564-3568.
Teramoto, Y. A., Kufe, D., and Schlom, J. (1977b). *J. Virol. 24,* 525-533.
Varmus, H. E., Bishop, J. M., Nowinski, R. C., Sarkar, N. (1972). *Nature New Biol. 238,* 189-191.
Varmus, H. E., Stavnezer, J., Medeiros, E., and Bishop, J. M. (1975). *In* "Comparative Leukemia Research 1973" (Y. Ito and R. M. Dutcher, eds.), Leukemogenosis, pp. 451-461. Univ. of Tokyo Press, Tokyo.
Verstraeten, A. A., van Nie, R., Kwa, H. G., and Hageman, Ph.C. (1975). *Int. J. Cancer 15,* 270-281.

GENETICAL ASPECTS OF ENDOGENOUS MAMMARY TUMOR VIRUS EXPRESSION IN MICE REINVESTIGATED

Peter Bentvelzen
Jan Brinkhof

Radiobiological Institute TNO
Rijswijk, The Netherlands

Joost Haaijman

Institute for Experimental Gerontology TNO
Rijswijk, The Netherlands

I. INTRODUCTION

Lwoff (1953) has speculated that murine mammary tumor virus (MuMTV) may have a special interaction with the mouse genome, comparable to lysogeny in bacteria. Moore (1963), like Dmochowski a champion of B-type virus particles as being MuMTV, invoked a lysogenic relationship as an explanation for the presence of B-type particles in tumors of presumed virus-free C3Hf mice. Several investigators in the mouse mammary carcinoma field then refused to accept B-type particles as being the MuMTV virions. An intellectual breakthrough has been the hypothesis by the Crgl-group in Berkeley, that the virus particles in C3Hf would represent a less oncogenic virus strain, which would be transmitted by either parent at conception (Pitelka *et al.*, 1964; Nandi and DeOme, 1965). Van Nie and Verstraeten (1975) demonstrated this phenomenon to be under single-genic control; they called this gene, which is located on chromosome 7, *Mtv-1*.

Mühlbock (1965) described a new high-mammary cancer mouse strain GR, in which a virulent MuMTV could be as effectively transmitted by the male as by the female. This property seemed to be controlled by a single dominant gene (Bentvelzen, 1968, 1972; Van Nie *et al.*, 1972, 1977; Van Nie and Hilgers, 1976).

ISBN 0-12-131150-3

This conclusion has been seriously challenged by Nandi and Helmich (1974) and Heston *et al*. (1976; Heston and Parks, 1977), as will be discussed below.

On the basis of the Crgl concept on the C3Hf strain and our findings in the GR strain we speculated that in these strains a MuMTV would be transmitted as a genetic factor of the host, i.e., that one of the chromosomes of these strains would contain a DNA copy of MuMTV-RNA. This copy (germinal provirus) could be transcribed in the mammary gland, giving rise to virus release and eventually to neoplastic transformation (Bentvelzen, 1968; Bentvelzen and Daams, 1969).

It was envisaged, that spontaneous virus release would be an abnormal situation, and it was also postulated that low cancer mouse strains might carry a MuMTV-provirus in their normal cellular DNA, but that transcription is normally repressed. Repression might be abrogated by treatment with environmental carcinogens. In the low-cancer strain 020 a potent MuMTV can be induced by the combination of X-rays and urethane in the drinking water (Timmermans *et al*., 1969).

All these considerations led to the model, which was presented as the most economic explanation for the phenomena studied by us (Bentvelzen, 1968; Bentvelzen and Daams, 1969). The model states that in all mouse strains studied at one and the same chromosomal site a single germinal MuMTV provirus would be present. Its transcription would normally be inhibited by a repressor produced by a neighboring regulator gene. Environmental carcinogens could interfere with this repression. A germinal mutation in the regulator gene of C3Hf would lead to a lack of repressor and a germinal mutation in the operator gene of the GR strain would make it insensitive to the repressor. In both cases, virus would be produced continuously.

This model proved to be too economical. Molecular hybridization studies showed the presence of multiple DNA copies of MuMTV-RNA in normal mouse DNA (Varmus *et al*., 1972; Scolnick *et al*., 1974; Michalides *et al*., 1976). The genetics of the endogenous viruses is more complicated than foreseen because of the presence of several MuMTV proviruses, but also because of different levels of control (see the chapter by Michalides *et al*., in this volume). The present status of genetic control will be discussed below, mainly on the basis of our recent investigations using a sensitive immunoassay (Haaijman and Brinkhof, 1977).

II. DESCRIPTION OF THE MOUSE STRAINS USED IN THIS INVESTIGATION

The last four years our research has concentrated on four mouse strains, which differ considerably in mammary tumor incidence and mammary tumor virus expression.

(A) BALB/c has been widely used in MuMTV research, because it was generally regarded as being virus free but highly susceptible to infection with any MuMTV strain. The strain has a moderate tumor incidence at a late age in breeding females (Deringer, 1965). In only four of 41 BALB/c tumors infectious MuMTV could be demonstrated (Bentvelzen, 1975). Occasionally a virulent MuMTV can be isolated from mammary glands of retired breeders (Hageman *et al.*, 1972). Viral antigens have never been detected in the milk of BALB/c mice of different age and parity. The BALB/c strain is highly sensitive to its own MuMTV, which seems to be antigenically different from the milkborne prototype MuMTV-S of C3H mice (Daams and Hageman, 1972). The BALB/c virus is called MuMTV-O; the O indicating overlooked. Chemically transformed kidney cells of BALB/c origin release a B-type virus which is highly oncogenic (Links *et al.*, 1972).

(B) C57BL has been the traditional low mammary-cancer strain for many years. It produces less than 1% mammary carcinomas in breeding females. The strain is refractory to milk-borne MuMTV-S, probably due to a poor replication of the virus (Mühlbock, 1956), but not to MuMTV of the GR or RIII mouse strain (Mühlbock and Dux, 1971; Moore *et al.*, 1974). An infectious MuMTV still remains to be isolated from C57BL, but at high parities small amounts of viral antigens can be found in the milk (Haaijman, 1977).

(C) C3Hf has been derived from the high-cancer strain C3H, which carries the milk-borne MuMTV-S, by foster nursing on C57BL. The C3Hf strain does not carry the virulent MuMTV-S, but releases another virus strain with a limited oncogenic potential. It produces a high incidence of mammary tumors in BALB/c mice but at a late age (Hageman *et al.*, 1972). The virus is therefore called MuMTV-L. The F1 hybrids of C3Hf and BALB/c also produce this MuMTV-L (Pitelka *et al.*, 1964; Van Nie and Verstraeten, 1975). However, in tumors of F1 hybrids of C3Hf with several low-cancer strains like C57BL, no B-type particles can be found (Boot, 1969; Hilgers and Bentvelzen, 1978).

We recently found that glucocorticoids could activate a highly potent MuMTV in kidney cultures of C3Hf mice. We had found earlier that dexamethasone could induce the appearance of MuMTV antigens in C3Hf kidney cultures (Bentvelzen, 1974, 1975). Also a few B-type particles were released. They were thought to represent MuMTV-L. However, they proved to induce mammary tumors at an early age in BALB/c mice (Table I).

TABLE I. In Vitro Activation of a Virulent MuMTV in C3Hf Kidney Cultures by Glucocorticoids

Inoculum	*Number of mice*	*Mice with tumors %*	*Tumor age (months)*
None	*20*	*5 (25)*	*20*
C3Hf tumor extract	*20*	*12 (60)*	*19*
C3Hf kidney culture	*18*	*3 (17)*	*18*
C3Hf kidney culture + dexamethasone	*20*	*20 (100)*	*9*
C3Hf kidney culture + hydrocortisone	*10*	*9 (90)*	*7*
C57BL kidney culture	*20*	*4 (20)*	*17*
C57BL kidney culture + dexamethasone	*10*	*3 (30)*	*21*

This virus, which we propose to call MuMTV-D, can also be activated *in vivo* by cortisone (LeMonde *et al.*, 1976).

(D) GR develops a mammary lesion, called plaques (Foulds, 1956) during the first pregnancy. Usually these tumors regress during parturition and reappear in the second half of the next pregnancy. Ultimately the tumors become fully hormone independent. When the virus of the GR (MuMTV-P) is introduced into other mouse strains the latency period is considerably lengthened. The duration of the hormone-dependency period is shortened, however. The virus is then also not transmitted by the male, indicating the very intimate relationship of the GR host and MuMTV-P with regard to this mode of transmission.

Of all mouse strains tested so far, the GR has the highest amount of MuMTV antigens in its milk (Noon *et al.*, 1975; Haaijman, 1977; Van Nie *et al.*, 1977). This property has even been used for genetic analysis (Van Nie *et al.*, 1977).

Van Nie *et al.* (1972, 1977; Van Nie and Hilgers, 1976) can induce with the steroid compound 17-α-ethynyl-19-nortestosterone mammary tumors within a few weeks in the GR strain and its hybrids. This property has been a very useful distinct phenotypic trait for genetic analysis. It proved to be controlled by a single dominant gene, which is also associated with abundant virus production. This gene has been called *Mtv-2* (Van Nie *et al.*, 1972, 1977; Van Nie and Hilgers, 1976) and is thought to represent the germinal provirus of MuMTV-P.

A congenic strain of the GR has been developed from which this *Mtv-2* gene has been eliminated. It does not produce early mammary tumors any longer, and the quantity of viral antigens in the milk is low (Van Nie and De Moes, 1977). Most likely another low-oncogenic MuMTV-strain is expressed in the GR.

III. GENETICS OF RELEASE OF MuMTV INTO THE MILK

By means of Sepharose bead immunofluorescence assay (Haaijman, 1977; Haaijman and Brinkhof, 1977) the amount of MuMTV antigens was determined in milk samples of the aforementioned mouse strains, their F1 hybrids and subsequent crosses (Table II). The method proved to be specific in that no reaction was found with Rauscher murine leukemia virus, normal mouse serum, normal BALB/c mammary gland extract, and ovalbumin. This technique is fairly sensitive: when purified MuMTV preparations were tested, the lowest detectable amount is 0.3 ng per sample of 50μl. Probably because of a specific binding of milk proteins to the beads, the sensitivity is considerably less for milk samples: 5 ng.

The specificity of the technique can also be concluded from the fact that the strains C57BL and BALB/c scored negative, as has been reported with radioimmunoassay (Noon *et al.*, 1975; Verstraeten *et al.*, 1975). The samples have been arbitrarily divided into three categories: negative, less than 5 mg/mg per mg milk protein, and more than 5 micrograms.

All F1 hybrids sired by a GR male had large amounts of MuMTV antigens in their milk. All (BALB/c × C3Hf)F1 hybrid mice were positive, as to be expected, but the majority of the (C57BL × C3Hf)F1 were negative for MuMTV antigens.

In three of the crosses involving the GR strain, an approximate 50% incidence is found, as to be expected on a single-gene basis. The high incidence in BALB/c × (C3Hf × GR)F1 is to be expected, because of virus production by either the MuMTV-L proviral genome of C3Hf or the MuMTV-P proviral genome of GR. In case both proviruses would be "allelic" a 100 % incidence must be anticipated.

The excess of MuMTV-positives in BALB/c × (BALB/c × GR)F1 is partly due to extrachromosomal male transmission, which is known to take place in the GR strain (Bentvelzen, 1968; Nandi and Helmich, 1974). In order to exclude this as much as possible the females used to produce the backcross generations and so on were mated only once with the GR-hybrid male. They were thereafter mated with a BALB/c male and allowed to raise a litter. The females were meanwhile milked once for immunoassay of MuMTV antigens.

TABLE II. *Presence of MuMTV-Antigens in the Milk of Inbred Mouse Strains and Their Hybrids as Detected by the Sepharose Bead Immunofluorescence Assay*

Female	Male	Number of animals	Number of positive milks	Percentage
C57BL	C57BL	28	0	0
BALB/c	BALB/c	24	0	0
C3Hf	C3Hf	14	14	100
GR	GR	21	21	100
C57BL	GR	31	31	100
BALB/c	GR	36	36	100
C3Hf	GR	27	27	100
C57BL	BALB/c	38	1	3
C57BL	C3Hf	28	4	14
BALB/c	C3Hf	31	31	100
C57BL	(C57BLxGR)F1	166	84	51
C57BL	(BALB/cxGR)F1	48	28	58
BALB/c	(BALB/cxGR)F1	103	88	85
BALB/c	(C57BLxGR)F1	135	79	59
BALB/c	(C3HfxGR)F1	192	156	81
BALB/c	(BALB/cxC3Hf)F1	277	121	44
C3Hf	(BALB/cxC3Hf)F1	104	95	91
C3Hf	(C57BLxC3Hf)F1	111	60	54
(C57BLxC3Hf)F1	(C57BLxC3Hf)F1	68	14	21
BALB/c	(C57BLxC3Hf)F1	84	17	20

The females in the resulting litter were also mated to a BALB/c male and tested for MuMTV antigen too. Both mother and offspring were then subjected to forced breeding. Early tumor production (before one year of age) was regarded as a sign of infection with MuMTV. From Table III can be concluded that infection sometimes only shows in the subsequent litter and not in the mother. However, the rate of infection seems to be relatively low and cannot explain the excess over 50% in BALB/c × (BALB/c × GR)Fl.

When the quantity of MuMTV antigens is taken into account it seems that in the groups with more than 5 μg, incidences are approximately 50%. In that case there seems to be a GR gene, associated with large amounts of MuMTV, and as will be outlined below, also with early tumor development. Other genes are associated with the release of small amounts of MuMTV. They can manifest themselves quite well in crosses with BALB/c but not with C57BL. This resembles the inhibition of MuMTV-L in (C57BL × C3Hf)Fl.

The crosses involving the C3Hf and the BALB/c strains yielded incidences compatible with the single-gene hypothesis of Van Nie and Verstraeten (1975) with regard to the release of MuMTV-L. It seems that a single dominant gene in C57BL inhibits MuMTV release in the Fl hybrid with C3Hf. This gene *Imv* (inhibition of mammary tumor virus release) segregates independently from *Mtv-1*, as can be concluded from the 20% incidence in the cross BALB/c × (C57BL × C3Hf)Fl. In Fig. 1 a scheme of the segregation of the two genes is given.

C3Hf: *Mtv-1*; $+^{Imv}$
C57BL: $+^{Mtv-1}$; *Imv*
BALB/c: $+^{Mtv-1}$; $+^{Imv}$

Test cross: BALB/c × (C57BL × C3Hf)Fl

$$+^{Mtv\text{-}1};\ +^{Imv} \times \frac{+^{Mtv\text{-}1};\ Imv}{Mtv\text{-}1\ \ +^{Imv}}$$

Expected phenotypes:

Mtv-1;Imv	*Mtv-1*;$+^{Imv}$	$+^{Mtv-1}$;*Imv*	$+^{Mtv-1}$;$+^{Imv}$
25%	25%	25%	25%

FIGURE 1. Scheme of segregation of the Imv and the Mtv-1 genes.

TABLE III. Tests for Extrachromosomal Male Transmission of MuMTV in Crosses Involving GR Hybrids

Strain female	GR-hybrid male first mated with	Number of females	Number with MuMTV antigen	Number with early tumors	Number with infected litters
C57BL	C57BL × GR	61	1	0	1
C57BL	BALB/c × GR	20	0	0	0
BALB/c	BALB/c × GR	36	4	2	4
BALB/c	C57BL × GR	53	4	3	6
BALB/c	C3Hf × GR	90	7	3	8

IV. MAMMARY TUMOR DEVELOPMENT IN RELATION TO MuMTV STATUS

After collection of the milk at first lactation, the mice in this study were subjected to forced breeding. In Table IV are given tumor incidences and tumor ages in months for the different mouse strains and their hybrids in relation to the quantity of MuMTV antigens in the milk at a relatively young age. There is a very clear-cut inverse relationship between virus quantity and tumor age.

An even more pronounced picture is seen in the progeny of several crosses, as presented in Table V. Those categories which have large quantities of MuMTV in their milk develop many tumors at an early age, while the corresponding group with low amounts of virus develop less tumors at a higher age. Although a lower tumor percentage and higher tumor age is found in the virus-negative categories, the incidences are yet substantial.

Of particular interest is the cross BALB/c × (BALB/c × GR)F1. The group with high virus levels develops mammary tumors before one year of age: only one animal developed a tumor after a year. The tumor incidence in the group of low virus levels is surprisingly high, but average tumor age is late. Only two animals in this category developed a tumor before one year of age.

In an elegant study, Nandi and Helmich (1974) found a tumor incidence of 100% and tumor age of seven months in (BALB/c × GR)F1. In the backcross to BALB/c they found 53% and in the F2 generation 75% at the same age. In both cases milk-borne transmission has been excluded. This result is in agreement with a single-gene postulate for early tumor development. At 12 months of age, they found in both groups a considerably higher incidence of mammary lesions, like hyperplastic nodules. These have been probably induced by another virus strain than MuMTV-P: A gene other than *Mtv-2* would control the expression of this less oncogenic virus.

V. PRESENCE OF INFECTIOUS MuMTV IN MAMMARY TUMORS

The tumors which arose in the genetic program outlined in the preceeding sections were stored in liquid nitrogen. From many of these tumors cell-free extracts were prepared and bioassayed in four-week old female BALB/c mice, which were then force bred. Due to limited facilities, such tumor testing could not be done simultaneously. This whole program lasted four years. At least every four months we subjected a group of 25 control female BALB/c mice to forced breeding. No significant changes in tumor incidence in the controls was noted.

TABLE IV. Mammary Tumor Incidences in Inbred Mouse Strains and Their Hybrids in Relation to Their MuMTV Status

Strain or hybrid	Number of animals	Total incidence	MuMTV-negative			Less than 5 μg			Greater than 5μg		
			number	tumor (%)	tumor[a] (age)	number	tumor (%)	tumor[a] (age)	number	tumor (%)	tumor[a] (age)
BALB/c	24		24	21	22						
C57BL	28		28	0							
C3Hf	14	50				2	0		12	58	18
GR	21	100				1	100	8	20	100	6
C57BL x BALB/c	38	18	37	16	24	1	100	19			
BALB/c x C3Hf	31	71				9	33	20	22	86	14
C57BL x C3Hf	28	25	24	13	26	3	100	22	1	100	18
BALB/c x GR	36	100				3	100	8	33	100	6
C57BL x GR	31	100				5	100	9	26	100	6
C3Hf x GR	27	100				4	100	11	23	100	6

[a]Tumor age in months.

TABLE V. *Mammary Tumor Incidences in the Offspring of Several Crosses in Relation to MuMTV Status*

Cross		Number of	Tumor	MuMTV-negative			Less than 5 μg viral antigens			Greater than 5 μg viral antigens		
Female	Male	animals	(%)	number	tumor (%)	tumor[a] (age)	number	tumor (%)	tumor[a] (age)	number	tumor (%)	tumor[a] (age)
C57BL	C57BL × GR	166	55	82	9	16	3	100	15	81	100	8
C57BL	BALB/c × GR	48	71	20	35	19	2	50	19	26	96	8
BALB/c	BALB/c × GR	103	78	15	20	21	39	74	20	48	100	7
BALB/c	C57BL × GR	135	75	56	50	22	18	67	19	61	100	7
BALB/c	C3Hf × GR	192	78	36	36	24	8	50	21	148	91	10
BALB/c	BALB/c × C3Hf	277	26	156	14	21	5	20	20	89	44	15
C3Hf	BALB/c × C3Hf	104	54	9	11	23	6	33	19	54	60	17
C3Hf	C57BL × C3Hf	111	26	51	14	21	6	16	22	54	39	18
C57BL × C3Hf	C57BL × C3Hf	68	34	54	20	23	1	0		13	69	20
BALB/c	C57BL × C3Hf	84	31	67	17	20	2	50	17	15	73	14

[a]Tumor age in months.

Unfortunately an epizootic with a virulent mycoplasma strain interfered with this assay part of the program; several groups of mice had to be killed before any information about the presence of an infectious MuMTV in an inoculum was obtained. However, as can be concluded from the summary in Table VI, sufficient information can be obtained from the remaining groups. In these experiments, a virulent MuMTV was defined as inducing at least 20 % tumors before one year in the BALB/c recipients; a late-oncogenic MuMTV, as not fulfilling the criteria for a virulent MuMTV but inducing at least 60 % tumors after two years.

Except for one, all early tumors in crosses involving the GR strain contained a virulent MuMTV, while only a few of the late tumors harbored such a virus. The majority of these tumors produced a late-oncogenic MuMTV, according to our standards. Unfortunately, this conclusion could not be followed up by serial passage of an avirulent virus, because of our gnotobiological problems. A few tumors coming up in mice, which were at the time of testing negative for MuMTV antigens in their milk, nevertheless contained infectious mammary tumor virus.

In the crosses, involving the C3Hf strain (except for the one in which the GR strain also takes part), a somewhat different pattern is found. This does not hold for those tumors, which developed in so-called virus-free mice. None of the tumors, which came up before one year of age in the aforementioned crosses, contained MuMTV, which was able to induce early tumors in BALB/c. This result strongly indicates that the combination of continuous expression of endogenous MuMTV-L of C3Hf in a BALB/c background may lead to early tumor development, but that exogenous infection, resulting in a somatic provirus with continuous virus expression, has less effect in this respect. The majority of late tumors in this category contain a late-oncogenic MuMTV.

It is a little bit difficult to combine the results of both groups of crosses. The conclusions which can be drawn, are that some tumors, which have arisen in so-called virus-free mice, nevertheless contain an infectious MuMTV. Second, that most late-appearing tumors harbor a virus which induces tumors at a late age in BALB/c mice. It does not make sense to combine results obtained with early tumors in either category.

TABLE VI. Presence of Infectious MuMTV in Mammary Tumors Developing in the Progeny of Several Crosses

	Number of tumors	*Number with virulent MuMTV*	*Number with late-oncogenic MuMTV*
GR crosses			
Tumors in virus-negative mice	*8*	*1*	*1*
Early tumors in virus-positive mice	*17*	*16*	*0*
Late tumors in virus-positive mice	*19*	*2*	*12*
C3HF crosses			
Tumors in virus-negative mice	*14*	*2*	*3*
Early tumors in virus-positive mice	*5*	*0*	*4*
Late tumors in virus-positive mice	*23*	*2*	*14*
Combined			
Tumors in virus-negative mice	*22*	*3*	*4*
Early tumors in virus-positive mice	*22*	*16*	*4*
Late tumors in virus-positive mice	*42*	*4*	*26*

VI. EXPRESSION OF MuMTV-gp52 IN MAMMARY TUMORS

A number of tumors, which had not been bioassayed in BALB/c mice because of our gnotobiological problems have been screened for the presence of the major MuMTV envelope glycoprotein with a molecular weight of 52,000 (gp52). This viral polypeptide has been isolated to complete purity in our laboratory (Westenbrink *et al.*, 1977). Antisera have been raised in rabbits to this antigen. After the usually needed absorption with fetal calf serum and normal mouse serum (J. Brinkhof, unpublished results), the antisera proved to be highly specific for MuMTV.

With the Sepharose bead immunofluorescence assay, as developed by Haaijman and Brinkhof (1977), it became obvious that organ extracts were very tricky; there was a great chance for false positives. Rat mammary carcinoma extracts did not show any obvious positive reaction with the antisera to MuMTV-gp52 but showed an unwanted high binding with the Sepharose beads coated with this antiserum. A mixture was then made of MuMTV-S and a rat mammary carcinoma extract and subsequently diluted in phosphate-buffered saline. We found a reliable titration curve of MuMTV combined with rat tumor, but the sensitivity of the method seemed to have decreased 10-fold as compared to the titration of milk samples. The most important findings in this study were (1) that 41 tumors which came up in animals with virus-positive milks in the aforementioned program, were also positive for MuMTV-gp52 and (2) that the majority of tumors (25 of 39), which arose in mice which were negative for MuMTV antigens in their milk when they were approximately six months of age, were positive for this MuMTV antigen. It is obvious that endogenous MuMTV can be switched on at a late age. Presumably, the age-dependent expression of MuMTV plays a major role in mammary carcinogenesis at a late age. It is tempting to speculate that the virus negative tumors result from the expression of only the "*mam*" gene of endogenous MuMTV (Hilgers and Bentvelzen, 1978).

VII. GENERAL DISCUSSION

In the past our studies on the genetic control of expression of endogenous MuMTV were concentrated on mammary tumor development, which is the ultimate concern of experimental cancer research but an unreliable phenotypical trait for genetical analysis, particularly in view of the great variation in tumor ages. The studies by Van Nie *et al.* (1972, 1977; Van Nie and Hilgers, 1976) in which tumor development was standardized in that mammary lesions would appear in a fixed surprisingly short period after hormonal stimulation, have confirmed our possibly premature conclusion of a single dominant gene in the GR controlling virus release and early tumor development. The lumping together of various mammary lesions, as done by Nandi and Helmich (1974), has led to erroneous conclusions.

The development of a tumor and how relevant it might be from an oncological point of view, is quite a remote phenomenon from the early events of regulation of MuMTV expression. The assay of viral antigens in the milk as done by Van Nie and Verstraeten (1975), Heston *et al.* (1976) and by us in this report, would provide somewhat more relevant information. It has become evident that a single dominant gene of the C3Hf, as compared to the BALB/c strain, controls the expression of a MuMTV. Bioassays of the virus produced in (C3Hf × BALB/c)F1 indicate it to be a late-oncogenic MuMTV strain (Hageman *et al.*, 1972). It follows that the aforementioned gene *Mtv-1* of the C3Hf only allows the release of a C3Hf-strain virus, which is late oncogenic, but not the virulent virus of C3Hf we could induce by glucocorticoid treatment, or the virulent virus occasionally released in old BALB/c mice. *Mtv-1* seems to be concerned with a single type of MuMTV, present in the same mouse strain. In case *Mtv-1* would represent a mutation in the controlling gene of the provirus coding for MuMTV-L, the corresponding allelic regulatory element must be closely linked to the germinal MuMTV-L provirus. Otherwise, a 25% incidence of virus-positive animals had to be expected in the backcross to BALB/c.

An alternative explanation is that *Mtv-1* would just represent MuMTV-L-provirus without any involvement of a neighboring regulatory gene. That such genes must exist, however, can be concluded from the relative lack of transcription of MuMTV proviruses in BALB/c mice (see Michalides *et al.*, this volume). The regulatory genes involved in this inhibition of transcription must have a very specific effect, because they do not affect expression of *Mtv-1* from C3Hf or *Mtv-2* from GR.

In our studies the C57BL strain seems to possess a gene *Imv*, which interferes with the expression of MuMTV-L. As this gene segregates independently from *Mtv-1*, it cannot be regarded as having an effect on only that provirus, to which it is closely linked. Since in C57BL mammary glands substantial amounts of MuMTV-RNA are produced but no MuMTV proteins are synthesized, it is attractive to postulate that *Imv* would interfere with translation of MuMTV messenger RNA molecules (Fig. 2). Its negative influence on the level of MuMTV-L production in (C57BL × C3Hf)F1 could be explained in this way.

Several other low-cancer strains like 020 or CBA/A inhibit the expression of MuMTV in hybrids with the C3Hf or DBAf strains (Boot, 1969; Hilgers and Bentvelzen, 1978). We are presently

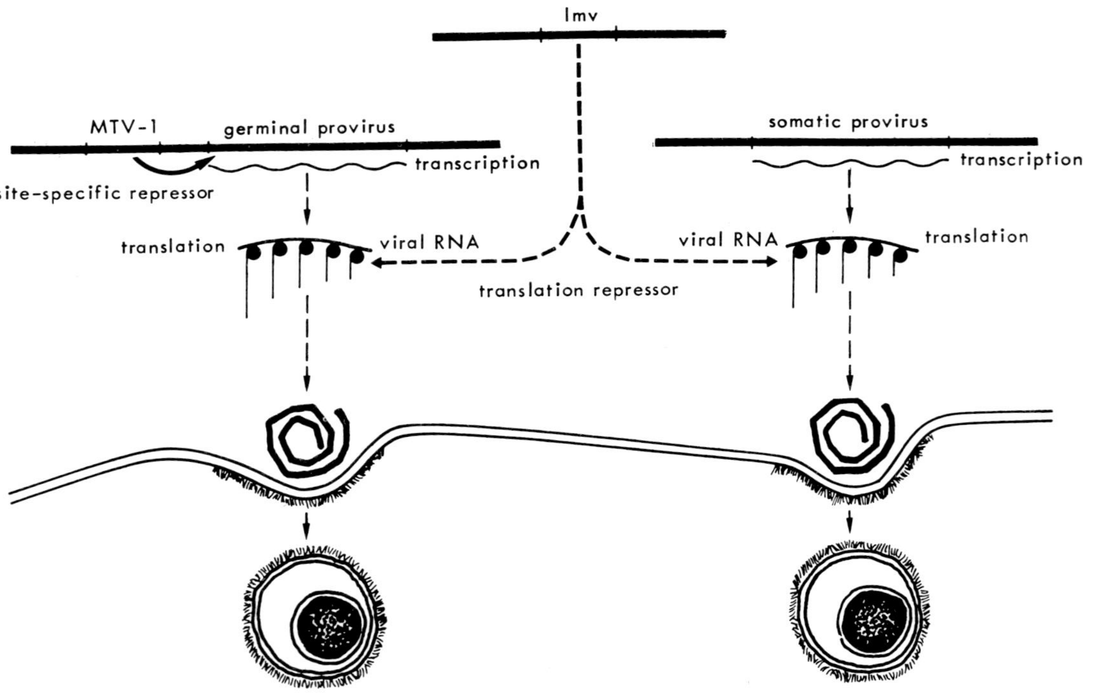

FIGURE 2. Presumed regulation of endogenous and exogenous MuMTV expression by the genes MTV-1 *and* Imv.

investigating the genetics of this inhibition, and are trying to establish whether these strains also carry the *Imv* gene.

Every mouse strain, derived from a high-cancer strain by foster nursing on a low-cancer strain, still release some B-type particles. These virus particles seem to have a low oncogenic potential. Genes like *Mtv-1* must control the release of the endogenous late oncogenic MuMTV-strains in strains like DBAf, RIIIf, and Af. We presently investigate whether such genes are allelic to *Mtv-1*. These strains obviously do not harbor the *Imv* gene, because virus production would then be inhibited.

There is an obvious correlation between spontaneous release of a late-oncogenic MuMTV and susceptibility to milk-borne MuMTV-S. This indicates that the *Imv* gene would also control susceptibility to exogenous MuMTV.

The C57BL mouse strain is susceptible to viruses of the MuMTV-P type. This corresponds with the observed noninterference by *Imv* with the expression of endogenous MuMTV-P of the GR strain.

In contrast to the studies by Heston *et al.* (1976); Heston and Parks, 1977) we have attempted to distinguish phenotypes on the basis of not only MuMTV positivity but also by the quantity of MuMTV antigens in the milk. The rather arbitrary division in this respect proved to be closely related to tumor age, on the basis of which very pronounced different classes could be recognized. In the backcross of GR to C57BL approximately 50% of the animals had large amounts of viral antigens in their milk and developed tumors at a relatively early age. Obviously the gene *Mtv-2* is responsible for this. Only a few tumors developed in the other animals.

In the backcross of GR to BALB/c also approximately 50% of the animals belonged to the category of high virus production and early tumors, but another substantial category was found with low virus production and significant tumor production but at a late age. It seems that the BALB/c genome not only allows the expression of *Mtv-2* but also of genes associated with other MuMTV proviruses. Most likely, the *Imv* gene of C57BL interferes with the expression of the late oncogenic viruses in GR.

Most of our studies have concentrated on the expression of endogenous MuMTV at a relatively young age. It became evident that at late ages repression of virus expression may break down, resulting in the presence of infectious MuMTV in late arising mammary carcinomas. Most likely, these viruses have been involved in the genesis of the tumors they have been isolated from.

As in the majority of the tumors appearing so-called virus-free mice gp52 can be found, it is tempting to speculate that the *mam*-gene of endogenous MuMTV has been expressed and involved in the neoplastic transformation of a mammary gland cell.

As only a minority of these tumors, which were positive for gp52, also contained infectious MuMTV in a test which is considerably more sensitive than any immunoassay, it seems that only partial expression of the endogenous MuMTV might have taken place. It is therefore an acceptable hypothesis, that in tumors, which do not contain detectable gp52, only the "*mam*" gene has been expressed. To test this hypothesis, reagents must be available for the detection of the *mam*-gene product.

In conclusion, there are genes which control the transcription of germinal proviruses of MuMTV. They probably only act upon the proviruses that they are closely linked to. There are also genes which control translation of MuMTV-RNA molecules. They seem to have an effect of several categories of both endogenous and exogenous MuMTV. Control of endogenous MuMTV may break down upon aging resulting in virus release and/or tumor development.

ACKNOWLEDGMENTS

From 1974 onwards our investigations on this problem have been financially supported by contract NO1-CP43328 within the Biological Carcinogenesis Branch of the US National Cancer Institute. Dr. R. Michalides is thanked for fruitful discussion of our concepts and making available the results of his molecular biological studies.

REFERENCES

Bentvelzen, P. (1968). "Genetical Control of the Vertical Transmission of the Mühlbock Mammary Tumour Virus in the GR Mouse Strain." Hollandia, Amsterdam.

Bentvelzen, P. (1972). *In* "RNA Viruses and Host Genome in Oncogenesis." (P. Emmelot and P. Bentvelzen, eds.), p. 309. North-Holland, Amsterdam.

Bentvelzen, P. (1974). *Biochim. Biophys. Acta 355,* 236.

Bentvelzen, P. (1975). *Cold Spring Harbor Symp. Quart. Biol. 39,* 1145.

Bentvelzen, P., and Daams, J. H. (1969). *J. Natl. Cancer Inst. 43,* 1025.

Boot, L. M. (1969). Ph.D. thesis, University of Amsterdam, North-Holland.

Daams, J. H., and Hageman, P. (1972). *In* "Fundamental Research on Mammary Cancer" (J. Mouriquand, ed.), p. 97, INSERM, Paris.

Deringer, M. K. (1965). *J. Natl. Cancer Inst. 35,* 1047.
Foulds, L. (1956). *J. Natl. Cancer Inst. 17,* 701.
Haaijman, J. J. (1977). "Quantitative Immunofluorescence Microscopy. Methods and Applications." TNO, the Hague.
Haaijman, J. J., and Brinkhof, J. (1977). *J. Immunol. Meth. 14,* 213.
Hageman, P., Calafat, J., and Daams, J. H. (1972). *In* "RNA Viruses and Host Genome in Oncogenesis" (P. Emmelot and P. Bentvelzen, eds.), p. 283. North-Holland, Amsterdam.
Heston, W. E., Smith, B., and Parks, W. P. (1976). *J. Exp. Med. 144,* 1022.
Heston, W. E., and Parks, W. P. (1977). *J. Exp. Med. 146,* 1206.
Hilgers, J., and Bentvelzen, P. (1978). *Adv. Cancer Res. 29,* 143.
LeMonde, P., Berthiaume, L., and Lussier, G. (1976). *Proc. Am. Assoc. Cancer Res. 17,* 223.
Links, J., Boys, F., and Tol, D. (1972). *In* "Fundamental Research on Mammary Cancer" (J. Mouriquand, ed.), p. 263. INSERM, Paris.
Lwoff, A. (1953). *Bacteriol. Rev. 17,* 269.
Michalides, R., Nusse, R., and Van Nie, R. This volume.
Michalides, R., Vlahakis, G., and Schlom, J. (1976). *Internat. J. Cancer 18,* 105.
Moore, D. H. (1963). *Nature (London) 198,* 429.
Moore, D. H., Chaney, J., and Holben, J. A. (1974). *J. Natl. Cancer Inst. 52,* 1757.
Mühlbock, O. (1956). *Acta Unio contra Cancrum 12,* 665.
Mühlbock, O. (1965). *Eur. J. Cancer 1,* 123.
Mühlbock, O., and Dux, A. (1971). *Transpl. Proc. 3,* 1247.
Nandi, S., and DeOme, K. B. (1965). *J. Natl. Cancer Inst. 35,* 299.
Nandi, S., and Helmich, C. (1974). *J. Natl. Cancer Inst. 52,* 1567.
Noon, M. C., Wolford, R. G., and Parks,, N. P. (1975). *J. Immunol. 115,* 653.
Pitelka, D. R., Bern, H. A., Nandi, S., and DeOme, K. B. (1964). *J. Natl. Cancer Inst. 33,* 867.
Scolnick, E. M., Parks, W., Kawakami, T., Kohne, D., Okabe, H., Gilden, R., and Hatanaka, M. (1974). *J. Virol. 13,* 363.
Timmermans, A., Bentvelzen, P., Hageman, P. C., and Calafat, J. (1969). *J. Gen. Virol. 4,* 619.
Van Nie, R., and De Moes, J. (1977). *Internat. J. Cancer 20,* 588.
Van Nie, R., and Hilgers, J. (1976). *J. Natl. Cancer Inst. 56,* 27.
Van Nie, R., and Verstraeten, A. A. (1975). *Internat. J. Cancer 16,* 922.

Van Nie, R., Hilgers, J., and Lenselink, M. (1972). *In* "Fundamental Research on Mammary Tumours" (J. Mouriquand, ed.), p. 21. INSERM, Paris.

Van Nie, R., Verstraeten, A. A., and De Moes, J. (1977). *Internat. J. Cancer 19,* 383.

Varmus, H. E., Bishop, J. M., Nowinski, R. C., and Sarkar, N. H. (1972). *Nature, New Biol. 238,* 189.

Verstraeten, A. A., Van Nie, R., Kwa, H. G., and Hageman, P. C. (1975). *Internat. J. Cancer 15,* 270.

Westenbrink, F., Koornstra, W., and Bentvelzen, P. (1977). *Eur. J. Biochem. 76,* 85.

THE STRUCTURAL PROTEINS OF MURINE MAMMARY TUMOR VIRUSES: MOLECULAR BASIS FOR GROUP- AND TYPE-SPECIFICITIES

Arnold S. Dion
Donald C. Farwell
Charlene J. Williams
and
Anthony A. Pomenti

Department of Molecular Biology
Institute for Medical Research
Camden, New Jersey

I. MURINE MAMMARY TUMOR VIRUS (MuMTV) STRUCTURAL PROTEINS: EVIDENCE FOR GROUP- AND TYPE-SPECIFICITIES

Following the usual chronology of virus nomenclature, MuMTVs were initially designated by the name of the investigator, e.g., Bittner agent (C3H-or A-MuMTV) and Mühlbock (GR-MuMTV). More definitive classifications ensued taking advantage of differences in MuMTVs with regard to oncogenic potential, histopathology of the viral-induced mammary tumors, and growth properties of the latter (Bentvelzen, 1972; Nandi and McGrath, 1973). Variations in growth properties of murine mammary tumors dependent on the infecting MuMTV are especially intriguing. For example, mammary tumors induced in the BALB/c strain fostered on C3H or RIII, i.e., BALB/cfC3H or BALB/cf RIII, have clinicopathological characteristics of the donor MuMTV strain (Squartini *et al.*, 1963). That both viral and host genetic information play a role in mammary tumor induction and progression has been extensively investigated and recently reviewed (Hilgers and Bentvelzen, 1977). Within this constellation of biological phenomena lies the widely variable susceptibilities of various inbred mouse strains dependent on the mouse strain of origin of the infecting MuMTV (Moore *et al.*, 1974). Taken *in toto*, these observations strongly indicate a pronounced viral and host genetic interplay in the onset and progression of murine mammary tumors, and, most importantly

ISBN 0-12-131150-3

relative to this discussion, that MuMTVs differ genetically. Direct evidence for the latter, obtained through nucleic acid hybridization assays, has been demonstrated by Schlom and collaborators and are amply reviewed in this volume. From the foregoing it is plausible to assume that similarities and differences also occur in the viral coded polypeptides of MuMTV dependent on the strain of origin.

Immunodiffusion studies (Blair, 1970, 1971) provided the first indication of possible type-specificities on antigens associated with various MuMTVs; however, the lack of definitive viral and immunological reagents, as well as lack of quantitation, impeded obtaining definitive conclusions regarding these suspected type-specificities. The application of competitive radioimmunoassays to the "typing" of MuMTVs has clearly corroborated group-specific antigenic sites associated with gp49-55, the major viral envelope glycoprotein of MuMTV (Parks *et al.*, 1974; Sarkar and Dion, 1975; Kimball *et al.*, 1976; Ritzi *et al.*, 1976; Sheffield *et al.*, 1977). Recently, however, evidence for type-specificities associated with the major envelope glycoproteins of various MuMTVs has accumulated. For example, the major viral glycoproteins (gp49-55) of highly oncogenic MuMTVs (RIII, GR, C3H) were found to possess both group- and type-specific reactivities (Teramoto *et al.*, 1977b). In addition, an expanded study (Teramoto *et al.*, 1977c) corroborated differences in type-specificities of isolated gp49-55s (RII, GR, C3H), and most importantly, group- and type-specificities were observed for milk-transmitted C3H-MuMTV and the endogenous MuMTV of the fostered strain, C3Hf-MuMTV.

Group- and type-antigenic determinants on a viral polypeptide strongly imply similarities and differences in the protein and/or carbohydrate moieties of the gp49-55s investigated above by radioimmunoassay which are amenable to biochemical analyses. The purpose of this investigation includes

(1) the establishment of reproducible protocols for the isolation of the major structural proteins of MuMTV;

(2) biochemical characterizations of all of the major structural proteins of RIII-MuMTV; and

(3) comparative biochemical study of the major envelope and core proteins of RIII- and A-MuMTV to establish a molecular basis for group- and type-specific determinants.

II. MuMTV STRUCTURAL PROTEIN

A. *Nomenclature and Relationship to Viral Structure*

By convention, the structural proteins of RNA tumor viruses (retroviridae) are designated as pN, where N is the molecular weight $\times 10^{-3}$; glycoproteins are denoted by the prefix gp. Regarding the latter, it should be emphasized that molecular weights are determined by sodium dodecyl sulfate-polyacrylamide gel electrophoresis (SDS-PAGE); therefore, molecular weights of glycoproteins are overestimates because of the decreased electrophoretic mobility resulting from the oligosaccharide moieties. In some instances, this decreased mobility may be further affected by neuraminic acid as the terminal residue of an oligosaccharide and/or by the sulfation of the latter. In addition, it is well known that molecular weight estimates of small polypeptides by SDS-PAGE are often incorrect and tend to be more affected by changes in electrophoretic conditions.

In view of these factors, purified MuMTVs from mouse milks of various strains or tissue culture sources possess similar major associated polypeptides (Dion and Moore, 1977) as shown in Fig. 1, and most of these determinations fall within the ±5 to 10% accuracy of this analytical assay. Grouping these MuMTV-associated polypeptides into various molecular weight classes by virtue of other common criteria, e.g., prevalence within the virus, glucosamine-labeling or periodic acid-Schiff (PAS) staining, etc., the following molecular weight ranges are obtained: gp58-70, gp49-55, gp34-38, p24-28, p17-18, p13-15 and p8-12. For convenience these ranges will be designated as gp68, gp55, gp34, p28, p18, p14, and p12. With regard to the data summarized in Fig. 1, two points should be emphasized which distinguish milk- from tissue culture-derived MuMTVs:

(1) milk-derived MuMTVs generally have many more associated proteins with molecular weights in excess of 70,000 than tissue culture virions, and these perhaps represent contamination with milk components; and

(2) MuMTVs from tissue culture sources usually have a resolved doublet in the gp34-38 region.

With regard to the localization of polypeptides within the viral structure, various strategies have been employed, including

(1) accessibility of viral proteins to enzymatic reactions (Witte *et al.*, 1973; Parks *et al.*, 1974; Sarkar and Dion, 1975; Sheffield and Daly, 1976; Schloemer *et al.*, 1976) or protease treatment (Sheffield *et al.*, 1976; Yagi and Compans, 1977);

(2) isolation of subviral components followed by SDS-PAGE analyses (Cardiff *et al.*, 1974; Sarkar *et al.*, 1976; Teramoto

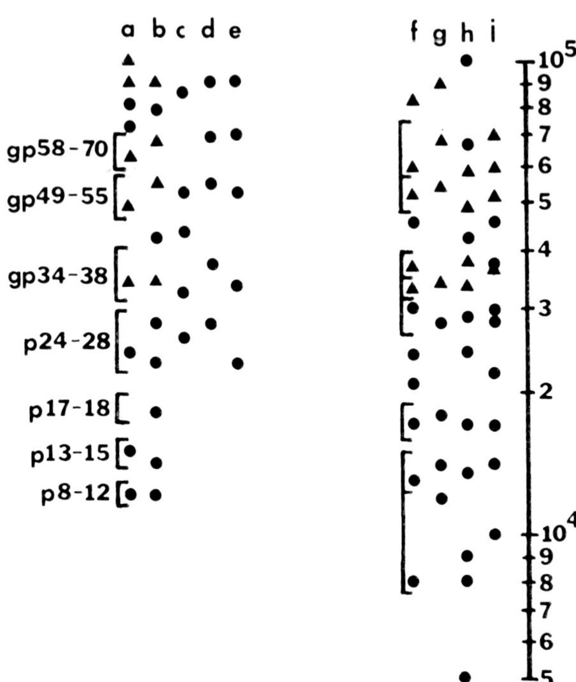

FIGURE 1. Schematic representation of the major proteins reported to be associated with MuMTV purified from mouse milks (a-e) or tissue culture supernates (f-i). (a) ICRC (Karande et al.*, 1978); (b) RIII (Sarkar and Dion, 1975); (c) BALB/cfC3H (Witte* et al.*, 1973); (d) RIII (Smith and Wivel, 1973); (e) C3H (Nowinski* et al.*, 1971); (f) MJY-alpha (Yagi and Compans, 1977); (g) BALB/cfC3H (Sarkar* et al.*, 1977); (h) BALB/cfC3H (Teramoto* et al.*, 1974); (i) BALB/cfC3H (Dickson and Skehel, 1974). Where determined, glycoproteins are denoted by triangles.*

et al., 1977a; Cardiff *et al.*, 1978); and

(3) immunoelectron microscopy (Sarkar and Dion, 1975).

From these studies it is possible to tentatively localize the major structural polypeptides of MuMTV. The glycoproteins (gp68, gp55, and gp34) are components of the viral envelope including the spikes or projections that protrude from the envelope. gp34 is relatively inaccessible and, therefore, probably constitutes a transmembrane protein of the envelope and gp55 is the major component of the viral projection; the localization of gp68 has not yet been clarified; however, it appears to be associated with the external surface of the viral envelope. The major nonglycosylated protein of MuMTV, viz. p28, is an internal viral component as are p18, p14, and p12. p28 is most probably localized within the core envelope and one or more of the lower molecular weight components forms the ribonucleoprotein complex.

B. *ISOLATION*

Techniques for the isolation of the structural polypeptides of MuMTV have included

(1) ion-exchange and gel permeation chromatography (Parks *et al.*,1974; Sarkar and Dion, 1975; Dion *et al.*, 1977b);

(2) ion-exchange, hydroxyapatite, and gel permeation chromatography (Zangerle *et al.*, 1977; Hendrick *et al.*, 1978);

(3) gel permeation chromatography of MuMTV proteins disrupted with SDS (SDS/Sephadex G-200 chromatography) or guanidinium hydrochloride (Dion *et al.*, 1977b);

(4) ion-exchange and lectin affinity binding chromatography (Ritzi *et al.*, 1976);

(5) preparative SDS-PAGE (Yagi *et al.*, 1978; Cardiff *et al.*, 1978); and

(6) hydrophobic binding chromatography (Marcus *et al.*, 1978).

In most instances, the above protocols only effected the purification of gp55 and p28 (Parks *et al.*, 1974; Sarkar and Dion, 1975; Ritzi *et al.*, 1976) or multiple MuMTV polypeptides in relatively low yield (Yagi *et al.*, 1978; Cardiff *et al.*, 1978). Because of the requirement for relatively large quantities of purified MuMTV proteins for chemical characterizations, we expanded the original protocols developed in this laboratory (Sarkar and Dion, 1975) to encompass the isolation of all of the major structural proteins of MuMTV in high yield by two protocols (Dion *et al.*, 1977b).

As shown in Fig. 2, the application of two isolation protocols (Dion *et al.*, 1977b) effects the purification of gp90, gp68, gp55, gp34, p28, p18, p14, and p12. Method 1, employing ion-exchange and molecular sieving chromatography, leads to the purification of gp68, gp55, p28, and p12 as well as RNA-directed DNA polymerase (Dion *et al.*, 1974; Dion *et al.*, 1977a). gp90, gp34, p18, and p14 are most easily purified by method 2, consisting of Sephadex G-200 chromotography of SDS-disrupted MuMTV. Criteria for the purity of these preparations, i.e., unique N-termini, tryptic peptide maps, etc., are given below.

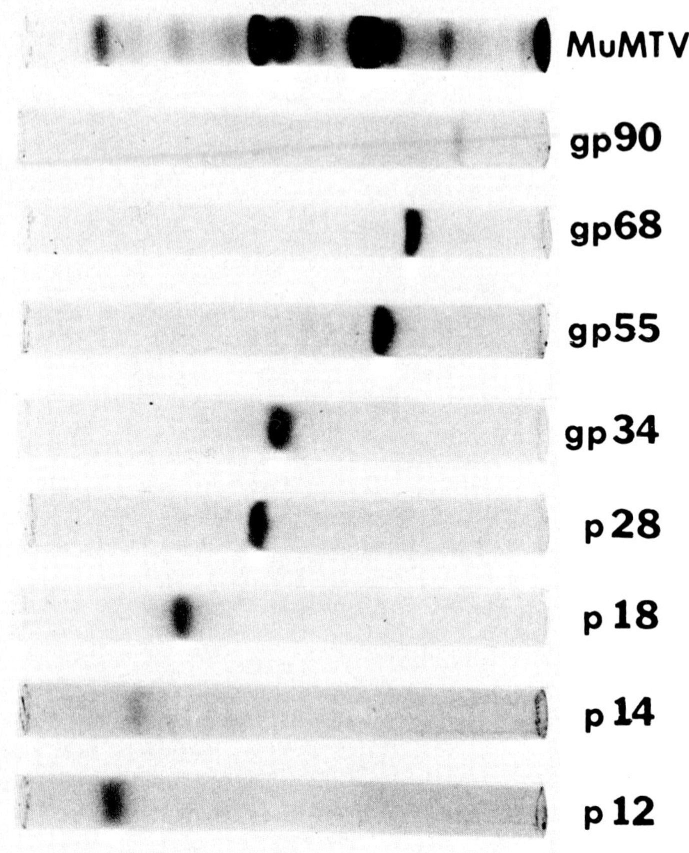

FIGURE 2. SDS-PAGE analyses of the major glycosylated and nonglycosylated proteins of RII-MuMTV isolated by techniques described in the text (Dion et al., *1977b).*

C. Biochemical Characterizations

1. Quantitative Amino Acid Analyses. By various criteria, e.g., SDS-PAGE, N-termini, quantitative amino acid analyses, tryptic peptide mapping, and immunodiffusion assays, each of the isolated major glycoproteins and proteins of RIII-MuMTV is unique. Quantitative amino acid analyses for each of the glycoproteins are presented in Table I with a summation of molecular weights of the protein moieties that correspond to those values established by SDS/Sephadex G-200 chromatography (Dion *et al.*, 1977b). The salient points with reference to Table I include

(1) relative to gp68 and gp55, the contents of arginine, threonine, serine, proline, and isoleucine in gp34, on a molar basis, are remarkably reduced with increased contents of lysine, histidine, half-cystine, methionine and phenylalanine;

(2) gp55 contains a high proportion of amino acids with a high frequency of occurrence in coil structures (proline, glycine, serine), which are known to disrupt α-helix and β-sheet protein structures (Chou and Fasman, 1974);

(3) gp34 contains low percentages of the latter with a high proportion of amino acid residues that participate to structure proteins.

TABLE I. Quantitative Amino Acid Composition of MuMTV Glycoproteins

	Residues/mole protein[a]		
Amino acid	*gp68*	*gp55*	*gp34*
Lys	*21*	*27*	*26*
His	*8*	*10*	*13*
Arg	*16*	*16*	*4*
Asp	*46*	*43*	*17*
Thr	*26*	*30*	*8*
Ser	*32*	*37*	*8*
Glu	*44*	*30*	*15*
Pro	*8*	*37*	*trace*
Gly	*41*	*31*	*15*
Ala	*32*	*24*	*22*
1/2 Cys	*4*	*8*	*34*
Val	*20*	*22*	*11*
Met	*2*	*3-4*	*9*
Ile	*17*	*23*	*6*
Leu	*37*	*36*	*13*
Tyr	*4*	*11*	*5*
Phe	*17*	*23*	*19*
Number of residues	*375*	*411*	*225*
Molecular weight:	*39,998*	*44,804*	*25,104*

[a]*Averages obtained from 24, 48, and 72 hr hydrolyses. Values for serine and threonine were corrected for hydrolytic losses.*

From the foregoing, it is plausible to assume that gp34 has a highly ordered tertiary structure; gp55 is predicted to be considerably less structured and gp68 is intermediate.

Similar analyses for the major, nonglycosylated proteins of RIII-MuMTV, i.e., p28, p18, p14, and p12, are presented in Table II. The major points to be emphasized from these data include (1) p18, p12, and possibly p14, are phosphorylated proteins and these observations have been corroborated by the ^{32}P-phosphate labeling (Dion *et al.*, 1979) of tissue culture-derived MuMTV from an established cell line of BALB/cfC3H

TABLE II. Quantitative Amino Acid Composition of Nonglycosylated MuMTV Protein

	Residues/mole protein[a]			
Amino acid	*p28*	*p18*	*p14*	*p12*
Lys	*19*	*12*	*8*	*4*
His	*4*	*3*	*3*	*4*
Arg	*12*	*5*	*4*	*4*
Asp	*22*	*11*	*11*	*9*
Thr	*15*	*13*	*13*	*7*
Ser	*22*	*11*	*10*	*12*
Glu	*32*	*17*	*13*	*8*
Pro	*17*	*5*	*3*	*3*
Gly	*32*	*17*	*16*	*26*
Ala	*20*	*11*	*9*	*9*
1/2 Cys	*8*	*8*	*2*	*5*
Val	*19*	*9*	*8*	*6*
Met	*5*	*3*	*2*	*5*
Ile	*11*	*10*	*6*	*4*
Leu	*22*	*15*	*10*	*5*
Tyr	*6*	*3*	*2*	*2*
Phe	*7*	*7*	*5*	*3*
Unknown	*23*	–	–	*6*
Number of residues	*296*	*160*	*125*	*123*
Molecular weight	*31,494*	*17,653*	*13,174*	*12,247*

[a]*Averages obtained from 24, 48, and 72 hr hydrolyses. Values for serine and threonine were corrected for hydrolytic losses.*

adenocarcinomas (Sarkar *et al.*, 1977); (2) p28 and p12 contain an unknown, ninhydrin-reactive component which elutes just prior to glycine, and attempts to characterize this component are in progress.

2. *Polarities of RIII-MuMTV Proteins.* Polarities of purified MuMTV proteins were estimated from percentages of occurrence (Table I and II) of amino acids within three classes, viz. polar, intermediate, and nonpolar (Capaldi and Vanderkooi, 1972) as illustrated in Table III. For the glycoproteins, the increase in apolar residues coincides with the localization of these proteins (cf. Section II, A), i.e., gp68 and gp55 are external components of the viral envelope while gp34 is embedded within the viral envelope. This internalization is consonant with the hydrophobicity of gp34 that has previously been observed to yield high molecular weight aggregates resistant to reducing conditions or the action of hydrogen bond disrupters (guanidinium.HCl and urea), but susceptible to ionic detergents (Dion *et al.*, 1977b). The postulated core shell protein p28 has an intermediate polarity while p18 and p12 are relatively apolar. Finally, it should be noted that these predicted polarities computed on the basis of amino acid frequencies are subject to alterations imposed by host-controlled, posttranslational modifications. For example, glycosylation (gp68, gp55, gp34) and phosphorylation (p18, p14, p12) would significantly increase the polarities of these modified proteins.

TABLE III. Polarities of MuMTV Structural Proteins

	Percent of total amino acids			
Protein	*Polar*[a]	*Intermediate*[b]	*Nonpolar*[c]	*Polar/nonpolar*
gp68	*33.9*	*29.6*	*36.5*	*0.93*
gp55	*28.2*	*29.0*	*42.9*	*0.66*
gp34	*27.6*	*21.8*	*50.7*	*0.54*
p28	*31.1*	*28.9*	*39.9*	*0.78*
p18	*28.1*	*29.4*	*42.5*	*0.66*
p14	*28.8*	*35.2*	*36.0*	*0.80*
p12	*21.5*	*44.0*	*34.5*	*0.62*

[a]*Polar: Lys, Arg, Asp, Asn, Glu, Gln (Asn and Gln included as Asp and Glu).*
[b]*Intermediate: His, Ser, Thr, Gly, Tyr.*
[c]*Nonpolar: Ala, Leu, Ile, Cys, Met, Pro, Phe, Val.*

3. Tryptic Peptide Mapping. Separation of peptides released by trypsin digestion offers a simple and rapid technique for comparative protein studies. Tryptic peptide maps of the glycosylated, viral membrane-associated proteins of MuMTV, i.e., gp68, gp55, and gp34, are illustrated in Fig. 3. For each of these glycoproteins, a distinctive peptide map was observed. Similar mapping studies also included the internal viral proteins of MuMTV as demonstrated in Fig. 4. Although some maps appear to contain similar patterns, e.g., p28, p18, and p14, distinct differences were noted with regard to the number of peptides released, intensities, and simultaneous analyses; therefore, none of the nonglycosylated proteins is identical by this assay. However, cochromatography of p14 and p18 yielded a map indicating that all of the p14 tryptic peptides were contained in the p18 map. From these data, and previous observations that both p14 and p18 contained blocked N-termini, we tentatively conclude that p14 arises from cleavage of p18 proximal to the carboxy terminus; however, definitive results will require partial sequence analyses.

III. COMPARATIVE STUDY OF RIII- AND A-MuMTV POLYPEPTIDES

A. *The Major Envelope Glycoproteins*

By protocols previously described (Section II, B), the major envelope glycoproteins of RIII- and A-MuMTVs, gp55 (RIII), and gp50 (A), were purified to apparent homogeneity. As indicated by their designations, the major glycoprotein of A-MuMTV possesses a lower molecular weight than the analogous protein derived from RIII-MuMTV. By both micro-Ouchterlony and radioimmunoassays (Dion *et al.*, in preparation), these proteins possess a high degree of immunological relatedness, corroborating group-specific determinants or sequence similarities on these MuMTV glycoproteins (Sarkar and Dion, 1975); however, it is also apparent from the molecular weight estimates that significant differences in the structure of these glycoproteins exist that may lead to type-specific reactivities, and the biochemical elucidation of the latter forms the basis of this investigation.

Gel-stabilized isoelectric focusing (Righetti and Drysdale, 1973) offers an extremely sensitive technique for monitoring heterogeneity within or between proteins. As illustrated in Table IV, both gp55 (RIII) and gp50 (A) are heterogenous, i.e., possess multiple isoelectric points, indicative of differential host-controlled, posttranslational modifications within each protein. Regarding the latter, heterogeneity within each protein is most probably due to differences in glycosylation. However, variations between gp55 (RIII) and gp50 (A) may arise

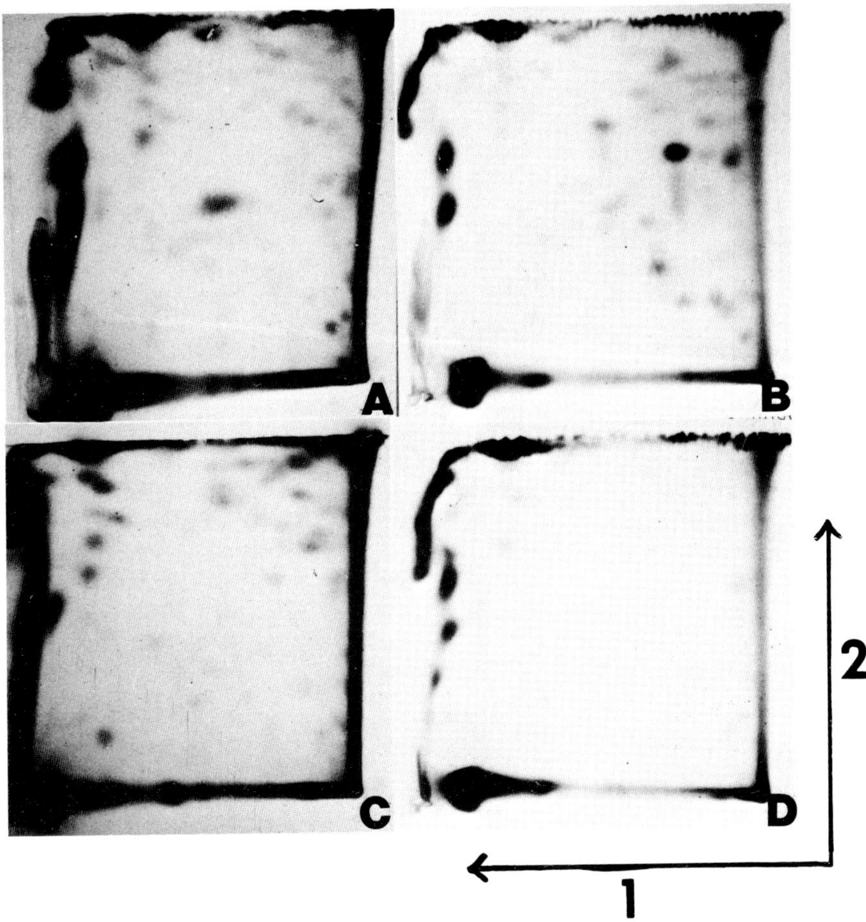

FIGURE 3. Radioautograms of ^{14}C-dansyl-labeled tryptic peptides of the major viral envelope-associated glycoproteins of RIII-MuMTV. Purified proteins were denatured and electrophoresed (SDS-PAGE), followed by staining with Coomassie blue. SDS and stain were removed from the stained band by maceration of the gel section in methanol/acetic acid, the gel fragments were lyophilized, and the protein was digested overnight with TPCK-trypsin at an enzyme to substrate ratio of 1:50 in 50 mM triethylamine·HCl(pH 8.8) containing 5.75 mM $CaCl_2$. After removal of the gel fragments by centrifugation, the released peptides were derivatized with ^{14}C-dansyl chloride (0.5 µg/µl; 62.2 mC/mmol) in 0.1 M $NaHCO_3$ at 37°C for 45 min. Labeled preparations were dried in a stream of nitrogen and resuspended in 95% ethanol. For two-dimensional analyses, samples were

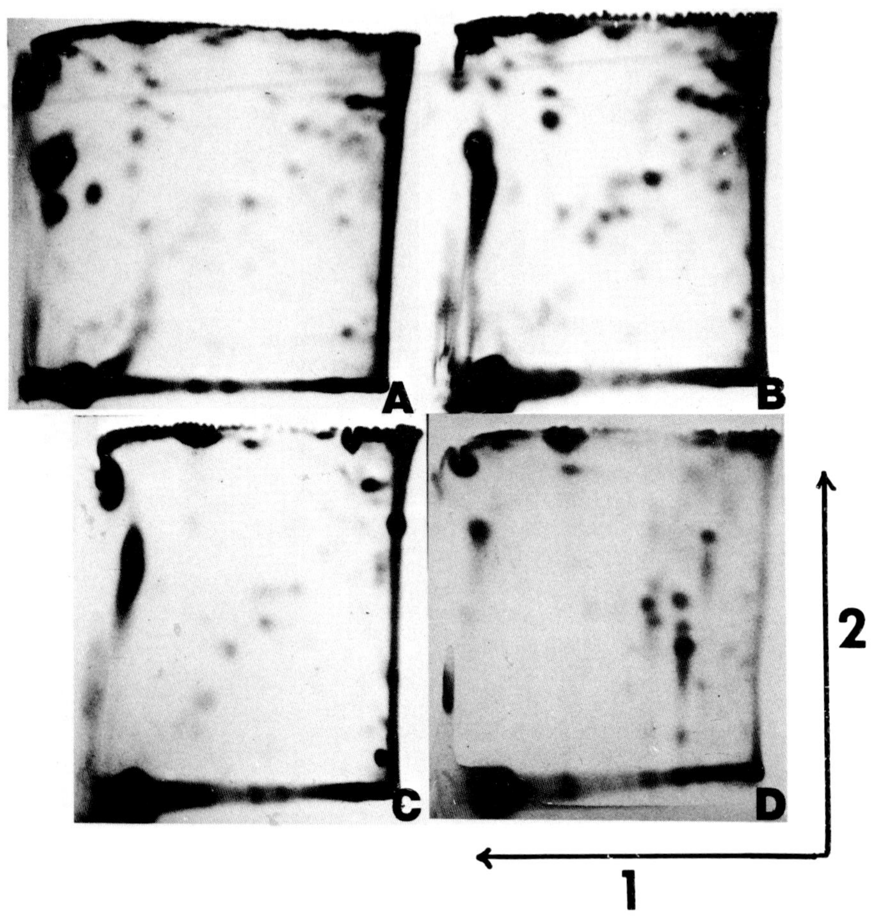

FIGURE 4. Radioautograms of ^{14}C-dansyl-labeled tryptic peptides of the major internal, nonglycosylated proteins of RIII-MuMTV. Conditions of trypsin digestion and techniques for peptide mapping are described in the legend to Fig. 3. A, p28; B, p18; C, p14, D, p12.

(Figure 3, cont.) spotted on polyamide plates (7.5 × 7.5 cm). First dimension, two times in 7.5% formic acid; second dimension, benzene/acetic acid (3:1). For radioautographic detection of labeled peptides, the chromotograms were directly apposed to Kodak NS-5T X-ray film. A, gp68; B, gp55; C, gp34; D, Blank.

TABLE IV. Isoelectric Points (pIs) of the Major Envelope and Core Proteins of RIII- and A-MuMTV

	Envelope glycoproteins	
	gp55(RIII)	gp50(A)
pI	7.32	8.10 (major)
	6.98	7.60
	6.82	7.80
	6.70 (major)	6.60
	Core proteins	
	p28(RIII)	p28(A)
	7.21	7.61
pI	6.72 (major)	7.55

from primary sequence differences coded by the virus or post-translational modifications under host control. As given below, it is possible to elucidate whether one or both of these mechanisms is operative to effect the observed variations.

A comparative study of the amino acid compositions of gp55 (RIII) and gp50(A) is given in Table V. From these assays, including a summation of molecular weights from the quantitative amino acid analyses, it is seen that gp50(A) possesses a smaller protein moiety than does gp55(RIII). In part, therefore, the lower apparent molecular weight for gp50(A) resides in a shorter polypeptide sequence that is reflected in reduced quantities of most amino acids of gp50(A) as compared to gp55(RIII). That further differences are also involved is indicated by the increased quantities of some amino acids in gp50(A), i.e., a simple deletion of part of the polypeptide chain would result in a depletion of many, if not all, of the amino acids of gp50(A). Therefore, an increase in certain amino acids of gp50(A), as compared to gp55(RIII), could only be effected by sequence differences in addition to sequence deletion.

The most evident host-controlled, posttranslational modification vis-a-vis glycoproteins involves glycosylation. Therefore, our comparative study has included quantitative carbohydrate analyses for gp55(RIII) and gp50(A) as demonstrated in Table VI. It should be emphasized that the isoelectric point heterogeneity indicated in Table IV is most probably the result of variable glycosylation; therefore, the values given in

TABLE V. Amino Acid Compositions of the Major Envelope Glycoproteins of RIII- and A-MuMTV

	Residues/mole protein[a]	
Amino acid	*gp55(RIII)*	*gp50(A)*
Lys	27	27
His	10	10
Arg	16	17
Asp	43	43
Thr	30	24
Ser	37	32
Glu	30	28
Pro	37	42
Gly	31	28
Ala	24	22
1/2 Cys	8	17
Val	22	22
Met	3-4	4
Ile	23	16
Leu	36	34
Tyr	11	9
Phe	23	22
Number of residues	411	397
Molecular weight	44,804	43,334

[a]*Averages obtained from 24, 48, and 72 low hydrolyses. Values for serine and threonine were corrected for hydrolytic losses.*

Table VI may represent averages for a relatively diverse population of glycosylated variants within each glycoprotein. For both gp55(RIII) and gp50(A), the numbers of sialic acid or neutral sugar components are similar; the most striking difference involves a considerably larger number of aminosugar residues per mole of gp50(A) protein as compared to gp55(RIII).

TABLE VI. Carbohydrate Compositions of the Major Envelope Glycoproteins of RIII- and A-MuMTV[a]

	Residues/mole protein	
Component	*gp55(RIII)*	*gp50(A)*
Sialic acid	5	4
Glucosamine	2	3
Galactosamine	1	2
Mannose	14	13
Galactose	5	7
Fucose	*ND*[b]	*ND*

[a]*Quantitative sialic acid determinations were estimated by the procedure of Hess and Rolde (1964). Aminosugar analyses were carried out by the technique of Farwell and Dion (1979). Quantitative assays of neutral sugars were performed on silyl derivatives by gas chromatography by Dr. Leonard Warren (Wistar Institute, Philadelphia).*

[b]*ND, not detectable.*

B The Major Core Proteins

The major core proteins of RIII- and A-MuMTV were isolated to homogeneity as previously described (Section II, B). In contrast to the molecular weight difference observed for the major glycoprotein of RIII- and A-MuMTV, no significant differences were observed between p28(RIII) and p28(A) when monitored by SDS-PAGE (coelectrophoresis) or Sephadex G-100 chromatography. That these core proteins are immunologically related was readily apparent from micro-Ouchterlony assays that demonstrated confluent lines of identity (not shown), corroborating group-specific determinants on the major core proteins of MuMTV as previously reported (Sarkar and Dion, 1975).

Although these data indicated that p28(RIII) and p28(A) were closely analogous, the determination of isoelectric points of these proteins by gel-stabilized isoelectric focusing indicated that they were not identical (Table IV). The observed heterogeneity within each protein is most likely the result of differential deamidination in the appearance of aspartic and glumatic acid residues from asparagine and glutamine, respectively. This mechanism may also be, in part, responsible for the differences between p28(RIII) and p28(A); however, the possibility of primary sequence differences may not be obviated in the absence of sequence data. Unless the major core proteins of MuMTV are highly conserved, it is probable that they too bear type-specificities as do the major envelope glycoproteins.

SUMMARY AND DISCUSSION

As described above, we have designed reproducible protocols for the purification of all of the major structural proteins of RIII-MuMTV, i.e., gp68, gp55, gp34, p28, p18, p14, and p12. During the course of biochemical characterizations of these proteins by N-termini, quantitative amino acid analyses, tryptic peptide mapping, etc., as described in the text, it became apparent that each protein was unique, i.e., no evidence for significant cross-contamination was observed. However, from tryptic peptide mapping studies, it is possible that p14 arises from p18 cleavage.

The polyprotein precursors of the envelope (env) and core (gag) proteins of MuMTV have reported molecular weight values of 75,000 (Schochetman *et al.*, 1977) and 77,000/75,000 (Dickson and Atterwill, 1978), respectively. The envelope precursor gives rise to gp55 and gp34 and the summation of the molecular weights of these proteins, as indicated in Table I, yields a value of 69,000, which is in reasonable agreement with the value reported for the env precursor that is glycosylated and, therefore, overestimated by SDS-PAGE. As previously noted, gp68 is not related to either gp55 or gp34; therefore, it most likely represents a host cell contaminant. However, the constant association of gp68 with MuMTV deserved consideration in order to eliminate it as a possible uncleaved env precursor associated with this virus. A similar summation of molecular weights of nonglycosylated RIII-MuMTV proteins (Table II) yields a molecular weight of 74,568, which is in excellent agreement with the gag-precursor value of 77,000/75,000 (Dickson and Atterwill, 1978).

From the foregoing, the development of reproducible isolation and characterization protocols for the structural polypeptides of RIII-MuMTV enabled us to conduct a comparative study of the major envelope and core proteins of RIII and A-MuMTV. In this investigation we observed both structural similarities and differences between gp55(RIII) and gp50(A) to establish a sound basis for group- and type-specificities, respectively. Regarding the latter, analyses of the protein moieties of these glycoproteins strongly indicate that both viral and host genetic factors, in this instance, play a role in determining type-specificities. In addition, the oligosaccharide moieties of these glycoproteins differed significantly, and might also play an important role in type-specific determinants on these antigens. The latter is even more probable in view of recent results, demonstrating a profound influence of oligosaccharide structure on the antigenicity of an envelope glycoprotein of avian myeloblastosis virus (Van Eldik *et al.*, 1978).

The results presented here might also have important implications with reference to a possible MuMTV-like agent associated with human breast carcinomas (Dion and Moore, 1977). For example, as measured by the leukocyte migration inhibition assay, specific cell-mediated immune responses have been elicited with gp55(RIII) with some human breast tumors (Black *et al.*, 1976, 1978); however, little or no response was obtained with gp50(A) (Zachrau *et al.*, 1978). Therefore it appears that elicitation of specific cellular-mediated responses is exquisitely sensitive to structural differences observed between gp55(RIII) and gp50(A) as investigated in this study. Through continued structural characterizations of these antigens, it should be possible to identify specific determinants responsible for the cellular-mediated immune responses noted above.

ACKNOWLEDGMENTS

This research was supported in part by Contract NO1-CP-81003 within the Virus Cancer Program of the National Cancer Institute and by a Biomedical Research Support Grant #5 SO7 RR05582-11.

REFERENCES

Bentvelzen, P. (1972). *Int. Rev. Exp. Pathol. 11,* 259-297.

Black, M. M., Zachrau, R. E., Dion, A. S., Shore, B., Fine, D. L., Leis, H. P., and Williams, C. J. (1976). *Cancer Res. 36,* 4137-4142.

Black, M. M., Zachrau, R. E., Shore, B., Dion, A. S., and Leis, H. P. (1978). *Cancer Res. 38,*2068-2076.

Blair, P. B. (1970). *Cancer Res. 30,* 625-631.

Blair, P. B. (1971). *Cancer Res. 31,* 1473-1477.

Capaldi, R. A., and Vanderkooi, G. (1972). *Proc. Natl. Acad. Sci. 69,* 930-932.

Cardiff, R. D., Puentes, M. J., Teramoto, Y. A., and Lund, J. K. (1974). *J. Virol. 14,* 1293-1303.

Cardiff, R. D., Puentes, M. J., Young, L. J. T., Smith, G. H., Teramoto, Y. A., Altrock, B. W., and Pratt, T. S. (1978). *Virology 85,* 157-167.

Chou, P. Y., and Fasman, G. D. (1974). *Biochemistry 13,* 211-222.

Dickson, C., and Atterwill, M. (1978). *J. Virol. 26,* 660-672.

Dickson, C., and Skehel, J. J. (1974). *Virology 58,* 387-395.

Dion, A. S., and Moore, D. H. (1977). *In* "Recent Advances in Cancer Research: Cell Biology, Molecular Biology, and Tumor Virology" (R. C. Gallo, ed.), Vol. II, pp. 69-87. CRC Press, Inc., Cleveland, Ohio.

Dion, A. S., Vaidya, A. B., Fout, G. S., and Moore, D. H. (1974). *J. Virol. 14,* 40-46.

Dion, A. S., Williams, C. J., and Moore, D. H. (1977a). *J. Virol. 22,* 187-193.

Dion, A. S., Williams, C. J., and Pomenti, A. A. (1977b). *Anal. Biochem. 82,* 18-28.

Dion, A. S., Fout, G. S., and Pomenti, A. A. (1979). *J. Gen. Virol..* (In press).

Farwell, D. C., and Dion, A. S. (1979). *Anal. Biochem. 95,* 533-539.

Hendrick, J. C., Francois, C., Carlberg-Bacq, C. M., Colin, C., Franchimont, P., Gosselin, L., Kozma, S., and Osterrieth, P. M. (1978). *Cancer Res. 38,* 1826-1831.

Hess, H. H., and Rolde, E. (1964). *J. Biol. Chem. 239,* 3215-3220.

Hilgers, J., and Bentvelzen, P. (1977). *Adv. Cancer Res. 26,* 143-195.

Karande, K. A., Joshi, B. J., Talageri, V. R., Dumaswala, R. V., and Ranadive, K. J. (1978). *Europ. J. Cancer 14,* 251-261.

Kimball, P. C., Truitt, M. B., Schochetman, G., and Schlom, J. (1976). *J. Natl. Cancer Inst. 56,* 111-117.

Marcus, S. L., Smith, S. W., Racevskis, J., and Sarkar, H. H. (1978). *Virology 86,* 398-412.

Moore, D. H., Charney, J., and Holben, J. A. (1974). *J. Natl. Cancer Inst. 52,* 1757-1761.

Nandi, S., and McGrath, C. M. (1973). *Adv. Cancer Res. 17,* 353-414.

Nowinski, R. C., Sarkar, N. H., Old, L. J., Moore, D. H., Scheer, D. I., and Hilgers, J. (1971). *Virology 46,* 21-38.

Parks, W. P., Howk, R. S., Scolnick, E. M., Oroszlan, S., and Gilden, R. V. (1974). *J. Virol. 13,* 1200-1210.

Righetti, P. G., and Drysdale, J. W. (1973). *In* "Isoelectric Focusing and Isotachophoresis" (N. Catsimpoolas, ed.), Vol. 209, pp. 163-186. Ann. N. Y. Acad. Sci., New York.

Ritzi, E., Baldi, A., and Spiegelman, S. (1976). *Virology 75,* 188-197.

Sarkar, N. H., and Dion, A. S. (1975). *Virology 64,* 471-491.

Sarkar, N. H., Taraschi, N. E., Pomenti, A. A., and Dion, A. S. (1976). *Virology 69,* 677-690.

Sarkar, N. H., Pomenti, A. A., and Dion, A. S. (1977). *Virology 77,* 12-30.

Schloemer, R. H., Schlom, J., Schochetman, G., Kimball, P., and Wagner, R. R. (1976). *J. Virol. 18,* 804-808.

Schochetman, G., Oroszlan, S., Arthur, L., and Fine, D. (1977). *Virology 83,* 72-83.

Sheffield, J. B., and Daly, T. M. (1976). *Virology 70,* 247-250.

Sheffield, J. B., Zacharchuk, C. M., Taraschi, N., and Daly, T. M. (1976). *J. Virol. 19,* 255-266.

Sheffield, J. B., Daly, T., Dion, A. S., and Taraschi, N. (1977). *Cancer Res. 37,* 1480-1485.

Smith, G. H., and Lee, B. K. (1975). *J. Natl. Cancer Inst. 55,* 493-496.

Smith, G. H., and Wivel, N. A. (1973). *J. Virol. 11,* 575-584.

Squartini, F., Rossi, G., and Paoletti, I. (1963). *Nature 197,* 505-506.

Tanaka, H. (1977). *Virology 76,* 835-850.

Teramoto, Y. A., Puentes, M. J., Young, L. J. T., and Cardiff, R. D. (1974). *J. Virol. 13,* 411-418.

Teramoto, Y. A., Cardiff, R. D., and Lund, J. K. (1977a). *Virology 77,* 135-148.

Teramoto, Y. A., Kufe, D., and Schlom, J. (1977b). *Proc. Natl. Acad. Sci. 74,* 3564-3568.

Teramoto, Y. A., Kufe, D., and Schlom, J. (1977c). *J. Virol. 24,* 525-533.

Tichy, H. (1975). *Anal. Biochem. 69,* 552-557.

Van Eldik, L. J., Paulson, J. C., Green, R. W., and Smith, R. E. (1978). *Virology 86,* 193-204.

Witte, O. N., Weissman, I. L., and Kaplan, H. S. (1973). *Acad. Sci. 70,* 36-40.

Yagi, M. J., and Compans, R. W. (1977). *Virology 76,* 751-766.

Yagi, M. J., Stutzman, R. E., Robertson, B. H., and Compans, R. W. (1978). *J. Virol. 26,* 448-456.

Zachrau, R. E., Black, M. M., Dion, A. S., Shore, B., Williams, C. J., and Leis, H. P. (1978). *Cancer Res. 38,* 3414-3420.

Zangerle, P. F., Carlberg-Bacq, C. M., Colin, C., Franchimont, P., Francois, C., Gosselin, L., Kozma, S., and Osterrieth, P. M. (1977). *Cancer Res. 37,* 4326-4331.

CHARACTERIZATION OF RIII MOUSE MAMMARY TUMOR VIRUS*

Francesco Squartini
Raffaele Pingitore
and
Maria Bistocchi

Laboratory of Experimental Oncology
Institute of Pathological Anatomy and Histology
University of Pisa
Italy

I. INTRODUCTION

The C3H and GR variants of murine mammary tumor virus (MTV) are indicated as prototypes of two different biologic behaviors. C3H MTV, referred to as MTV S (standard), induces preneoplastic hyperplastic alveolar nodules and fast-growing pregnancy-independent mammary tumors. GR MTV, referred to as MTV P (plaque forming), induces palpable ductular growths in form of plaques and pregnancy-dependent mammary tumors (Bentvelzen and Daams, 1969).

In various recent papers the RIII MTV has differently been quoted as MTV S (Schlom *et al.*, 1977), PS (Schlom *et al.*, 1973; Bentvelzen, 1974) or P (Ringold *et al.*, 1976; Squartini and Bistocchi, 1977). A further characterization of RIII MTV seems appropriate in this respect. During a series of experiments, the RIII MTV has been compared with the standard C3H MTV after transfer of both into the same genetic environment (susceptible BALB/c mice) by foster nursing. Some preliminary data have already been published (Squartini and Bistocchi, 1977; Bistocchi *et al.*, 1977b) but a complete survey is given here.

Supported by contract no. 78.00401.84 from the National Research Council, Rome, Progetto Finalizzato CNR "Virus."

ISBN 0-12-131150-3

II. MATERIALS AND METHODS

The following mice and procedures were used throughout the experiments.

Noduligenic test. Forty three BALB/cfC3H (BALB/cfC3H/Cb/Se substrain) and 45 BALB/cfRIII (Squartini *et al.*, 1974) virgin females were submitted to the noduligenic test (Nandi, 1963).

Spontaneous tumorigenesis. (a) Virgin females: 40 BALB/cf C3H and 41 BALB/cfRIII virgin females were observed until age 20 months for the occurrence of spontaneous mammary tumors.

(b) Breeding females: 71 BALB/cfC3H breeding females, 29 normally bred plus 42 force-bred, and 80 BALB/cfRIII breeding females, 34 normally bred plus 46 force-bred were also observed till death for the occurrence of spontaneous mammary tumors.

(c) Procedure: Records were kept of the reproductive histories of each mouse and of the occurrence of all palpable mammary tumors. During life, palpable tumors were measured weekly. At autopsy, tumors were removed for histologic examination.

MTV in milk. Quantitative determinations of MTV release have been carried out in milk samples collected at identical times from six BALB/cfC3H and six BALB/cfRIII breeding females standardized for age at delivery and size of litters. Milk samples from six MTV negative BALB/c controls have also been analyzed and used as blank, according to the method previously described (Bistocchi *et al.*, 1977a) based on the light-scattering measure of partially purified MTV. All the experimental mice were kept in plastic cages, 1-3 per cage, fed with pellets and given water ad libitum.

III. RESULTS

1. Virgin Females.

Data are summarized in Table I. The average number of mammary hyperplastic alveolar nodules per mouse after noduligenic test was 20.1 in BALB/cfC3H and 10.7 in BALB/cfRIII females. Mammary tumor incidence at 20 months of age was 47.5% in BALB/cfC3H and 14.6% in BALB/cfRIII virgin females. The frequency of lung metastases in mammary tumor-bearing mice was 63.1% in BALB/cfC3H and 16.6% in BALB/cfRIII virgin females. The differences found were significant.

TABLE I. *Mammary Noduligenesis and Tumorigenesis in BALB/cfC3H and BALB/cfRIII Virgin Female Mice*

A. *Hyperplastic alveolar nodules after noduligenic test*

Substrain	No. mice	No. nodules	Nodules per mouse
BALB/cfC3H	43	863	20.1
BALB/cfRIII	45	438	10.7

$T = 3.46$; $P < 0.01$

B. *Spontaneous mammary tumors after 20 months*

Substrain	No. mice	With tumors	Tumor %
BALB/cfC3H	40	19	47.5
BALB/cfRIII	41	6	14.6

$X^2 = 10.25$; $P < 0.01$

C. *Lung metastases in mammary tumor-bearing mice*

Substrain	No. mice	With lung metastases	Metastases %
BALB/cfC3H	19	12	63.1
BALB/cfRIII	6	1	16.6

$X^2 = 3.95$; $P < 0.05$

2. Breeding Females.

The cumulative mammary tumor incidence of normally and force-bred females was 96% in both BALB/cfC3H and BALB/cfRIII mice. The average age at onset of first palpable tumor was also comparable: 285 days in BALB/cfC3H and 292 days in BALB/cfRIII females. The total number of mammary tumors developed was 205 in BALB/cfC3H (average 2.9 per mouse) and 176 in BALB/cfRIII (average 2.2 per mouse). The behavior of these mammary tumors is summarized in Table II. Tumors occurring during pregnancies were classified as pregnancy-dependent (total regression after delivery), pregnancy-responsive (partial regression after delivery), or pregnancy-independent (no regression after delivery).

In BALB/cfRIII females, the number of pregnancy-dependent mammary tumors (18.2%) is six times that in BALB/cfC3H females (2.9%). The number of pregnancy-responsive mammary tumors is also three times more in BALB/cfRIII females (13.1%) compared to BALB/cfC3H females (4.4%). The differences are highly significant. A larger number of mammary tumors in BALB/cfRIII females occur during pregnancies (43.8% versus 31.7%) and appear earlier (271 days versus 290 days). Conversely, tumors occurring out of pregnancies are less (56.2% versus 68.3%) and appear later (343 days versus 312 days) in BALB/cfRIII females. The clinical duration of tumors is in any case longer in BALB/cfRIII females (Table II).

The peculiar aspects of this different tumor behavior are illustrated and compared in Figs. 1-3. The appearance of mammary tumors in BALB/cfRIII females is strongly influenced by the events of pregnancy (Fig. 1). Of 77 tumors occurring during pregnancies in this strain, three were palpated during the first five days of pregnancy, i.e., from the 20th to the 16th day before delivery, 13 from the 15th to the 11th day before delivery, 20 from the 10th to the 6th day before delivery, and 41 during the last five days of pregnancy with peak just at delivery. The enhancing effect of delivery on mammary tumor appearance is much less pronounced in BALB/cfC3H females (Fig. 1).

Pregnancy-dependent and pregnancy-responsive tumors occur in BALB/cfRIII females from the third to the 12th pregnancy, whereas in BALB/cfC3H females they occur only from the sixth to the ninth pregnancy (Fig. 2). Pregnancy-independent tumors and tumors occurring out of pregnancies may occur at any time after first delivery but develop later in BALB/cfRIII females (Fig. 3).

The histologic analysis of mammary tumors has shown a significantly higher cystic component in the structure of BALB/cf RIII as compared to BALB/cfC3H tumors.

TABLE II. Occurrence and Behavior of Mammary Tumors in BALB/cfC3H and BALB/cfRIII Breeding Females Normally and Force-Bred[a]

Mammary tumors		Number	Percent (%)	Onset	Duration
A. BALB/cfC3H females: 71					
Occurring during pregnancies					
Pregnancy-dependent	PD	6	2.9	261 D.	72 D.
Pregnancy-responsive	PR	9	4.4	285	32
Pregnancy-independent	PI	50	24.4	295	17
Subtotal		65	31.7	290	24
Occurring out of pregnancies		140	68.3	312	34
Total		205	100.0	305	31
B. BALB/cfRIII females: 80					
Occurring during pregnancies					
Pregnancy-dependent	PD	32	18.2	253 D.	115 D.
Pregnancy-responsive	PR	23	13.1	264	70
Pregnancy-independent	PI	22	12.5	305	44
Subtotal		77	43.8	271	81
Occurring out of pregnancies		99	56.2	343	56
Total		176	100.0	312	67

[a]PD + PR/PI CHI SQUARE: 33,240; $P < 0.00001$ - D = days

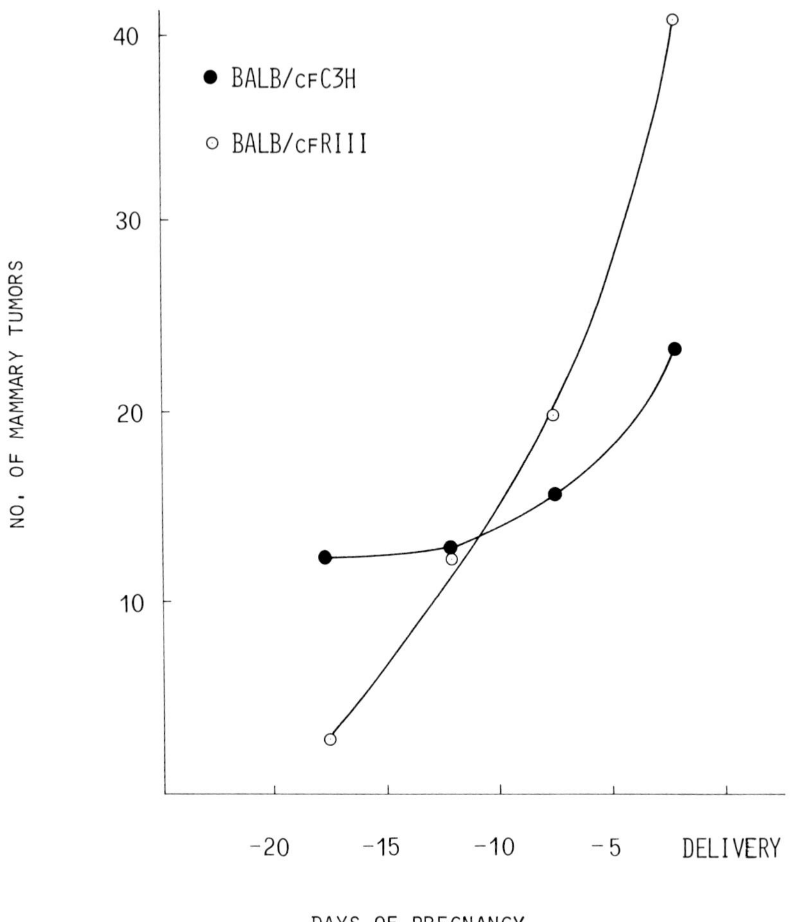

FIGURE 1. Appearance of palpable mammary tumors during the various stages of pregnancy in BALB/cfC3H and BALB/cfRIII breeding females, normally and force-bred.

3. Release of MTV in Milk

A difference in release through BALB/c milk during lactation periods has been found between C3H and RIII MTV. Data are illustrated in Table III. The 1st, 2nd, 3rd and 6th lactation periods were tested in BALB/cfC3H and BALB/cfRIII females, and the amount of MTV released was expressed for comparison as light-scattering units. These measure the optical density at 260 nm of the gradient fractions corresponding to the density of 1.15-1.20 gm/ml, referred to 100 mg of proteins in the whole milk, after subtraction of the average values obtained from the

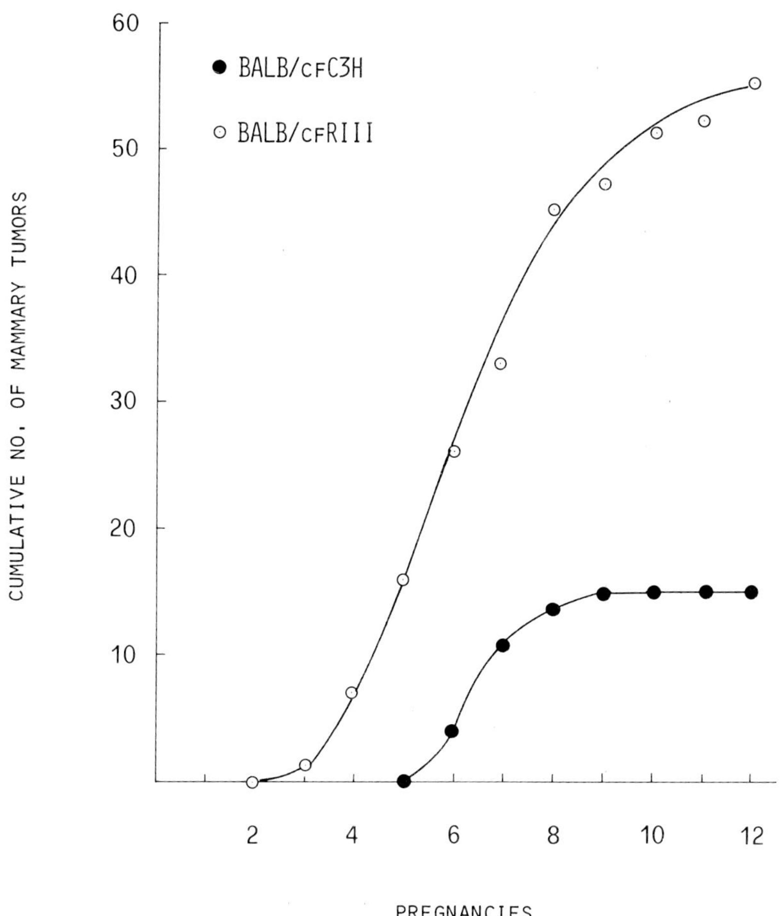

FIGURE 2. Cumulative number of pregnancy-dependent + pregnancy-responsive mammary tumors according to the pregnancy of appearance in BALB/cfC3H and BALB/cfRIII breeding females, normally and force-bred.

same fractions of MTV-negative BALBc milk samples at the respective lactation periods (Bistocchi *et al.*, 1977a). In Table 3 the light-scattering units of MTV in milk are expressed as BALB/cfRIII:BALB/cfC3H ratio, and it is apparent that release of RIII MTV in BALB/c milk is more than double that of C3H MTV.

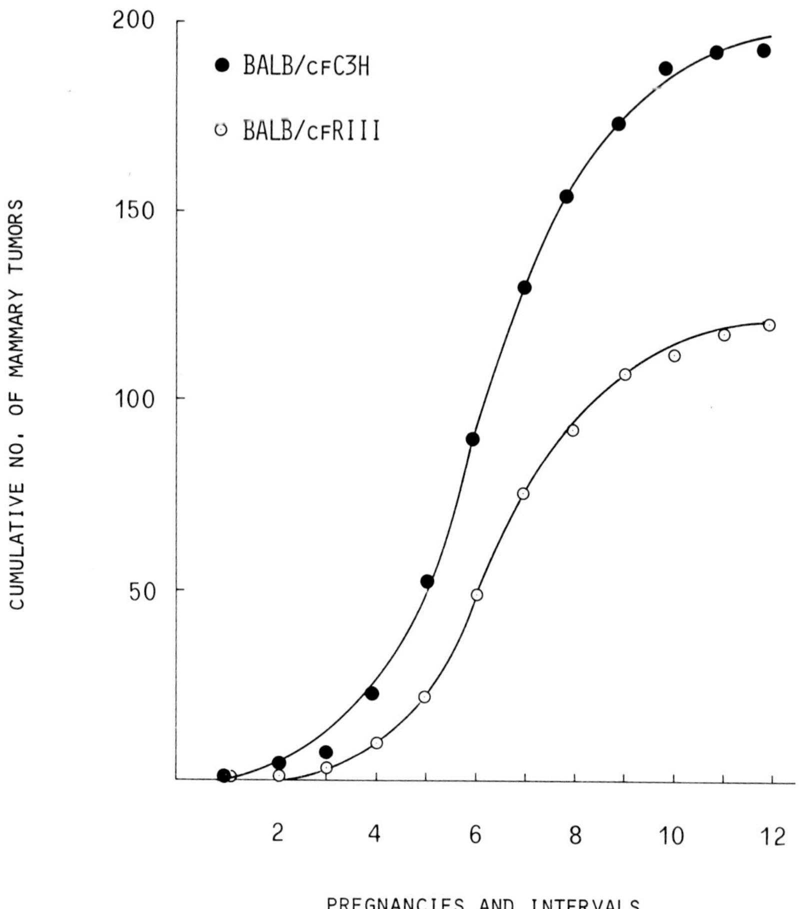

FIGURE 3. Cumulative number of pregnancy-independent mammary tumors and mammary tumors occurring out of pregnancies according to the pregnancy or interval of appearance in BALB/cfC3H and BALB/cfRIII breeding females, normally and force-bred.

IV. DISCUSSION

The first clear description of one mammary tumor followed for 313 days that grew and disappeared through two successive pregnancies was given in Paris by Dobrovolskaja-Zavadskaja (Dobrovolskaja-Zavadskaja, 1930a) while raising the original RIII strain (Dobrovolskaja-Zavadskaja, 1930b). The first de-

TABLE III. Release of C3H and RIII Mammary Tumor Viruses Through BALB/c Milk During Lactation Periods (as Light-Scattering Units: 46 Determinations)

Lactation periods	*Ratio:* $\frac{BALB/cfRIII}{BALB/cfC3H}$
1	*2.40*
2	*1.92*
3	*2.20*
6	*2.55*
Total	*2.26*

tailed report on pregnancy-dependent mouse mammary tumors and "plaques" was provided by Foulds (1949b, 1956) using force-bred female mice RIII x C57BL and reciprocal hybrids that harbour MTV received from their RIII high cancer parents (Foulds, 1949a). The first mention of pregnancy-dependent mammary tumors (Squartini and Rossi, 1959a) and plaques (Squartini and Rossi, 1959b) in inbred mice concerned RIII breeding females (Squartini, 1962). In successive experiments, transfer of pregnancy-dependent mammary tumors from RIII to BALB/c female mice by foster nursing was successfully achieved, showing that pregnancy-dependence is a tumor character to some extent controlled by the MTV RNA (Squartini *et al.*, 1963).

The present data provide a further characterization of the activities of RIII MTV in BALB/c mice indicating that, when compared to C3H MTV, it shows (a) lower virulence, (b) higher release in milk, and (c) pregnancy-dependent mammary tumors as a rule: 3/4 of mammary tumors occurring during pregnancies are dependent or responsive in BALB/cfRIII females, compared with 1/4 in BALB/cfC3H females. Although it is known that the genetic environment of host mice may influence the bioactivity of MTV (Moore *et al.*, 1974), the behaviors found in BALB/c fostered strains are closely similar to those observed in the strains of respective MTV origin, namely, RIII and C3H (Squartini, 1961, 1962; Squartini and Severi, 1962; Squartini *et al.*, 1964). Therefore, the conclusion is that the differences in mammary tumor behavior found between BALB/cfC3H and BALB/cfRIII females express to a large extent differences in bioactivity of the respective MTVs.

On the basis of biologic behavior, the RIII MTV tested here displays a good resemblance with the prototype plaque-forming MTV of the GR strain. In some American sublines of the RIII strain, however, the resident MTV has lost its ability to induce plaques, while it has gained in virulence (Bentvelzen, 1969). Therefore, different RIII MTV strains may have a different behavior.

The higher release of RIII MTV is somewhat surprising, since RIII MTV is less effective than C3H MTV. This finding is in agreement with recent data concerning MTV production in tissue cultures of mouse mammary tumor cells. The MTV produced by cultures of RIII mammary tumor cells was found to be approximately double that produced by BALB/cfC3H mammary tumor cells or by other mammary tumor cells (GR, DD) carrying P-type MTV (Kimball *et al.*, 1976).

Although rare with C3H MTV, a few plaques and pregnancy-dependent tumors are observed in BALB/cfC3H and even in C3H mice (Squartini *et al.*, 1964; Squartini and Rossi, 1960). Conversely, a few pregnancy-independent tumors are induced by RIII MTV. Whether this means coexistence in inbred mouse strains of mixtures of MTV S and P, with absolute prevalence of one or the other in the different strains, it is unknown at present and it remains a problem for future investigation.

V. SUMMARY

The RIII MTV has been compared with the standard C3H MTV after transfer of both into the same genetic environment (susceptible BALB/c mice) by foster nursing. In this comparison the RIII MTV has shown the following significant differences from C3H MTV:

(1) Lower nodule-inducing capability in virgins;

(2) Lower mammary tumor-inducing capability in virgins;

(3) Lower number of mammary tumors occurring out of pregnancies (during intervals or after fertile life) in breeders;

(4) Later occurrence of tumors in these conditions;

(5) Lower malignancy of tumors (based on lung metastases and survival time);

(6) Higher replication and release of MTV during lactation periods (at least double);

(7) Higher number of mammary tumors occurring during pregnancies in breeders;

(8) Higher number of pregnancy-dependent tumors (3/4 versus 1/4);

(9) Earlier occurrence of pregnancy-dependent tumors or plaques (from the third pregnancy onwards);

(10) Higher cystic component in the structure of tumors.

REFERENCES

Bentvelzen, P. (1974). *Biochem. Biophys. Acta 355,* 236-259.

Bentvelzen, P., and Daams, J. H. (1969). *J. Natl. Cancer Inst. 43,* 1025-1035.

Bistocchi, M., Bevilacqua, G., and Nuti, M. (1977a). *Tumori 63,* 525-534.

Bistocchi, M., Nuti, M., and Squartini, F. (1977b). *Tumori 63,* 535-542.

Dobrovolskaja-Zavadskaja, N. (1930a). *Compt. Rend. Soc. Biol. 103,* 994-996.

Dobrovolskaja-Zavadskaja, N. (1930b). *Compt. Rend. Soc. Biol. 104,* 1191-1193.

Foulds, L. (1949a). *Brit. J. Cancer 3,* 230-239.

Foulds, L. (1949b). *Brit. J. Cancer 3,* 345-375.

Foulds, L. (1956). *J. Natl. Cancer Inst. 17,* 713-753.

Kimball, P. C., Michalides, R., Colcher, D., and Schlom, J. (1976). *J. Natl. Cancer Inst. 56,* 119-124.

Moore, D. H., Charney, J., and Holben, J. A. (1974). *J. Natl. Cancer Inst. 52,* 1757-1761.

Nandi, S. (1963). *J. Natl. Cancer Inst. 31,* 57-73.

Ringold, G. M., Blair, P. B., Bishop, J. M., and Varmus, H. E. (1976). *Virology 70,* 550-553.

Schlom, J., Michalides, R., Kufe, D., Helmann, R., Spiegelman, S., Bentvelzen, P., and Hageman, P. (1973). *J. Natl. Cancer Inst. 51,* 541-551.

Schlom, J., Colcher, D., Drohan, W., Kettmann, R., Michalides, R., Vlahakis, G., and Young, J. (1977). *Cancer 39,* 2727-2733.

Squartini, F. (1961). *J. Natl. Cancer Inst. 26,* 813-828.

Squartini, F. (1962). *J. Natl. Cancer Inst. 28,* 911-926.

Squartini, F., and Bistocchi, M. (1977). *J. Natl. Cancer Inst. 58,* 1845-1847.

Squartini, F., and Rossi, G. (1959a). *Lav. Anat. Pat. Perugia 19,* 105-124.

Squartini, F., and Rossi, G. (1959b). *Lav. Anat. Pat. Perugia 19,* 165-214.

Squartini, F., and Rossi, G. (1960). *Lav. Anat. Pat. Perugia 20,* 133-165.

Squartini, F., and Severi, L. (1962). *In* "A Ciba Foundation Symposium on Tumour Viruses of Murine Origin," (G. E. Wolstenholme and M. O'Connor, eds.), pp. 82-106. Churchill Ltd., London.

Squartini, F., Rossi, G., and Paoletti, I. (1963). *Nature 197,* 505-506.

Squartini, F., Barola, E., Paoletti, I., and Rossi, G. (1964). *Lav. Anat. Pat. Perugia 24,* 29-37.

Squartini, F., Bolis, G. B., and Rossi, G. (1974). *J. Natl. Cancer Inst. 52,* 1635-1641.

HUMAN BREAST CARCINOMAS CONTAIN AN ANTIGEN IMMUNOLOGICALLY RELATED TO A GLYCOPROTEIN OF THE MOUSE MAMMARY TUMOR VIRUS

S. Spiegelman

Institute of Cancer Research
College of Physicians and Surgeons
of Columbia University

R. Mesa-Tejada

Institute of Cancer Research
and
Department of Pathology
College of Physicians and Surgeons
of Columbia University

I. Keydar
M. Ramanarayanan
T. Ohno

Institute of Cancer Research
College of Physicians and Surgeons
of Columbia University

C. Fenoglio

Department of Pathology
College of Physicians and Surgeons
of Columbia University

ISBN 0-12-131150-3

I. THE MOUSE MAMMARY TUMOR VIRUS AND HUMAN BREAST CANCER

The description by Bittner (1936) of a "milk factor" in high cancer strains of mice capable of initiating mammary tumors, and its subsequent identification as a B-type RNA virus (Lyons and Moore, 1962), stimulated considerable speculation as to the possibility that a similar agent could be associated with human breast cancer. The subsequent search for a putative agent led to the ultrastructural finding of particles resembling murine B-type and C-type viruses in human breast cancer tissues (Seman *et al.*, 1971) as well as in human milk (Sarkar and Moore, 1972). The eventual isolation and biochemical and biophysical analysis of these particles (Michalides *et al.*, 1975) revealed further similarities, principally the presence of RNA-dependent DNA polymerase (reverse transcriptase) complexed to a 70S RNA molecule. In addition, molecular hybridization studies have demonstrated a partial homology between RNA molecules found in human breast tumors and the RNA genome of the mouse mammary tumor virus (MMTV) (Axel *et al.*, 1972a,b; Spiegelman *et al.*, 1972; Vaidya *et al.*, 1974).

Although at present it is futile to dwell on the etiologic implications of these findings, the presence of these particles provides a novel opportunity to generate information of potentially practical importance for the diagnosis and management of human breast cancer. Thus, if one or several of the particle proteins appear in the circulation, these could serve as systemic signals of the presence of the corresponding tumor. The feasibility of this approach was explored and established in our laboratory with the mouse mammary tumor model in which a 52,000 dalton viral glycoprotein (gp52) was found to be an excellent indicator of disease status. Plasma levels of gp52, measured by radioimmunoassay, could be accurately correlated with the existence (Ritzi *et al.*, 1976a), size (Ritzi *et al.*, 1976b) and recurrence of mouse mammary tumors after surgical excision (Ritzi *et al.*, 1977), frequently in the absence of gross physical signs of the disease.

At the same time, considerable experimental evidence has accumulated strongly suggesting an antigenic relationship between MMTV proteins and components in human breast cancer. Thus, studies with sera of breast cancer patients have demonstrated the presence in such sera of antibodies capable of neutralizing MMTV (Charney and Moore, 1971) and of localizing antigens in the mouse mammary tumors by immunofluorescence (Müller *et al.*,1972, 1973), and ultrastructurally, by immunoferritin (Holder *et al.*, 1976) and immunoperoxidase (Bowen *et al.*, 1976; Hoshino and Dmochowski, 1973) techniques. In addition, migration inhibition studies of leucocytes from breast cancer patients suggest a cross-reactivity between the major glycoprotein of MMTV and a protein component eluted from human breast cancer tissues (Black *et al.*, 1976). Finally, MMTV cross-reactive antigens have been detected in two human breast carcinoma cell lines, namely, MCF-7 (Yang *et al.*, 1977) and T47D (Keydar *et al.*, 1978b).

In the light of all these experimental data, we have of late concentrated our effort in searching for a specific tumor marker in human breast cancer through the exploitation of its possible antigenic relationship to MMTV. In considering the question of where and how to look for such antigens in humans, however, it is important to recognize logistical and quantitative limitations in transferring certain technologies from mice to humans. Thus, it is unlikely that attempts to set up radio immunoassays for cross-reacting proteins in human plasma (Zangerle *et al.*, 1977) will produce much information due to the 1000-fold blood volume difference between mice and humans. Even if a human tumor is as effective, on a gram basis, as a mouse tumor in producing a protein antigen detectable in the blood, one would still have to cope with the fact that the signal would be diluted 1000-fold in the human as compared with the mouse. For this and other reasons, we decided to focus on the tumor itself as the most plausible site to initiate the search for a cross-reactive protein, and we again turned to the murine model to develop a convenient, reliable, and sensitive microscopic method for finding such an antigen.

II. IMMUNOHISTOCHEMICAL LOCALIZATION OF MMTV IN MOUSE MAMMARY TUMORS

Most previous investigators (Hilgers *et al.*, 1973; Zotter *et al.*, Tanaka *et al.*, 1974; Gillette, 1977) have used immunofluorescence as the detecting device in the localization of MMTV proteins in mouse mammary tumor tissues. The numerous limitations and disadvantages inherent to the routine use of this immunohistologic technique led us to explore the application of the immunoperoxidase method, which appeared more suitable to our present and future needs.

Aside from its applicability to immunoelectron microscopy, the immunoperoxidase procedure has three major advantages that make it an exceddingly attractive method for antigen localization using conventional bright field microscopy (Mesa-Tejada *et al.*, 1977). Briefly, these are as follows:

(a) The positive staining reaction appears as a brown precipitate that, in combination with an appropriate contrasting counterstain, provides sufficient histologic detail to permit precise cytological identification and localization.

(b) The stained preparations do not fade and thus can be filed as permanent records for future comparison.

(c) Paraffin sections can be used if the antigenic determinants of the substance being localized are not appreciably altered by the routine fixation and embedding required.

In view of our ultimate goal to transfer this technology to human material, the possibility of using paraffin sections was particularly intriguing. We immediately compared the stainability of MMTV antigens in parallel paraffin and frozen sections cut from the same tumor, using an indirect immunoperoxidase method and rabbit anti-MMTV IgG as previously described (Keydar *et al.*, 1978a; Mesa-Tejada *et al.*, 1978b). In agreement with previous experience (Mesa-Tejada *et al.*, 1977) with other antigens, we found that localization of the MMTV antigens in the mammary tumor is visualized with greater precision and sensitivity in paraffin than in frozen sections. This last finding may be attributed to the superior fixation and preservation of cytologic integrity by paraffin embedding compared to frozen sections in which diffusion of antigens and cellular disruption occurs more readily.

A representative example of the type of staining observed in the mouse mammary tumors is illustrated in Fig. 1. In this typical Paris RIII mammary adenocarcinoma, localization of MMTV antigens can be seen in most cells and within the lumina of tumor glands. The intracellular stain varies from coarsely granular to diffuse and, in the case of cells lining tumor glands, staining is most common along the apical, intraluminal border of the cells (Fig. 1b). In agreement with the immunofluorescent studies of Zotter *et al.* (1974), the staining pattern varies according to the degree of histologic differentiation of the tumor. Thus, in areas of poor differentiation, as in the nest of cells in Fig. 1b, the staining is sparse to absent, while wherever the tumor forms glands, a greater amount of reaction product is noted in the cells and in secretions within these glands (Fig. 1b). Similar reactions, varying somewhat in intensity, were noted in all of the Paris RIII and $CD8F_1$ mammary tumors tested in these studies. The specificity of the reaction was determined by the complete absence of reaction product after absorption of anti-MMTV with whole disrupted MMTV (Fig. 1c).

In eight tumor-bearing mice examined for metastatic lesions, four were found (one hepatic, three pulmonary) and an example of the staining reaction in these lesions is illustrated in Figs. 2 and 3. The smaller pulmonary metastases (Fig. 2) were microscopic findings consisting of small clusters of intensely stained cells within peribronchiolar vessels. The relatively large liver metastasis (Fig. 3) was typically surrounded by compressed liver tissue and does not differ substantially from the primary tumor in its staining characteristics.

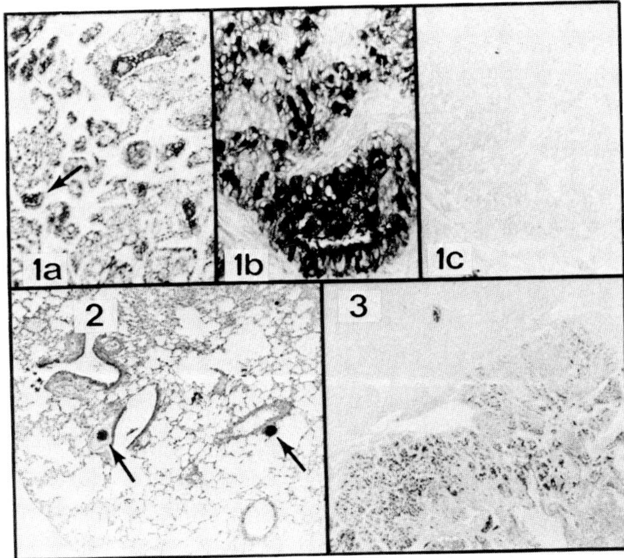

FIGURE 1. (a) Immunoperoxidase stain of mammary adenocarcinoma from Paris RIII mouse using anti-MMTV as primary antibody. (b) High magnification of small field in 1a (arrow) illustrates differences in intensity and pattern of stain in tumor glands as compared to adjacent cluster of cells. (c) Identical field in adjacent serial section stained with anti-MMTV previously absorbed with MMTV. (Methylene blue counterstain; a, X88; b and c, X550.) Copyright (c) 1978, The Histochemical Society, Inc.

Figures 2 and 3. Mammary tumor metastases in lung (2) and liver (3) of $CD8F_1$ mice stained with anti-MMTV. Note in Fig. 2 the microscopic metastasis in peribronchiolar vessel (left arrow) and in Fig. 3 unstained liver tissue surrounding tumor. (Methylene blue counterstain; Fig. 2, X88; Fig. 3, X55.)

Before terminating the discussion of the mouse tumors, it should be noted that we deliberately chose highly infected mouse strains (Ritzi *et al.*, 1976b) in order to optimize our method of MMTV antigen localization. Nevertheless, even in these mouse mammary tumors, MMTV antigen could not be detected in numerous tumor cells. This cellular variability of antigen expression, frequently observed in human tumors with respect to other tumor-associated antigens (Pascal *et al.*, 1977) was found to be even greater in several x-ray and urathane-induced mammary tumors (provided by Dr. Anna Goldfeder), which we have also stained by this same method (unpublished observations). It is interesting to note that in some of these last tumors in which antigen has been localized, a thorough ultrastructural search for virus particles has been unsuccessful (Goldfeder, A., personal communication).

III. IMMUNOPEROXIDASE STAINING OF HUMAN BENIGN AND MALIGNANT TISSUES WITH ANTI-MMTV

The successful application of the immunoperoxidase technique to the localization of MMTV antigens in sections of paraffin-embedded mouse mammary tumor tissues made possible the extensive, primarily retrospective studies described below. While eliminating the need for fresh tissue in our search for a cross-reacting human antigen, we also had at our disposal the same tissues received by the pathology laboratory, which we could then test without interfering with the diagnostic activities of the Pathology Department.

Serial sections for immunohistochemical staining were cut from the paraffin blocks of tissues used for diagnostic purposes, selected from the files of the divisions of surgical, gynecologic, and anatomic pathology of the College of Physicians and Surgeons of Columbia University, as previously described (Mesa-Tejada *et al.*, 1978a). Additional breast cancer cases were received from Dr. Marvin Rich (Michigan Cancer Foundation), Dr. Maurice M. Black (New York Medical Colledge), and from Dr. Y. Hirschaut (The Memorial Sloan-Kettering Cancer Center), either in the form of unstained paraffin sections or as fresh tumor tissue (to be used primarily for antigen isolation studies) from which a small section was processed for immunohistochemical staining (Mesa-Tejada *et al.*, 1978b).

A detailed description of the purification and characterization of the anti-MMTV IgG preparations used in these studies, as well as of the preparation of immunoperoxidase conjugated antibodies, is reported elsewhere (Mesa-Tejada *et al.*, 1978a, b).

A. Malignant Breast Tissues

A positive-staining reaction has been observed in 149 (44.5%) of 335 cases of human breast carcinomas tested, including all cases received from other institutions (Table I). Table II summarizes the positive staining reactions seen in the 238 Columbia-Presbyterian breast cancer cases classified according to histopathologic type. The larger percentage of the positive cases in the intraductal and invasive group reflects a trend noted in our original report of 131 cases (Mesa-Tejada *et al.*, 1978a), which suggests a significant correlation in this en-

TABLE I. Immunoperoxidase Staining of Carcinoma of the Breast: Total Cases Classified as to Source

Source	*Cases*	*Positives*	*%Positive*
Columbia-Presbyterian	*238*	*110*	*46.2*
Michigan Cancer Foundation	*56*	*26*	*45.4*
New York Medical College	*17*	*5*	*29.4*
Memorial Sloan-Kettering	*24*	*8*	*33.3*
Total	*335*	*149*	*44.5*

TABLE II. Immunoperoxidase Staining of Carcinoma of the Breast: Histopathologic Classification of Columbia-Presbyterian Cases

Type	*Cases*	*Positives*	*%Positive*
Intraductal	*22*	*8*	*36.3*
Intraductal and Invasive	*61*	*39*	*63.9*
Invasive[a]	*101*	*47*	*46.5*
Medullary	*15*	*5*	*33.3*
Metastatic[b]	*39*	*11*	*28.2*
Total	*238*	*110*	*46.2*

[a]*Includes all types of invasive carcinoma (e.g., tubular, lobular, small cell, etc.) except those with predominantly medullary features or associated with intraductal lesions.*

[b]*Includes metastases to lymph nodes, lungs, liver, adrenal gland, and ovaries in proven cases of primary carcinoma of the breast.*

larged series. It appears, therefore, that an invasive carcinoma associated with an intraductal component is more likely to contain a cross-reacting antigen than either a pure intraductal or invasive tumor.

The pattern of immunohistochemical staining in human breast tumors tends to be focal, intracellular, and cytoplasmic with considerable variability even within the same tumor (Figs. 4-8). For example, in the intraductal carcinoma illustrated in Fig. 4,

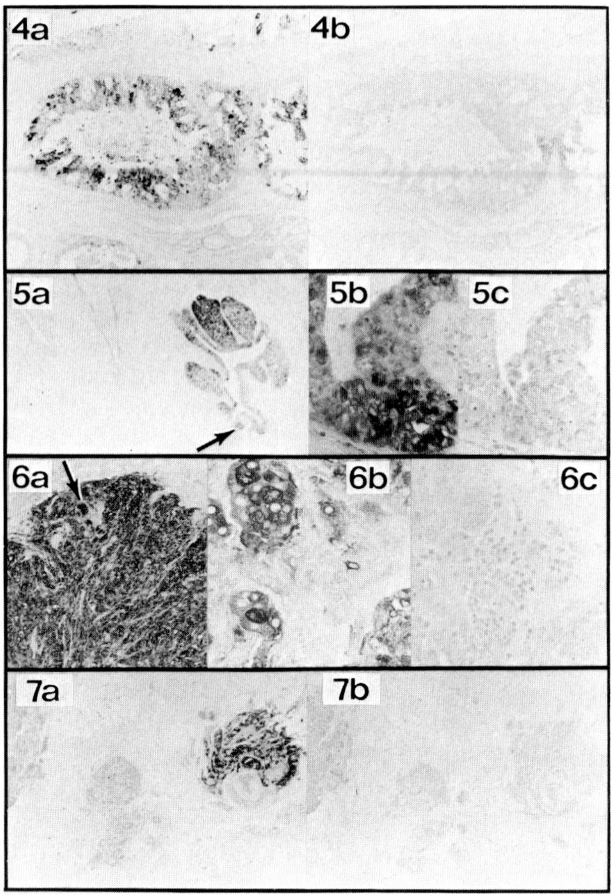

FIGURE 4. Immunoperoxidase stain of human intraductal breast carcinoma with anti-MMTV (a) and anti-MMTV after absorption with gp52 (b). Note in (a) that reaction product is not found in all of the cells nor in all of the intraductal lesions. (Methylene blue counterstain; X88.) Copyright (c) 1978, The Histochemical Society.

FIGURE 5. (a) Immunoperoxidase stain with anti-MMTV of transverse section of nipple ducts in a case of human intraductal and invasive carcinoma illustrating antigen localization only in duct with in situ *carcinoma. (b) Detail of field (indicated by arrow in 5a) showing that practically all cells contain some reaction product. (c) Same field in adjacent serial section stained with anti-MMTV absorbed with gp52. (Methylene blue counterstain; a, X35, b and c, X550.) Copyright (c) 1978, The Histochemical Society.*

only some of the intraductal lesions, and not all of the cells in these, contain reaction product. On the other hand, Fig. 5 illustrates a nipple duct involved by *in situ* carcinoma (from a case of intraductral carcinoma associated with invasive small cell carcinoma) in which all of the malignant cells show some degree of staining. In other sections of tumor from this same case, however, staining was not universal and was even completely absent in some intraductal lesions that were surrounded by strongly reacting invasive cells.

The invasive tumor illustrated in Fig. 6 represents the strongest staining reaction we have yet observed in a human tumor. As can be seen in the higher magnification (Fig. 6b), essentially every tumor cell contains reaction product, although the central group of lymphocytes is not stained. Likewise, in another microscopic field of the same section (Fig. 7), the staining reaction is confined to a small focus of invasive carcinoma, while no reaction product is noted in either the surrounding dense fibrous tissue or in the neighboring morphologically benign epithelial tissue such as the adjacent foci of adenosis.

Fig. 8 illustrates a positive reaction in several metastatic breast cancer cells found in a surgically resected ovary. Both regional (axillary) and distant metastatic lesions present more or less the same degree of variability in the expression of detectable cross-reactive antigen as the primary tumors themselves. However, we have not as yet tested a sufficient number of cases of primary and corresponding metastatic carcinoma to be able to deduce the presence or absence of a correlation in antigen expression between the primary carcinoma and its regional and/or distant metastases.

FIGURE 6. Immunoperoxidase stain of invasive breast carcinoma with anti-MMTV before (a, b) and after (c) absorption with gp52. Note in (b) [detail of area indicated by arrow in (a)] strong reaction in practically all tumor cells, and absence of stain in central area consisting mostly of lymphocytic infiltrate. Sparse extracellular reaction product may be due to antigen diffusion before fixation. (Methylene blue counterstain; a, X57; b and c, X354.)

FIGURE 7. Another field in same section as Fig. 6 showing staining of small focus of invasive carcinoma and lack of reaction in nearby foci of adenosis (a) as well as complete elimination of the former reaction after absorption with gp52 (b). (Methylene blue counterstain; X57.)

After reviewing these few examples of positive-staining reactions, it should be emphasized that there is considerable sampling error inherent in our testing procedure, and therefore the percentages given in Tables I and II represent, at best, minimal values. This conclusion is based on the following facts:

(1) Diagnostic tissue blocks of a given case are usually representative, but seldom include the entire tumor.

(2) These studies were limited to an average of less than three (one, in cases from other institutions) representative blocks per case and, as previously noted, a considerable variability in antigen localization was noted among and within sections of positive cases.

(3) In contrast to *in vitro* methods, where a given tissue can be assayed in bulk, our test is limited to 5 μ sections, which represent only a minute fraction of the entire tumor.

B. Normal and Benign Breast Tissue

Normal (resting and lactating) and benign (cystic disease, fibroadenoma, intraductal papilloma, gynecomastia) breast tissues from 137 patients, were also tested, with negative results (Table III, Figs. 9 and 10). It is noteworthy that 74 of these

TABLE III. Immunoperoxidase Staining of Benign and Normal Breast Tissues

Type	*Cases*	*Associated with breast carcinoma*[a]	*Positives*
Cystic disease[b]	*81*	*60*	*0*
Fibroadenoma	*19*	*4*	*0*
Intraductal papilloma	*10*	*10*	*0*
Gynecomastia	*9*	*0*	*0*
Resting gland (normal)	*9*	*0*	*0*
Lactating gland (normal)	*9*	*0*	*0*
Total	*137*	*74*	*0*

[a] *In the same breast.*

[b] *Excluding foci of apocrine metaplasia; the peculiar immunologic specificity of this reaction is discussed in Section IV.*

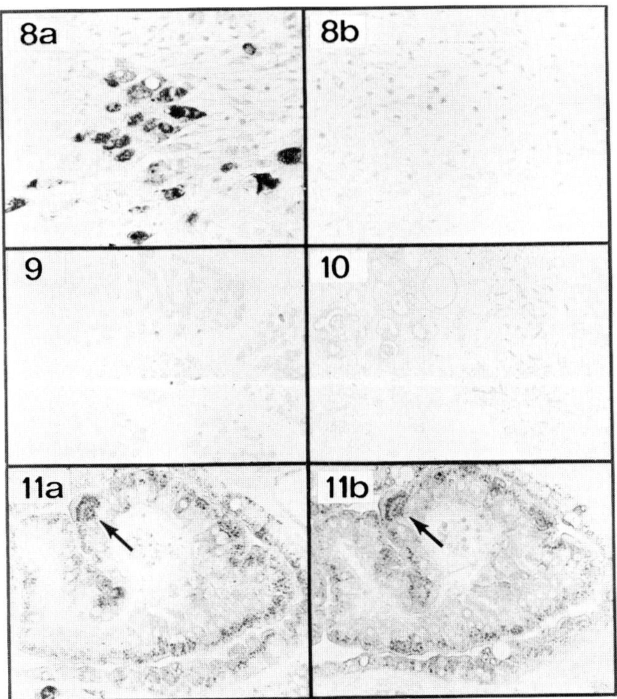

FIGURE 8. Immunoperoxidase stain of metastatic breast carcinoma cells in ovary with anti-MMTV (a) and adjacent serial section stained with anti-MMTV absorbed with gp52 (b). Methylene blue counterstain; X354).

FIGURES 9 and 10. Complete absence of reaction product in normal breast lobules (9) and area of cystic disease (10) stained with anti-MMTV. Occasional dark spots are due to counterstain. (Methylene blue counterstain; Fig. 9, X92; Fig. 10, X58.)

FIGURE 11. Area of apocrine metaplasia stained with anti-MMTV (a) showing typical coarsely granular stain towards apex of columnar apocrine cells (arrow). The reaction is essentially the same in adjacent section stained with anti-MMTV absorbed with MMTV after removal of sugar residues with endoglycosidase H. (Methylene blue counterstain; X354.)

negatively staining benign lesions coincided with the presence of carcinoma in the same breast, frequently in the same section, and some of these carcinomas gave a positive staining reaction.

1. Apocrine Metaplasia. The only exception to the absence of staining reaction in nonmalignant breast tissue was the staining of foci of apocrine metaplasia (Fig. 11), one of the microscopic features of cystic disease. This reaction, which is shared by the morphologically and histochemically indistinguishable (Ahmed, 1975; Tremblay, 1968) epithelium of apocrine glands of the axilla and perineum, appears to differ in specificity from the reaction observed in the carcinomas as discussed below in Section IV.

C. Malignancies Other than Breast Carcinomas

The specificity of the reaction for breast carcinoma was determined by testing 99 carcinomas from other organs and eight cases of cystosarcoma phyllodes (Table IV). Only one of these 107 tumors, a mucoepidermoid carcinoma of the parotid gland, gave a positive reaction; two other parotid carcinomas of the

TABLE IV. Immunoperoxidase Staining of Malignancies Other than Breast Carcinomas[a]

Malignancy	*Cases*	*Positive*
Colon	12	0
Stomach	3	0
Pancreas	3	0
Liver	4	0
Lung	9	0
Endometrium	22	0
Ovary	20	0
Prostate	8	0
Kidney	5	0
Urinary bladder	4	0
Skin	2	0
Thyroid gland	4	0
Parotid gland	3	1
Cystosarcoma phyllodes	8	0
Total	107	1

[a]Primary sites of non-breast carcinomas stained with α-MMTV. Cystosarcoma phyllodes is also listed because it is the most common noncarcinomatous malignancy of the breast.

same histopathologic type were negative. It is therefore clear that the antigen being detected by the anti-MMTV in human breast carcinomas is confined principally to this neoplastic disease.

IV. THE SPECIFICITY OF THE REACTION IN HUMAN BREAST CARCINOMAS

In the previous section we discussed the tissue specificity of the staining reaction observed in human tissues. Thus, a positive reaction is confined to the cytoplasm of breast carcinoma cells, with the one exception of the previously mentioned mucoepidermoid carcinoma of the parotid gland, and apocrine epithelium.

A precise evaluation of the immunologic specificity of staining reactions observed in immunohistochemistry, however, demands meticulous specific absorptions of the primary antibodies, not only with homologous antigen, but also with related and unrelated antigens which might be responsible for undesirable cross-reactive phenomena (Swaab *et al.*, 1977). A list of the immunoabsorbants we have used in these studies is shown in Table V. Their preparation and absorption modalities are reported elsewhere (Mesa-Tejada *et al.*, 1978a).

One outstanding difference between the mouse and human tumors with respect to antigen localization with anti-MMTV is readily apparent. In contrast to the mouse tumors, where only absorption with whole disrupted MMTV completely eliminates the staining reaction (see Section II; Fig. 1c), absorption with purified gp52 alone was sufficient to obliterate the reaction in positively staining human tumors (Figs. 4b, 5c, 6c, 7b, and 8b). We therefore consider a reaction in human tissues to be positive only when definite staining is seen, even in occasional cells, which is completely absent in an adjacent serial section stained with the same antibody preparation previously absorbed with gp52.

The specificity of this staining reaction was further explored by absorption with the various preparations of MMTV and gp52 listed in Table V. All of these blocked the staining reaction, indicating that the species differences that have been previously reported (Teramoto *et al.*, 1977a,b) for gp52 of the CD8 and RIII MMTV do not play a role in this reaction. On the other hand, absorption with different virus preparations (RLV, SSV, MMTV, and BEV) and with several possible cross-reacting substances, also listed in Table V, failed to eliminate the staining reaction.

These absorptions also led us to the conclusion that the staining reaction observed in apocrine epithelium (Section

TABLE V. *Absorption Specificity Tests of Immunoperoxidase Staining of Human Breast Carcinomas with α-MMTV*[a]

Completely eliminated by	Not eliminated by
MMTV (RIII) from milk	Viruses
MMTV (C_3H) from MM5T	Rauscher leukemia virus
MMTV (C_3H) from CrFeK	Simian sarcoma virus
gp52 (RIII) purified by concanavalin A	Mason-Pfizer monkey virus
gp52 (C_3H) affinity chromatography	Baboon endogenous virus
gp52 (RIII) purified by guanidium	Human
gp52 (C_3H) chloride chromatography	normal plasma
	normal leukocytes
	collagen
	actin
	hyaluronic acid
	milk
	normal breast tissue
	Bovine
	mucin
	fetal calf serum
	Sheep erythrocytes

[a]The absorptions were done by using these agents either in the soluble or insolubilized form.

III,B,1; Fig. 11) differs in specificity from the reaction observed in the carcinomas as evidenced by

(1) absorption with gp52 blocks only part of the reaction in the apocrine glands and metaplasia while it completely eliminates the reaction in the carcinomas; if this absorption is done with gp52 which has not previously been extracted with ether, both reactions are completely blocked;

(2) absorption with mucin almost completely eliminates the reaction in the apocrine epithelium while it does not interfere with the staining of the carcinoma;

(3) absorption with the isolated sugar residues of gp52 partially eliminates the apocrine reaction while it does not diminish the staining in the carcinomas;

(4) absorption with MMTV from which the sugar residues have been removed by treatment with endoglycosidase H hardly interferes with the reaction in apocrine metaplasia (Fig. 11b), while it completely abolishes the reaction observed in human breast carcinomas.

From the above it is also evident that the antibodies responsible for the staining reaction in the human breast carcinomas are those specifically directed at the polypeptide moiety of gp52. A more complete discussion of experiments directed toward defining the nature and differences of the reactions seen in the human tumor and the apocrine epithelium by separation of the sugar and protein moieties of the MMTV glycoproteins is in preparation and will be reported elsewhere (Ohno *et al.*, 1979).

V. IMPLICATIONS

It is of course gratifying to have extended to the protein level a relation between human breast cancer and the mouse mammary tumor virus that was discovered (Axel *et al.*, 1972a,b) in terms of nucleic acid sequence homology. But again, the etiologic implications are not our immediate concern, but rather the possibility that these findings can be used to generate clinically useful information. To this end, the resolution of the following issues assumes first priority:

(1) Can any clinically useful correlations be drawn between antigen localization in tissues and the natural history of the disease?

(2) What is the chemical nature of the gp52 cross-reacting antigen found in human breast cancer cells?

(3) Can additional specific antigens be detected by using antisera to other oncorna-viruses (for example, Mason-Pfizer monkey virus) with suspected (Colcher *et al.*, 1974; Ohno and Spiegelman, 1977) cross-reactivities?

An answer to the first question is being actively pursued both in our institution and through a cooperative study with Dr. Marvin Rich and the Michigan Cancer Foundation. A resolution of the second question will require purification to homogeneity of the relevant human breast cancer antigen. Its availability will also make possible the production of the immunologic reagents needed to develop the heterologous radioimmunoassays that can hope to attain the sensitivities required for the measurement of a systemic signal in the human disease.

ACKNOWLEDGMENTS

This investigation was supported by Grant CA-02332 and Contract N01-CP7-1016 awarded by the National Cancer Institute.

REFERENCES

Ahmed, A. (1975). *J. Pathol. 115,* 211.

Axel, R., Gulati, S. C., and Spiegelman, S. (1972a). *Proc. Natl. Acad. Sci. 69,* 3133.

Axel, R., Schlom, J., and Spiegelman, S. (1972b). *Nature 235,* 32.

Bittner, J. J. (1936). *Science 184,* 162.

Black, M. M., Zachrau, R. E., Dion, A. S., Shore, B., Fine, D. L., Leis, H. P., Jr., and Williams, C. (1976). *Cancer Res. 36,* 4137.

Bowen, J. M., Dmochowski, L., Miller, M. F., Priori, E. S., Seman, G., Dodson, M. L., and Maruyama, K. (1976). *Cancer Res. 36,* 759.

Charney, J., and Moore, D. H. (1971). *Nature 229,* 627.

Colcher, D., Spiegelman, S., and Schlom, J. (1974). *Proc. Natl. Acad. Sci. 71,* 4975.

Gillette, R. W. (1977). *J. Natl. Cancer Inst. 58,* 1629.

Hilgers, J. H. M., Theuns, G. J., and Van Nie, R. (1973) *Int. J. Cancer 12,* 568.

Holder, W. D., Jr., Peer, G. W., Bolognesi, D. P., and Wells, S. A. Jr. (1976). *Surgical Forum 27,* 102.

Hoshino, M., and Dmochowski, L. (1973). *Cancer Res. 33,* 2551.

Keydar, I., Mesa-Tejada, R., Ramanarayanan, M., Ohno, T., Fenoglio, C., Hu, R., and Spiegelman, S. (1978a). *Proc. Natl. Acad. Sci. USA 75,* 1524.

Keydar, I., Chen, L., Karby, S., Delarea, Y., Ramanarayanan, M., Mesa-Tejada, R., Spiegelman, S., Hager, J. C., and Calabresi, P. (1978b). Poster Abstract. Presented at *11th meeting on Mammary Cancer in Experimental Animals and Man,* Detroit, Michigan, June 25-28, 1978, p. 66.
Lyons, M. J., and Moore, D. H. (1962). *Nature 194,* 1141.
Mesa-Tejada, R., Pascal, R. R., and Fenoglio, C. M. (1977). *Human Pathol. 8,* 313.
Mesa-Tejada, R., Keydar, K., Ramanarayanan, M., Ohno, T., Fenoglio, C., and Spiegelman, S. (1978a). *Proc. Natl. Acad. Sci. 75,* 1529.
Mesa-Tejada, R., Keydar, I., Ramanarayanan, M., Ohno, T., Fenoglio, C., and Spiegelman, S. (1978b). *J. Histochem. Cytochem. 26,* 532.
Michalides, R., Spiegelman, S., and Schlom, J. (1975). *Cancer Res. 35,* 1003.
Müller, M., Zotter, S., Grossmann, H., and Kemmer, C. (1972). *Arch. Geschwulstforsch 40,* 285.
Müller, M., Kemmer, C., Zotter, S., Grossmann, H., and Michael, B. (1973). *Arch. Geschwulstforsch 41,* 100.
Ohno, T., and Spiegelman, S. (1977). *Proc. Natl. Acad. Sci. 74,* 2144.
Ohno, T., Mesa-Tejada, R. Keydar, I., Ramanarayanan, M., Bausch, J., and Spiegelman, S. (1979). *Proc. Natl. Acad. Sci., 76,* 2460.
Pascal, R. R., Mesa-Tejada, R., Bennett, S., Garces, A., and Fenoglio, C. M. (1977). *Arch. Pathol. Lab. Med. 101,* 568.
Ritzi, E., Baldi, A., and Spiegelman, S. (1976a). *Virology 75,* 188.
Ritzi, E., Martin, D. S., Stolfi, R. L., and Spiegelman, S. (1976b). *Proc. Natl. Acad. Sci. 73,* 4190.
Ritzi, E., Martin, D. S., Stolfi, R. L., and Spiegelman, S. (1977). *J. Exp. Med. 145,* 999.
Sarkar, N. H., and Moore, D. H. (1972). *Nature 233,* 103.
Seman, G., Gallagher, H. S., Lukeman, J. M., and Dmochowski, L. (1971). *Cancer 28,* 1431.
Spiegelman, S., Axel, R., and Schlom, J. (1972). *J. Natl. Cancer Inst. 48,* 1205.
Swaab, D. F., Pool, W. W., and Van Leeuwen, F. W. (1977). *J. Histochem. Cytochem. 25,* 388.
Tanaka, H., Tsujimura, D., and Nakamura, K. (1974). *Cancer Res. 34,* 1465.
Teramoto, Y. A., Kufe, D., and Schlom, J. (1977a). *Proc. Natl. Acad. Sci. 74,* 3564.
Teramoto, Y. A., Kufe, D., and Schlom, J. (1977b). *J. Virol. 24,* 525.
Tremblay, G. (1968). *J. Invest. Derm. 50,* 238.
Vaidya, A. B., Black, M. M., Dion, A. S., and Moore, D. H. (1974). *Nature 249,* 565.

Yang, N. -S., Soule, H. D., and McGrath, C. M. (1977). *J. Natl. Can. Inst. 59*, 1357.

Zangerle, P. F., Calberg-Bacq, C. -M., Colin, C., Franchimont, P., Francois, C., Gosselin, L., Kizma, S., and Osterreith, P. M. (1977). *Cancer Res. 37*, 4326.

Zotter, S., Müller, M., and Kemmer, C. (1974). *Arch. Geschwulstforsch 44*, 212.

TOWARD ESTABLISHING ETIOLOGIC SIGNIFICANCE OF MuMTV gp52-RELATED DETERMINANT EXPRESSION IN MAN

Ning-Sun Yang
Philip Furmanski
and
Charles M. McGrath

Department of Biology
Michigan Cancer Foundation
Detroit, Michigan

Sequences have been detected in the RNA of some human breast cancers which are homologous to the genomic RNA of the mouse mammary tumor virus (MuMTV) (Axel *et al.*, 1974; Vaidya *et al.*, 1974). Translation of these MuMTV-related sequences in the tumor cells is presumed to occur because antigens which are crossreactive with virion structural proteins specified by the MuMTV genome can be demonstrated in human breast cancer cells (McGrath *et al.*, 1974; Yang *et al.*, 1977; Zauchrau *et al.*, 1976; Black *et al.*, 1974, 1976). Individuals who develop breast cancer often show specific immunological reactivity against MuMTV antigenic determinants (Black *et al.*, 1976; McCoy *et al.*, 1977) and the presence of this reactivity has been associated with a favorable prognosis for the patient.

Thus MuMTV, a human homolog of this agent, or its gene products may be significant factors in the etiology or progression of human breast carcinomas and the ability of the host to respond against and control the disease.

To extend these results and to determine the specific role of MuMTV-related information in human mammary carcinogenesis, two questions need to be addressed;

(1) What is the identity of the MuMTV-related antigen(s) expressed in human breast cancer cells?

(2) Are similar antigens detectable in normal human mammary epithelial cells?

We have approached these questions by testing for expres-

ISBN 0-12-131150-3

sion of MuMTV-related antigens in cultures of normal and malignant human breast cells. Our laboratories have previously reported the development of a bona fide human breast carcinoma cell line, MCF (Soule *et al.*, 1973), and methods for the establishment of cultures of proliferating normal mammary epithelial cells derived from human milk and breast fluids (Furmanski *et al.*, 1974). These test cells were chosen because they represent pure populations of mammary epithelium in similar conditions of cell growth and physiology. Previous studies (Axel *et al.*, 1974; Vaidya *et al.*, 1974; Zauchrau *et al.*, 1976; Black *et al.*, 1976; Schlom *et al.*, 1971; Axel *et al.*, 1972) comparing normal and malignant breast tissues have used primarily autopsy, mastectomy, or mammoplasty samples, which are notoriously heterogeneous and, for the normals, consist almost entirely of nonepithelial nondividing cells.

Cultures of the malignant and normal human mammary epithelial cells were prepared as previously described Yang *et al.*, 1977; Soule *et al.*, 1973). The normal cells were obtained from breast milk and fluid samples from women who were actively lactating or who had just weaned their infants. The cells were grown in a modified Dulbecco's medium, pH 6.8, containing insulin (10 μg/ml), prolactin (5 μg/ml), and in some cases, 15 mM Hepes. This medium has proven highly efficacious in generating, from the fluid samples, large islands of confluent epithelial cells which possess all of the ultrastructural and histochemical features of normal mammary epithelium (Russo *et al.*, 1976).

Using fixed-cell indirect immunofluorescence assays (Yang *et al.*, 1977), we have shown that MCF-7 cells express antigens cross reactive with MuMTV structural proteins, but not with murine leukemia virus (MuLV) antigens or the major internal protein of the Mahson-Pfizer monkey virus (MPMV). A variety of cell and adsorption controls were used to establish that the cross reactive antigens in MCF-7 cells were MuMTV specific.

To identify the MuMTV polypeptide(s) responsible for the cross reactivity detected in the human breast cancer cell line, we tested the cells in the same indirect immunofluorescence assay using high-titered monovalent antisera to each of the major MuMTV structural proteins and glycoproteins. We found that the only monospecific serum which reacted with the MCF-7 cells was antiserum prepared against the major external glycoprotein of the virion, gp52 (Fig. 1). All of the antisera reacted with GR, MuMTV-produced mouse mammary tumor cells, and none of the sera reacted with the control mouse cells (D_2), normal human fibroblasts (D-549) or human non-breast epithelial tumor cells (D-562). Adsorption of the anti-gp52 with highly purified MuMTV removed essentially all of the reactivity against the MCF-7 cells.

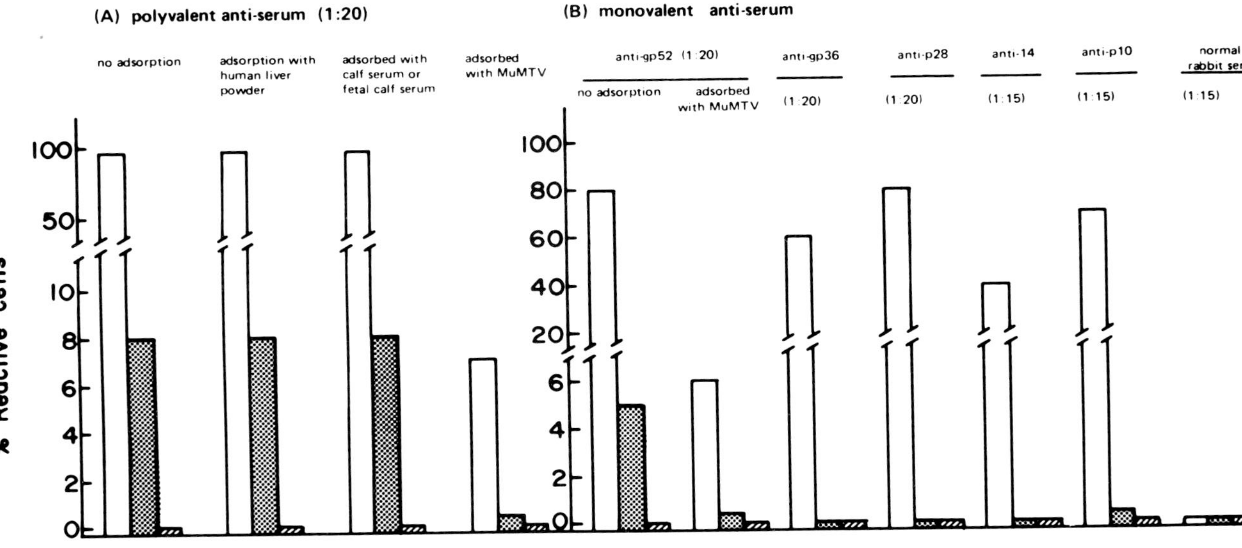

FIGURE 1. Identification of antigenic determinants responsible for cross reactivity against anti-MuMTV sera in human mammary carcinoma cells MCF-7. Polyvalent and monovalent anti-MuMTV sera were obtained from R. Cardiff and L. Young. The preparation and specificity of these antisera have been detailed by Cardiff (1973). Details of the immunofluorescence assay method on fixed cells, adsorption of antisera and scoring of positive cells have been described previously by Yang et al. *(1977).*

To determine whether similar MuMTV-related antigen(s) are expressed in normal human mammary epithelial cells, the same indirect immunofluorescence assays were applied to the epithelial colonies grown out from human milks and breast fluids. No reactivity was detected in the normal human mammary epithelial cell cultures using any of the polyvalent or monovalent anti-MuMTV sera. Each of the antisera was tested in a dilution series and no reactivity was observed in the normal cells even at antibody concentrations several fold higher than that required to detect fluorescence in MCF-7 cells or the mouse GR cells (Fig. 2). The reactivity of anti-MuMTV-gp52 serum with MCF-7 cells and normal human mammary epithelial cells in an immunofluorescence assay is shown in Fig. 3.

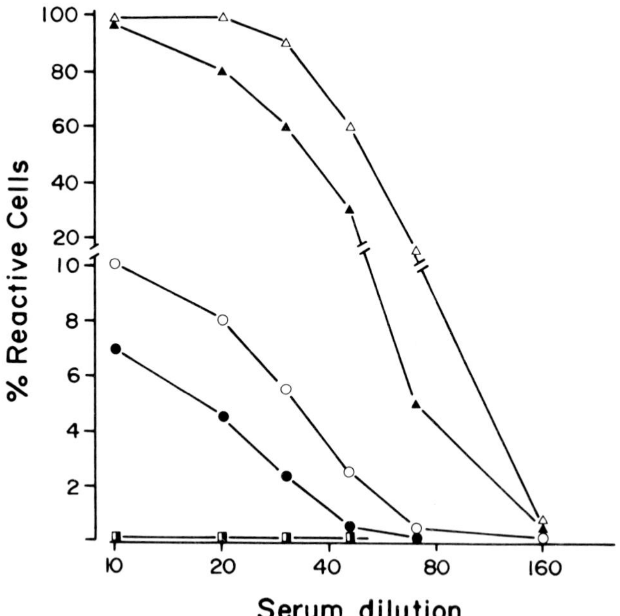

FIGURE 2. Immunofluorescence reactivity in MCF-7 and normal human mammary epithelial cells at various dilutions of polyvalent anti-MuMTV serum and monovalent anti-MuMTV-gp52 serum. △——△, O——O, and □——□ are reactivities in GR, MCF-7 and normal human mammary epithelial cells, respectively, with the polyvalent serum; ▲——▲, ●——●, and ■——■, are the reactivities in these cells with the anti-gp52 serum.

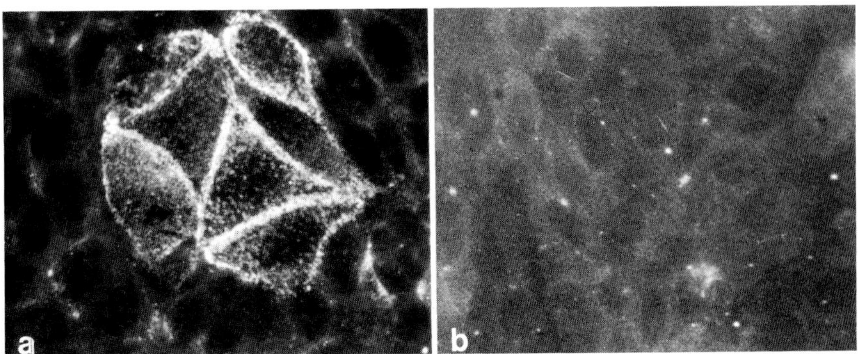

FIGURE 3. MCF-7 cells (a) and normal human mammary epithelial cells (b) stained with anti-MuMTV-gp52 serum (1:20 dilution) in immunofluorescence assay. The photograph of the normal cells was overexposed to show the autofluorescence and morphology of these cells.

The normal human mammary epithelial cells used in these experiments were obtained from a total of 41 different cancer-free donors. Cultures were initiated from samples obtained during active lactation, at weaning or postweaning. Replicate cultures from some donors were tested in early log phase through late log and stationary phase. Primary cultures obtained from 15 donors were treated with dexamethasone (10^{-5} M) and/or progesterone (10^{-8} M) for three to nine days in an attempt to augment MuMTV-related antigen synthesis, as has been reported for mouse cells (Park *et al.*, 1974; Ringold *et al.*, 1975; Dickson *et al.*, 1974) and MCF-7 cells (Yang *et al.*, 1977). In every case, the normal human mammary epithelial cells were negative in the immunofluorescence assays under conditions in which MuMTV-related antigens were readily detectable in the human breast carcinoma cells (MCF-7).

Our results show, therefore, that human breast cancer cells express an antigen related to gp52, the major external glycoprotein of MuMTV and, under the same conditions of cell growth *in vitro,* this antigen is not detectable in normal human mammary epithelial cells, nor is it inducible with a mammotropic hormone which induced antigen expression in malignant cells.

Mesa-Tejada *et al.* (1978) have reported that the gp52-related antigen was present in the primary human breast cancers tested. These investigators have used immunoperoxidase staining in fixed paraffin sections of the tumors as a test system.

Sections of normal breast tissue, non-breast cancers, or benign breast diseases did not show reactivity with the anti-gp52 serum. Our results are in accord with those findings.

In addition to the potential significance to studies on the etiology of human breast cancer, the finding of an MuMTV-related antigen in human mammary carcinomas and its absence in the normal counterpart of these cells, may provide new approaches to the diagnosis of the disease. The presence of the antigen in only a portion of the breast cancer population could serve to distinguish the tumors for prognostic or therapeutic purposes.

ACKNOWLEDGMENTS

Supported by Public Health Service (PHS) contract N01-CP33347 from the Division of Cancer Cause and Prevention and an institutional grant from the United Foundation of Greater Detroit.

REFERENCES

Axel, R., Gulati, S. C., and Spiegelman, S. (1972). *Proc. Natl. Acad. Sci. 69,* 3133-3137.

Axel, R., Schlom, J., and Spiegelman, S. (1974). *Nature (London) 235,* 32-36.

Black, M. M., Moore, D. H., Shore, B., Zaucharau, R. E., and Leis, H. P., Jr. (1974). *Cancer Res. 34,* 1054-1060.

Black, M. M., Zauchrau, R. E., Dion, A. S., Shore, B., Fine, D. G., Leis, H. P., Jr., and Williams, C. J. (1976). *Cancer Res. 36,* 4137-4142.

Cardiff, R. D. (1973). *J. Immunol. 111,* 1722-1729.

Dickson, C., Haslam, S., and Nandi, S. (1974). *Virology 62,* 242-252.

Furmanski, P., Longley, C., Fouchey, D., and Rich, M. A. (1974). *J. Natl. Cancer Inst. 52,* 975-977.

McCoy, J. L., Dean, J. H., and Herberman, R. B. (1977). *Proc. Am. Assoc. Cancer Res. 18,* 177.

Mesa-Tejada, R., Keydar, I., Ramanarayanan, M., Ohno, T., Fenoglio, C., and Spiegelman, S. (1978). *Proc. Natl. Acad. Sci. 75,* 1529-1533.

McGrath, C. M., Grant, P. M., Soule, H. D., and Rich, M. A. (1974). *Nature (London) 252,* 247-250.

Park, W. P., Scolnick, E., and Kozikowski, E. (1974). *Science 184,* 158-160.

Ringold, G., Lasfargues, E. Y., Bishop, J. M., and Varmus, H. E. (1975). *Virology 65,* 135-147.

Russo, J., Furmanski, P., Bradley, R., Wells, P., and Rich, M. A. (1976). *Am. J. Anat. 145,* 57-58.

Schlom, J., Spiegelman, S., and Moore, D. H. (1971). *Nature (London) 231,* 97-100.

Soule, H. D., Vasquez, J., Long, A., Albert, S., and Brennan, M. (1973). *J. Natl. Cancer Inst. 51,* 1409-1416.

Vaidya, A. B., Black, M. M., Dion, A. S., and Moore, D. H. (1974). *Nature (London) 249,* 565-567.

Yang, N. -S., Soule, H. D., and McGrath, C. M. (1977). *J. Natl. Cancer Inst. 59,* 1357-1367.

Zauchrau, R. E., Black, M. M., and Dion, A. S. (1976). *Cancer Res. 36,* 3143-3146.

REGULATION OF THE EXPRESSION OF THE MOUSE MAMMARY TUMOR VIRUS

Rob Michalides
Roeland Nusse
and
Robertha van Nie

Department of Virology and Genetics
Antoni van Leeuwenhoek-Huis
The Netherlands Cancer Institute
Amsterdam, The Netherlands

I. INTRODUCTION

The mouse mammary tumor virus (MTV) is a B-type tumor virus which causes mammary tumors in susceptible mice. It is an enveloped virus containing a DNA polymerase and an RNA genome encapsulated within a core. It replicates by means of a DNA intermediate (provirus). The genetic information of the MTV is encoded in a single-stranded RNA molecule with a molecular weight of approximately 3×10^6 (Dion *et al.*, 1977). As with C-type RNA tumor viruses (Eiseman and Vogt, 1978), this RNA contains at least three loci for gene products termed *gag*, *pol*, and *env*. The product of the *gag* gene results in the internal MTV proteins, the *pol* gene codes for the DNA polymerase while the *env* gene product specifies the external proteins of the MTV. No gene for a transformation-causing protein has yet been identified within the MTV genome. This transforming gene, termed *sarc*, is present in the genome of sarcoma RNA tumor viruses (Frankel and Fischinger, 1976; Stehelin *et al.*, 1976).

The MTV viral RNA is in infected cells present in at least two pools, one with RNA destined for incorporation into budding B-type virus particles and the other with RNA serving as messenger RNA to synthesize the viral proteins. The regulation of MTV expression involves mechanisms influencing the synthesis of this viral RNA and the viral proteins.

ISBN 0-12-131150-3

II. TRANSMISSION OF THE MTV

Endogenous and exogenous mammary tumor viruses are present in various inbred strains of mice (Bentvelzen, 1974). The exogenous MTV is transmitted mainly via the milk at nursing and is responsible for the early appearance of mammary tumors in susceptible strains of mice. The endogenous MTV is transmitted in its MTV-DNA proviral form as a gene, being part of the genetic make up of the mouse strain. The high mammary tumor strain C3H, for instance, contains an exogenous via a milk-nursing transmitted MTV variant which causes early mammary tumors in almost all of the C3H females. Removal of this exogenous MTV from the C3H strain by foster nursing newborns on mothers without the milk-transmitted MTV variant leaves a C3Hf mouse strain with a low frequency of late-onset mammary tumors. This C3Hf contains only the endogenous MTV variant, while C3H mice contain the exogenous MTV in addition to the endogenous MTV variant.

These routes of transmission of the MTV are reflected in the MTV-DNA proviral content of murine cellular DNA. All inbred strains of *Mus musculus* studied so far contain per haploid genome 2-4 MTV proviral DNA copies of the endogenous MTV variant in the DNA of all their cells (Michalides *et al.*, 1976; Morris *et al.*, 1977). Only cells which became infected with the exogenous MTV variant contain an extra number of MTV-DNA copies of the exogenous MTV. Thus, mammary tumors which have been originated by the exogenous MTV variant contain in their DNA 2-4 MTV proviral DNA copies of the endogenous MTV plus a variable number of MTV-DNA copies of the exogenous MTV, see Fig. 1.

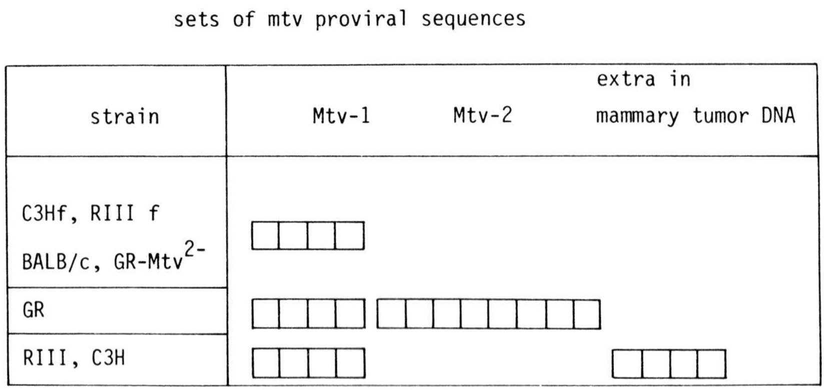

sets of mtv proviral sequences

strain	Mtv-1	Mtv-2	extra in mammary tumor DNA
C3Hf, RIII f BALB/c, GR-Mtv^{2-}	□□□□		
GR	□□□□	□□□□□□□□	
RIII, C3H	□□□□		□□□□

FIGURE 1. Sets of MTV proviral DNA sequences in cellular DNA of inbred strains of mice. The number of MTV-DNA copies per haploid genome is given. (From Michalides et al., *1976, 1978a.)*

The European high mammary tumor strain GR S/A (Mühlbock, 1965) is an exception, it contains the same number of MTV-DNA copies in mammary tumors as in the other cells of the animal. Twelve MTV-DNA copies are present in the haploid genome of all cells of the GR mouse (Michalides and Schlom, 1975; Morris *et al.*, 1977; Drohan *et al.*, 1977).

III. INDUCTION GENES OF MTV EXPRESSION

The C3Hf mouse strain carries a dominant MTV induction gene, termed *Mtv-1* which is responsible for the presence of viral antigens in the milk of C3Hf mice (Van Nie and Verstraeten, 1975). This gene is linked with the albino locus situated on chromosome 7. A gene similar to *Mtv-1* controls the expression of MTV antigens in the milk of another low mammary tumor strain, DBAf (Verstraeten and Van Nie, 1978).

The European high mammary tumor strain GR contains the MTV induction gene *Mtv-2* (Van Nie *et al.*, 1977) controlling the early appearance of pregnancy-dependent mammary tumors and the early expression of MTV-antigens in the milk. A congenic GR mouse strain without this locus was created by introducing genetic material of the C57BL/10 mouse strain using the cross-intercross system (Van Nie and De Moes, 1977). The offspring was selected for the absence of characteristics of the *Mtv-2* locus, i.e., early appearing mammary tumors and MTV-antigens in the milk. This GR-Mtv^{2-} strain lacks the early expression of MTV antigens in the milk and does not develop early and pregnancy-dependent mammary tumors, but keeps its genetic background of the GR mouse. Comparison of the number of MTV-DNA copies in the cellular genome of GR and GR-Mtv^{2-} mice revealed that the selective loss of the *Mtv*^{2} gene from the GR mouse strain in this GR-Mtv^{2-} strain was accompanied by a loss of 8 MTV-DNA copies (Michalides *et al.*, 1978a). We therefore associate the MTV induction gene *Mtv-2* with eight MTV-DNA copies present in the GR mouse genome.

Three sets of MTV proviral DNA sequences are now distinguishable in the cellular genome of inbred strains of mice (Fig. 1).

(a) Approximately four copies are present in the DNA of all mouse strains studied so far. It is tempting to associate these four MTV-DNA copies in the mouse strains C3Hf and DBAf with the MTV induction gene *Mtv-1*.
(b) Approximately eight extra copies are present in the DNA of only the GR mouse, these copies are associated with the MTV induction gene *Mtv-2*.

(c) Mammary tumors of high mammary tumor strains carrying a milk transmitted MTV, such as RIII and C3H, contain in their DNA an extra number of MTV-DNA copies as a consequence of infection by the exogenous MTV.

The regulation of the MTV expression concerns the regulation of expression of these three various sets of MTV-DNA sequences. The various levels at which this regulation of MTV expression might occur, are depicted in Fig. 2.

IV. REGULATION OF EXPRESSION OF THE EXOGENOUS MTV

From the foregoing it might be clear that regulation mechanisms for the expression of the exogenous and endogenous MTVs are different. The exogenous MTV has at first to enter the

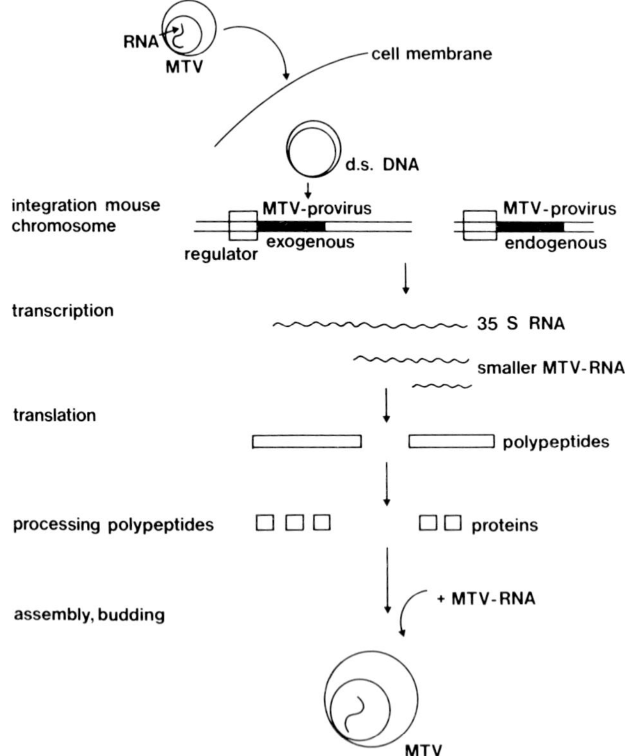

FIGURE 2. Levels of regulation in MTV expression.

animal and its final expression in this mouse depends on a successful infection of the target cells. The infection route of the exogenous MTV in the mouse is not quite resolved. Hageman *et al.* (1972) provided evidence that the MTV is absorbed in the white blood cells which could carry the exogenous MTV to its target cells in the mammary gland. More firm data have to be obtained to elucidate the infection route of the exogenous MTV. The outcome of an infection of a mouse by the exogenous MTV is determined by the following factors.

(a) The dose of MTV obtained. Milk at first lactation contains less MTV than is present at later lactations (Verstraeten *et al.*, 1975). For instance, first litters of RIII develop less mammary tumors than do later litters (Squartini and Bistocchi, 1978).
(b) The age of the animal. MTV infections of animals are less successful at later age. Whether this phenomenon is determined by the state of differentiation of the target cells or by the development of the immune system is unknown.
(c) Genetic factors of both the host and the virus, which influence the host-virus interaction (Bentvelzen, 1974). The best identified factor is the histocompatibility complex H-2. Genes in or near the D end of the H-2 locus determine the susceptibility to infection with MVT-(C3H), the subloci $H2D^b$ and $H2D^q$ determine resistance and $H2D^d$ and $H2D^f$ high susceptibility (Mühlbock and Dux, 1974).

Once the exogenous MTV has infected its target cells, proviral MTV-DNA has to be synthesized and become integrated into the genome of the host cell. This step of the viral infection is in the murine leukemia C-type virus system influenced by the *Fv-1* gene (Lilly and Pincus, 1973). Such a gene is unknown in the B-type mouse mammary tumor virus system. The site of integration of the provirus DNA into the host genome might be very important. Various models for the integration of exogenous viral DNA have arisen from studies on other viral systems. There appear to be various integration sites for the SV40 genome in SV40 transformed 3T3 cells (Botchan *et al.*, 1976), the avian RNA tumor virus AMV aligns its provirus next to the proviral sequences of the endogenous chicken RNA tumor virus (Shoyab *et al.*, 1976). In the system developed by Jaenish (1976), in which the Moloney leukemia virus (MoLV) has been genetically integrated in the BALB/c mouse by infecting embryonic stages with this virus, this MoLV appears to be integrated at a particular site (on chromosome 7). In leukemia cells of those animals this MoLV provirus is found at multiple sites, suggesting that a spread of MoLV proviral DNA sequences is associating the leukemogenesis (Jaenish, 1978).

Varmus and co-workers reported in a preliminary note (Varmus *et al.*, 1978) that BALB/c mice infected with MTV-(C3H) contain additional MTV-DNA proviral sequences at different sites in the genome of mammary gland cells. Mammary tumors of these mice were reported to contain additional MTV-DNA copies at various sites of the genome. These data indicate that in mammary tumors and mammary gland cells of MTV infected mice the proviral MTV-DNA sequences of the exogenous MTV are integrated at sites different from that of the endogenous MTV. They might thereby not be influenced by the regulation system of the mouse controlling the expression of the endogenous MTV.

V. REGULATION OF THE RNA EXPRESSION OF THE ENDOGENOUS MTV

The regulation of the expression of the endogenous MTV is poorly understood. Various authors have reported on the presence or induction of MTV-RNA, MTV proteins, and/or MTV particles in various low mammary tumor mouse strains (Timmermans *et al.*, 1968; Schlom *et al.*, 1974; Links *et al.*, 1977). Bentvelzen (1972) adopted the regulation mechanism controlling the bacteriophage interaction to propose a model for the regulation of the endogenous MTV expression. This expression would usually be strongly inhibited by regulator gene products (see Fig. 2), but virus or viral expression might be accidentally released. The degree of tightness of this control over the expression of the endogenous MTV would be different in each mouse strain.

This is also illustrated in Fig. 3. Two low mammary tumor strains, C57BL.B10 and GR-Mtv^{2-}, each containing four MTV-DNA proviral copies per haploid cellular genome, showed different amounts of MTV-RNA in the mammary glands at first lactation. The GR-Mtv^{2-} mouse strain contains approximately 10-fold more MTV-RNA than the C57BL mice, while the amount of MTV-RNA in the F1 cross between GR-Mtv^{2-} and C57BL.B10 is intermediate to the parental values. These data indicate that there are different regulation systems of MTV-RNA expression in the GR-Mtv^{2-} and C57BL.B10 mouse strains, and that neither regulation system behaves as a dominant trait in this F1 cross.

The data summarized in Table I show that there is a great variation in amounts of MTV-RNA present in the mammary glands at first lactation in low mammary tumor strains. The high mammary tumor strains GR and C3H contain large amounts of MTV-RNA in the cytoplasmic RNA of mammary glands at first lactation. The data presented in Table I represent average amounts of MTV-RNA present, because pools of mammary glands had to be taken in order to obtain enough cellular RNA.

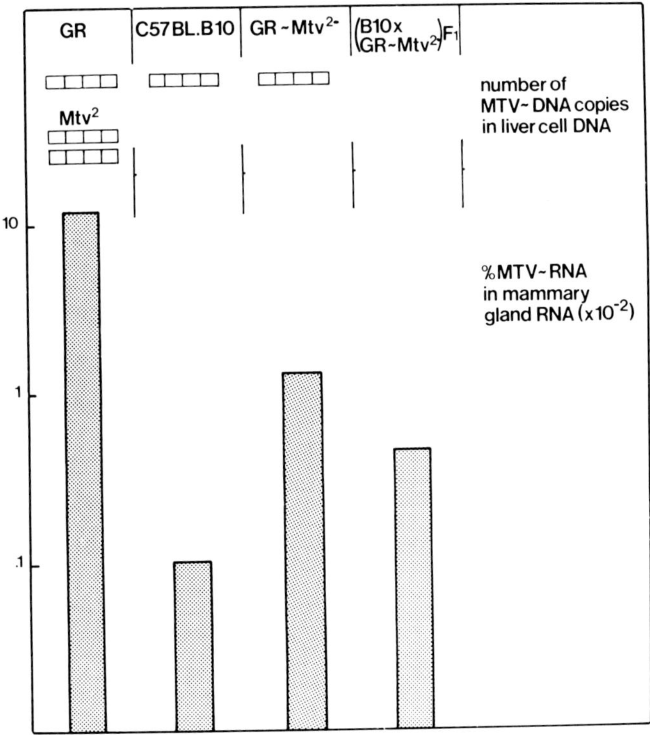

FIGURE 3. Amounts of MTV-RNA in mammary glands at first lactation of GR C57BL, GR.Mtv^{2-}, and (B10 x GR.Mtv^{2-})F1 mice. (From Michalides et al.*, 1978a).*

TABLE I. Amount of MTV-RNA (%x10^{-4}) Present in Cytoplasmic RNA[a]

	Mammary glands	*Spleens*
GR	*1,430*	*0.006*
C3H	*300*	*1.9*
GR-Mtv^{2-}	*160*	<[b]
C57BL.B10	*10*	<
(GR-Mtv^{2-} x C57BL.B10)	*45*	<
C3Hf	*4.8*	<
020	<	<
BALB/c	<	<

[a]*The amount of MTV-RNA was determined in mammary glands at first lactation. From Michalides* et al. *(1978b).*

[b]*Less than 10^{-7}%.*

The data from Table I and from others (see review Nandi and McGrath, 1973) also demonstrate an organ-specific expression of the MTV-RNA. This is mainly expressed in the mammary glands.

We can indicate the different controls on the expression of the endogenous MTV from measuring different MTV-RNA levels expressed in the various low mammary tumor strains. Other indications for the existence of such control mechanisms can be obtained by manipulating the MTV expression in the animal. This can be done by treating the mice with hormones and carcinogens or by altering the H2 haplotype of the animal.

A. Treatment with Hormones

Mammary tumors can be induced in low mammary tumor mouse strains by implantation of multiple hypophyseal isografts in these mice (Mühlbock and Boot, 1959). Prolactin is then continuously released and the excessive amount of this lactogenic hormone causes high mammary tumor frequences in almost all mouse strains (Boot and Röpcke, 1966). Comparison of MVT-RNA amounts present in mammary glands and mammary tumors of prolactin-stimulated mice and controls revealed the following, see Table II.

(1) In the strains C3Hf and 020 this prolactin stimulation resulted in an increase of MTV-RNA expression in the mammary glands, this did not occur in the C57BL strain.

TABLE II. Amount of MTV-RNA (%x10^{-4}) Present in Cytoplasmic RNA[a]

	Mammary glands	*Mammary tumors*
C3H	*300*	*3300*
C3Hf	*4.8*	*4.8*
C3Hf + H[b]	*300*	*16*
020	< [c]	-
020 + H	*0.008*	<
C57BL	*16*	-
C57BL + H	*11.1*	*.1*

[a]*The amount of MTV-RNA was determined in mammary glands at first lactation. From Michalides* et al. *(1978b).*

[b]*These mice received a hypophyseal isograft as described by Boot and Röpcke (1966).*

[c]*Less than 10^{-7}%.*

(2) The enhanced MTV-RNA expression in the stimulated mammary glands was not maintained in the hormone-induced mammary tumors in these three strains.

The difference in stimulation of MTV-RNA expression between C57BL and the two responsive strains 020 and C3Hf might be explained by different amounts of prolactin receptors in the mammary gland cells. Sheth *et al.* (1974) reported that membrane preparations from C3H mammary glands (so, likely also from C3Hf) bind more human placental lactogen, a hormone nearly identical to prolactin, than did similar membrane preparations from C57BL mice. This would imply a relationship between the number of prolactin hormone receptors on target cells and viral RNA production after hormonal stimulation. *In vitro,* such a relationship was found for glucocorticoid receptors of dexamethasone and MTV production after stimulation (Shymala and Dickson, 1976). In this way the regulation of the endogenous MTV might be influenced by genes controlling the production of hormones and by those influencing the sensitivity to hormones, as was already suggested by Bittner (1942).

B. *Treatment with Carcinogens*

The abrogation of the control over the expression of the endogenous MTV by treatments with carcinogens and/or irradiation *in vivo* and *in vitro* has been reported by various investigators (Timmermans *et al.*, 1968; Bentvelzen, 1972; Links *et al.*, 1977). The expression of this MTV proviral DNA would usually be suppressed by a regulator gene product (see Fig. 2), but this would become inactivated by the carcinogenic treatment. Our studies on the expression of the endogenous MTV in various organs of BALB/c mice treated either with 100 R whole-body irradiation at four weeks of age or with 0.5% urethane in the drinking water during the whole lifespan or with a combination of both (see Fig. 4), revealed the following,

(1) Only BALB/c mice which developed mammary tumors as a result of the carcinogenic treatment showed expression of the endogenous MTV. This RNA expression of the endogenous MTV over background values was observed in mammary tumors, mammary glands, and in spleens, but not in livers, of these animals.

(2) The combined treatment of urethane and irradiation was most efficient in inducing the synthesis of endogenous MTV-RNA. Mammary tumors induced by this treatment contained even more MTV-RNA than was present in mammary tumors induced by the exogenous MTV(C3H).

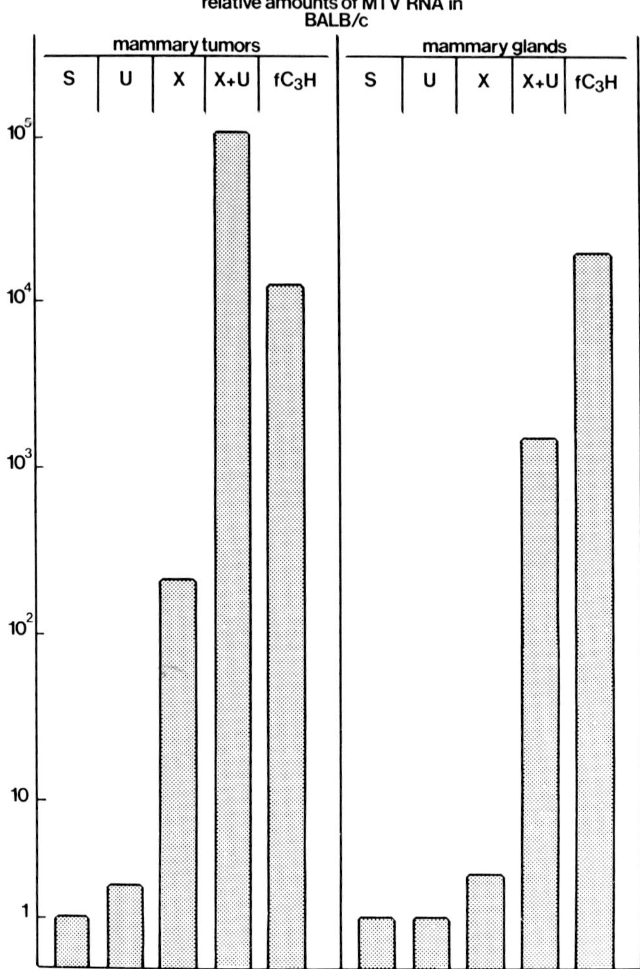

FIGURE 4. Amounts of MTV-RNA in mammary glands and mammary tumors of BALB/c mice. S---spontaneous mammary tumors; U---mammary tumors induced by treatment with urethane, 0.5% in drinking water; X---mammary tumors induced by treatment with irradiation, 100 R whole-body irradiation at four weeks of age; X+U---combined treatment of X+U; fC3H---mammary tumors induced by MTV(C3H). The amount of MTV-RNA present in spontaneous mammary tumors ($4x10^{-6}$ % of the cytoplasmic RNA) is put as 1.

Surprisingly, the mammary tumors of BALB/c mice treated with urethane and irradiation contained very low amounts of MTV proteins; per ng protein they contained 1.4 ng p27 (internal

MTV protein with molecular weight of 27,000) and 0.5 ng gp52 (external MTV protein with molecular weight of 52,000). By electronmicroscopy these tumors did not contain B-type particles, nor were they produced when these tumors were placed in tissue culture. This indicates that although this carcinogenic treatment in the BALB/c mouse has lifted the block on the transcription of the proviral sequences of the endogenous MTV, there still remains another regulating system preventing the translation of the MTV-(BALB/c) RNA, which is affected by the carcinogenic treatment.

However, the release of the RNA expression of the endogenous MTV-(BALB/c) by the carcinogenic treatment indicates the presence of a regulation system which under natural conditions suppresses the expression of endogenous MTV-RNA.

C. *Influence of the H-2 Haplotype on the Expression of the Endogenous MTV*

The H-2 locus belongs to the histocompatibility system of the mouse. The H-2 locus influences the resistency to the exogenous MTV (see Section IV). We also observed a difference in endogenous MTV expression between two strains which differ in the H-2 haplotype. The 020 mouse strain carries the H-2 haplotype $H\text{-}2^{pz}$, the OIR strain carrying the H-2 haplotype $H\text{-}2^{q}$ has been derived from the 020 mouse strain by only once introducing genetic material of the DBAf mouse and by subsequent selective breeding in which only animals rejecting 020 grafts were used for the next generation. Molecular hybridizations between a radioactive-labeled MTV-cDNA and cellular RNA from mammary glands at first lactation showed a marked difference in the amounts of MTV-RNA between the mammary glands of these two strains (see Fig. 5). The 020 mouse strain contains a low amount of MTV-RNA in the mammary glands, the OIR mammary glands on the other hand contain large amounts of MTV-RNA. Because these two strains differ only in the H-2 haplotype, it is likely that the H-2 haplotype influences the expression of the endogenous MTV in this system. A similar influence of the H-2 haplotype on the expression of the murine leukemia virus has recently been reported (Freedman *et al.*, 1978).

In general, the regulation of the expression of the endogenous MTV occurs at the level of transcription. The amounts of MTV proteins gp52 and p27 in various tissues, detected by sensitive radioimmunoassay, agree in general terms with the amounts of MTV-RNA in those tissues (data not shown). The few exceptions are discussed below.

In cells infected with murine sarcoma virus three distinct viral messenger RNAs have been found, with sedimentation values

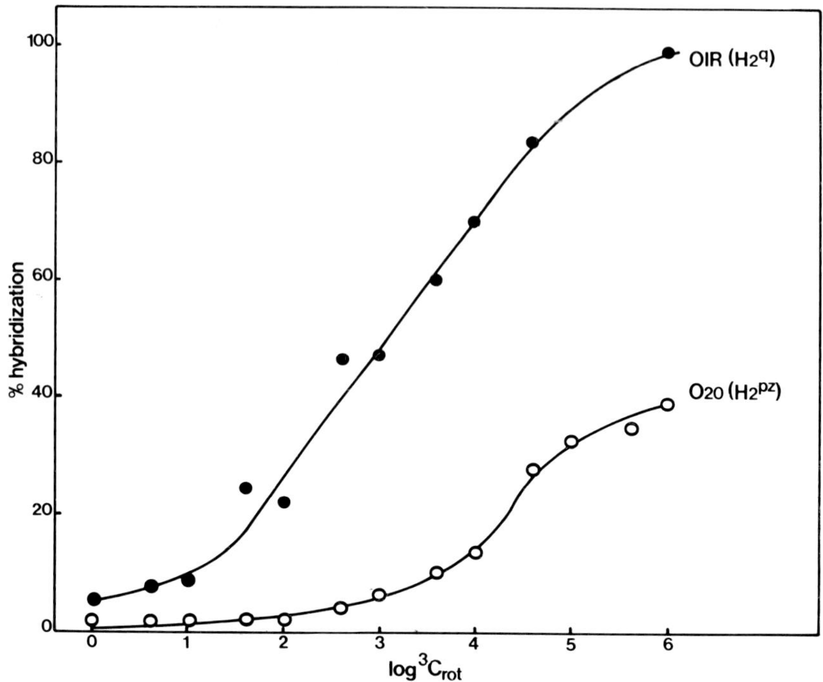

FIGURE 5. Molecular hybridization between MTV-³HcDNA and cellular RNA from mammary glands at first lactation of 020 and OIR mice. Hybridization conditions were described in Michalides et al. *(1978b).*

of respectively 35, 20, and 14S (Eiseman and Vogt, 1978). *In vitro* translation of these mRNAs revealed that the 35S mRNA functions as messenger RNA for the *gag* proteins (internal proteins), the 20S mRNA for the *env* proteins (external proteins), while the 14S mRNA directs the synthesis of the transformation causing protein, termed *sarc*. Similar studies are being performed to show the presence of distinct classes of intracellular mRNAs of MTV. It has been recently shown (Nusse *et al.*, 1978) that the virion 35S RNA instructs the synthesis of only the MTV *gag* protein in an *in vitro* translation system, indicating a similarity to the murine C-type virus system.

VI. REGULATION OF MTV EXPRESSION AT POSTTRANSCRIPTIONAL LEVELS

Posttranscriptional levels at which the expression of the endogenous MTV could be affected include translation of the viral messenger RNA, the processing of viral polypeptides and the assembly of the virion at the cell membrane.

1. Regulation at the Level of Translation. This might occur in two ways: quantitatively, in which the amounts of MTV proteins are being regulated, and qualitatively in which only certain MTV proteins are being synthesized. Both types of regulation do occur in the MTV system.

(a) *Quantitative control.* Evidence for such a control mechanism can only be obtained by comparing amounts of MTV-RNA and MTV-proteins between tissues of different strains of mice. Such a comparison between mammary tumors of C3Hf and of BALB/c mice treated with urethane and irradiation (Fig. 4) shows that BALB/c mammary tumors contain more MTV-RNA than those of C3Hf, but contain much less protein. Those BALB/c mammary tumors contain per mg protein 1.4-ng p27 and 0.5 ng gp52, C3Hf mammary tumors contain between 100-200-ng p27 and 50-100 ng gp52. This indicates a restriction on the synthesis of MTV proteins of the endogenous MTV (BALB/c). Such a restriction is also apparent in C57BL mice. Mammary glands of C57BL do contain more MTV-RNA than those of C3Hf (Table I), while the amounts of MTV-protein are less than 10-ng gp52 and p27 per mg protein of mammary glands of C57BL and between 300-400-ng gp52 and p27 in one mg of C3Hf mammary glands at first lactation.

(b) Qualitative control. In all murine tissues we have studied so far, there appeared a coordinate expression of the MTV viral protein of the *gag* gene, p27, and of the *env* gene, gp52. Only two exceptions have been found: mammary glands of GR-Mtv^{2-} and 020 mice do contain p27, but lack gp52. This might indicate either a partial expression of the MTV-proteins in these two mouse strains or a substantial difference between the gp52s in those strains and the standard gp52 of MTV (C3H) which was used in the radioimmunoassay.

2. Regulation of the Endogenous MTV Expression at the Level of Processing of Viral Polypeptides. The MTV proteins as they are present in the virion are derived from precursor polypeptides. The internal proteins, among which p14 and p27, are cleaved from a nonglycosylated precursor with a molecular weight of 75,000 (Schochetman *et al.*, 1978), which is encoded for by the *gag* gene. The external MTV proteins gp52 and gp36 (glycosylated proteins with molecular weights of 52,000 and

36,000) are cleaved from a precursor polypeptide of 73,000 D containing sugar residues (Dickson *et al.*, 1975), which is encoded for by the *env* gene. Both precursors are being synthesized independently (Schochetman and Schlom, 1976). This complex cleavage pattern of precursor polypeptides requires a precise cleavage mechanism in order to obtain the right proteins, how this is being done is unknown. From the study by Nusse *et al.* (1978) one might conclude that cellular modifications of the precursor polypeptides, as phosphorylation, are required for the processing of these polyproteins.

That this processing of precursor polypeptides is regulated in some way is evident from the exceptions in which this processing does not occur: Transplantable leukemias of strains DBAf and GR do contain large amounts of intracytoplasmic A particles (Tanaka, 1977; Calafat *et al.*, 1974), but no complete B-type particles are being synthesized. These intracytoplasmic A particles are pronucleocapsids of B particles which contain antigens crossreacting with the three major internal proteins of MTV. The major protein of the A particles, with a molecular weight of approximately 70,000, becomes processed into proteins with molecular weight values equivalent to those of the internal MTV proteins upon incubation with trypsin (Smith and Lee, 1975). This indicates that the MTV-precursor *gag* protein of the A particles of spontaneous leukemias is not processed at all or at a much lower rate than in MTV producing cells. Since the other MTV proteins, the *env* proteins, are present in these cells, it is likely that the retarded processing of the *gag* precursor delays the assembly of MTV virions.

VII. MTV EXPRESSION RELATED TO MURINE MAMMARY TUMORIGENESIS

The oncogenic capacity of MTV is derived from its ability to induce mammary tumors by infection of susceptible mice. The mammary tumor incidence in high mammary tumor strains such as C3H and RIII, for instance, is greatly reduced when the exogenous MTV is removed by foster nursing newborns on mothers without MTV in their milk. Strictly speaking the transforming MTV should fulfill two requirements.

(a) Temperature-sensitive mutations in the transforming locus should induce temperature-sensitive transformation of infected cells.

(b) All MTV-transformed cells should carry the information of a virally coded transformation gene. These two requirements have not been met yet because no *in vitro* transformation has been obtained with MTV. Still, the transforming capability of the exogenous MTV is generally accepted.

The involvement of the endogenous MTV in the murine mammary tumorigenesis is more troublesome. The various systems provide the following information.

(1) There is a clear connection between MTV-inducing genes *Mtv-1* and *Mtv-2* and the appearance of mammary tumors (see Section III). The strongest argument favoring the involvement of the endogenous MTV in mammary tumorigenesis in GR mice is that the development of a GR-Mtv^{2-} strain without early tumors is accompanied by a loss of MTV-DNA proviral sequences (see Section III).

(2) The presence of MTV-RNA in mammary tumors induced by carcinogens and irradiation (see Section V.B). Treatment of BALB/c mice with these agents induces mammary tumors (see Fig. 6). The combined treatment of urethane and irradiation provided the best procedure for inducing mammary tumors and resulted in the greatest release of MTV-RNA in these tumors (Fig. 4). However, urethane alone was almost as efficient in

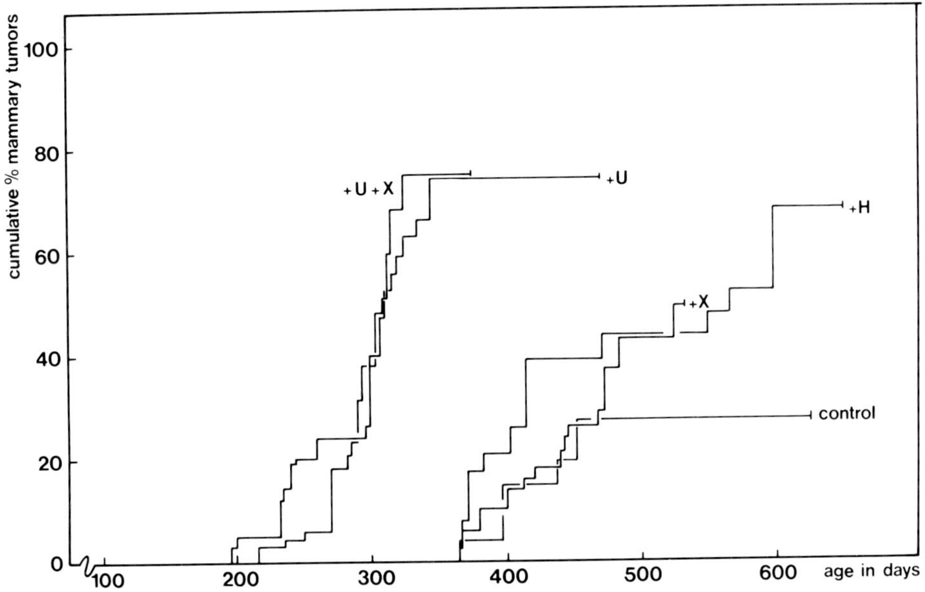

FIGURE 6. Mammary tumor incidence in BALB/c mice. +H---these mice obtained a hypophyseal isograft as described by Boot and Röpcke (1966). U---mammary tumors induced by treatment with urethane, 0.5% in drinking water; X---mammary tumors induced by treatment with X-irradiation.

inducing mammary tumors, while much less MTV-RNA was detectable in these tumors. One might therefore argue that the sensitivity to carcinogenic treatment coincides with the release of MTV information in these mice, instead of concluding a relationship between MTV expression and tumor development.

(3) Mammary tumor virus variants have been isolated from spontaneous C3Hf mammary tumors and mammary glands of old BALB/c mice, and have been shown to be oncogenic by injection in susceptible mice (Hageman *et al.*, 1972). These findings do not prove that these MTVs are instrumental in the spontaneous mammary tumorigenesis. By changing the endogenous MTV into an exogenous MTV variant, one also changes its transmission route and thereby the integration sites of the MTV-DNA proviral sequences in the murine cellular DNA (see Section IV). In spontaneous, chemically or hormone-induced mammary tumors we did not detect an amplification of MTV-DNA sequences, while such an addition of MTV-DNA sequences to the murine cellular genome occurs in mammary tumors which originated from an infection by MTV, either exogenous or endogenous from origin (Michalides *et al.*, 1978a,b).

(4) No expression of MTV at all occurs in spontaneous mammary tumors of BALB/c mice (Michalides *et al.*, 1978b). This argues against any involement of MTV in the development of spontaneous mammary tumors in BALB/c mice.

(5) The decrease or absence of MTV expression in prolactin-induced mammary tumors in C3Hf, 020, and C57BL mice (see Table II) compared to the amount of MTV-RNA in the mammary glands of these mice. The possibility arises that the MTV expression in these mammary glands is transient or that cell types which do not contain MTV-RNA proliferate from mammary glands to tumor cells. In any case, continued MTV expression does not seem necessary to maintain these hormone-induced mammary tumors in a transformed state.

(6) The increase in MTV expression in the OIR strain compared to 020 mice, which differ only in H2 haplotype (Fig. 5), is not correlated with an increase in the mammary tumor frequency (Dux, personal communication).

It is evident from these data that there are various patterns in the transformation of mammary glands to mammary tumors, even within one mouse strain. The endogenous MTV participates in some of those, might play a secondary role in others or is sometimes not involved at all.

REFERENCES

Bentvelzen, P. (1972). *In* "RNA Viruses and Host Genome in Oncogenesis" (P. Emmelot and P. Bentvelzen, eds.), pp. 309-337. North-Holland, Amsterdam.

Bentvelzen, P. (1974). *Biochem. Biphys. Acta 51,* 236-259.

Bittner, J. J. (1942). *Cancer Res. 2,* 710.

Boot, L. M., and Röpcke, G. (1966). *Cancer Res. 26,* 1492-1496.

Botchan, M., Topp, W., and Sambrook, J. (1976). *Cell 9,* 269-287.

Calafat, J., Buys, F., Hageman, Ph., Links, J., Hilgers, J., and Hekman, A. (1974). *J. Natl. Cancer Inst. 53,* 977-991.

Dickson, C., Puma, J. P., and Nandi, S. (1975). *Virology 58,* 387-395.

Dion, A. S., Heine, U., Pomenti, A., Korb, J., and Weber, G. H. (1977). *J. Virol. 22,* 822-825.

Drohan, W., Kettmann, R., Colcher, D., and Schlom, J. (1977). *J. Virol. 21,* 987-995.

Eiseman, R. N., and Vogt, V. M. (1978). *Biochem. Biophys. Acta 473,* 187-239.

Frankel, A. E., and Fischinger, P. J. (1976). *Proc. Natl. Acad. Sci. 73,* 3705-3709.

Freedman, H. A., Lilly, F., Strand, M., and August, J. F. (1978). *Cell 13,* 33-40.

Hageman, Ph., Calafat, J., and Daams, J. H. (1972). *In* "RNA Viruses and Host Genome in Oncogenesis" (P. Emmelot and P. Bentvelzen, eds.), pp. 283-300. North-Holland, Amsterdam.

Jaenish, R. (1976). *Proc. Natl. Acad. Sci. 73,* 1260-1264.

Jaenish, R. (1978). *In* "Abstracts XIth Meeting of the European Tumor Virus Group," p. 181, Balatonfüred, Hungary.

Lilly, F., and Pincus, T. (1973). *Adv. Cancer Res. 17,* 231-277.

Links, J., Calafat, J., Buys, F., and Tol, O. (1977). *Eur. J. Cancer 13,* 577-587.

Michalides, R., and Schlom, J. (1975). *Proc. Natl. Acad. Sci. 72,* 4635-4639.

Michalides, R., Vlahakis, G., and Schlom, J. (1976). *Internat. J. Cancer 18,* 105-115.

Michalides, R., Van Deemter, L., Nusse, R., and Van Nie, R. (1978a). *Proc. Natl. Acad. Sci. 75,* 2368-2372.

Michalides, R., Van Deemter, L., Nusse, R., Röpcke, G., and Boot, L. (1978b). *J. Virol. 27,* 551-559.

Morris, V., Medeiros, E., Ringold, G. M., Bishop, J. M., and Varmus, H. E. (1977). *J. Mol. Biol. 114,* 73-91.

Mühlbock, O., and Boot, L. M. (1959). *Cancer Res. 19,* 402-412.

Mühlbock, O. (1965). *Eur. J. Cancer 1,* 123-124.

Mühlbock, O., and Dux, A. (1974). *J. Natl. Cancer Inst. 53,* 993-996.

Nandi, S., and McGrath, C. M. (1973). *Adv. Cancer Res. 17,* 353-414.

Nusse, R., Asselbergs, F., Salden, M., Michalides, R., and Bloemendal, H. (1978). *Virology 91,* 106-115.

Schochetman, G., and Schlom, J. (1976). *Virology 73,* 431.

Schochetman, G., Long, C. W., Orozlan, S., Arthur, L., and Fine, D. F. (1978). *Virology 85,* 168-174.

Schlom, J., Michalides, R., Kufe, D., Hehlman, R., Spiegelman, S., Bentvelzen, P. and Hageman, Ph. (1974). *J. Natl. Cancer Inst. 51,* 541.

Shyamala, G., and Dickson, C. (1976). *Nature (London) 262,* 107-112.

Sheth, N. A., Ranadive, K. J., and Sheth, A. R. (1974). *Eur. J. Cancer 10,* 653-660.

Shoyab, M., Dastoor, M. N., and Baluda, M. A. (1976). *Proc. Natl. Acad. Sci. 73,* 1749-1753.

Smith, G. H., and Lee, B. K. (1975). *J. Natl. Cancer Inst. 55,* 493-496.

Squartini, F., and Bistocchi, M. (1978). *In* "Abstracts XIth Meeting of the European Tumor Virus Group," p. 193. Balatonfüred, Hungary.

Stehelin, D., Guntaka, R. V., Varmus, H. E., and Bishop. J. M. (1976). *J. Mol. Biol. 101,* 349-365.

Tanaka, H. (1977). *Virology 76,* 835-850.

Timmermans, A., Bentvelzen, P., Hageman, Ph., and Calafat, J. (1968). *J. Gen. Virol. 4,* 619-621.

Van Nie, R., and Verstraeten, A. A. (1975). *Internat. J. Cancer 16,* 922-931.

Van Nie, R., Verstraeten, A. A., and De Moes, J. (1977). *Internat. J. Cancer 19,* 383-390.

Van Nie, R., and De Moes, J. (1977). *Internat. J. Cancer 20,* 588-594.

Varmus, H. E., Cohen, J. G., Ringold, G. M., Shank, P. R., Morris, V. L., Cardiff, R., and Yamamoto, K. R. (1978). *J. Supramol. Struct.* Suppl. 2, p. 224.

Verstraeten, A. A., Van Nie, R., Kwa, H. G., and Hageman, Ph.C. (1975). *Internat. J. Cancer 15,* 270-281.

Verstraeten, A. A., and Van Nie, R. (1978). *Internat. J. Cancer 21,* 473-475.

RETROVIRUS RNA EXPRESSION IN DMBA-INDUCED RAT MAMMARY ADENOCARCINOMAS*

Howard A. Young
Edward M. Scolnick

Division of Cancer Cause and Prevention
Laboratory of Tumor Virus Genetics
National Cancer Institute

Martin L. Wenk

Microbiological Associates,
Bethesda, Maryland

Dawn G. Goodman

Division of Cancer Cause and Prevention
Tumor Pathology Branch
National Cancer Institute

With the technical assistance
of

John Vere, Jr. and Robert Shores

This work has been supported in part by contract NO1-CP-43236 of the Virus Cancer Program to Meloy Laboratories, Rockville, Maryland and by contract NO1-CP-02199 from the National Cancer Institute to Microbiological Associates, Bethesda, Maryland.

ISBN 0-12-131150-3

I. INTRODUCTION

Laboratories have been investigating for a number of years the mechanisms underlying the transformation of mammalian cells by type-C retroviruses. Recent studies utilizing rat cells as a model system have shown that all rat cells contain a replication-defective endogenous retrovirus (Scolnick *et al.*, 1976a,b) and that expression of this endogenous genome as RNA occurs in many naturally occurring rat tumors (Anderson and Robbins, 1976). These studies have led us to investigate the possible relationship between chemical transformation of cells and the expression of the replication-defective retrovirus.

7,12-Dimethylbenz(a)anthracene (DMBA) has been known for many years to be a potent inducer of mammary tumors in the female rat (Huggins *et al.*, 1959, 1961). This carcinogen is most effective when given to 50-day old rats and produces primarily mammary adenocarcinomas, following a latent period of 4-6 mos after administration. Many investigators have attempted to correlate biochemical and histological changes with tumor development (Stevens *et al.*, 1965; Archer and Orlando, 1968; Hilf *et al.*, 1969, 1970; McGuire and Julian, 1971; Boylan *et al.*, 1977; Hawkins *et al.*, 1977). To date these studies have produced limited markers for tumor development, and no clear correlation of endogenous viral markers and tumor formation has been reported. Up until now, the only model for viral involvement in breast cancer has been the mouse. In this model the presence of a type-B viral particle, the mouse mammary tumor virus, has been clearly associated with mammary tumor development (Bentvelzen and Daams, 1969; Nandi and McGrath, 1973: Bentvelzen, 1974; Heston and Parks, 1975). Knowledge of endogenous retroviruses associated with the rat is more limited, but has expanded in recent years. Type-C retroviruses have been isolated from a variety of rat tissue culture cell lines (Cremer *et al.*, 1970; Gazzolo *et al.*, 1971; Bergs *et al.*, 1972; Klement *et al.*, 1972, 1973; Sarma *et al.*, 1973; Benveniste and Todaro, 1973; Rasheed *et al.*, 1976) as well as chemically induced (Bergs *et al.*, 1970; Weinstein *et al.*, 1972; Rhim *et al.*, 1973) and transplantable rat tumors (Engle *et al.*, 1969; Chopra *et al.*, 1970). Though these viruses are from different strains of rats, they all appear similar to typical type-C helper independent retroviruses with the exception that only ecotropic viruses have been described (i.e., their host range appears limited only to rat cells). Another retrovirus present in the rat genome is replication-defective; its genome does not code for any known structural proteins, and helper type-C virus functions are needed in order to package this RNA into complete virus particles (Scolnick *et al.*, 1976a,b) and transmit this RNA to non-rat cells (Scolnick *et al.*, 1979). Interestingly, a homologue of this endogenous replication-defective virus has been found to be a part of both the Kirsten and Harvey sarcoma viruses (Scolnick *et al.*, 1974; Roy-Burman and Klement, 1975), which were isolated after passage of murine leukemia viruses in rats (Harvey, 1964; Kirsten and Mayer, 1967). These sarcoma viruses have recently been shown to be recombinant viruses containing both the replication-defective rat type-C virus and particular portions of the parental helper mouse leukemia virus (Shih *et al.*, 1978). This relationship between the replication-defective rat virus and known transforming viruses makes investigation of the expression of these sequences during a more natural oncogenic process in rats potentially of interest.

Other investigators have studied the expression of the endogenous rat retroviruses as RNA in a variety of rat tumors and tissues (Anderson and Robbins, 1976). These studies, however, involved only a limited number of any single type of tumor, involved tumors many generations removed from initial small tumors, and the results did not show a clear pattern of expression of either the helper-independent type-C virus or the replication-defective retrovirus in the tumors. We have investigated the expression of RNA of endogenous type-C retroviruses in chemically induced rat mammary tumors to determine if enhanced expression of an endogenous retrovirus can be correlated with the induction of mammary tumors and how this expression relates to the hormonal dependence of these tumors. In addition, attempts have been made to establish a tissue culture model for these tumors in order to further characterize the RNA of the endogenous retroviruses.

II. MATERIAL AND METHODS

A. Animals

Female Sprague-Dawley rats were purchased from Charles River Breeding Farms (Wilmington, Massachusetts) at five weeks of age. Animals were housed three per 13 x 15 in. polycarbonate cage on 1/8 in. corncob bedding with Purina lab chow and water available *ad libitum*. Each animal was individually identified by ear mark and assigned unique consecutive numbers. At 50 days of age experimental animals received a single 1.0 ml intragastric administration of a 20 mg/ml solution of 7, 12-dimethylbenz(a)anthracene (Eastman Organic Chemical) in laboratory grade sesame oil (Fisher Scientific). Control animals received a single 1.0 ml intragastric dose of sesame oil only. Animals were monitored weekly and animals bearing tumors of random size were designated for immediate sacrifice, ovariectomy, or ovariectomy and estrogen replacement. Those animals that were ovariectomized were anesthetized with 1.5 ml/100 gm body weight of a 10 mg/ml solution of sodium pentobarbitol injected intraperitoneally. Both ovaries were removed after ligating the uteri through bilaterial incisions in the dorsal wall of the peritoneal cavity. Those animals designated for hormone replacement (i.e., those bearing tumors that regressed following surgery) received 5 μg of 17 β-estradiol (Sigma Chemical) three times a week as a subcutaneous injection in 0.2 ml of sesame oil. Hormone-dependent tumors were those classified as decreasing in size for two consecutive weeks following ovariectomy or increasing in size for two consecutive weeks following hormone replacement. At the time of sacrifice a small section of tumor, liver, spleen, lung, and uterus from selected animals were removed for histological examination. These sections were placed immediately in 10% phosphate buffered formalin and the tissue was then embedded in parafin, 5-6 μm thick sections removed and stained with hematoxylin and eosin. The remaining tumor, liver, spleen, lungs, and uterus were immediately frozen.

B. RNA Estraction

Tumors were minced into fine pieces and homogenized in 0.01*M* Tris pH 7.2, 0.1*M* NaCl, 0.001*M* EDTA, and 0.5% sodium dodecyl sulfate (SDS). For those tumors weighing more than 3 gm, 2-3 gm portion were removed and extracted. Proteinase K was added to a final concentration of 100 μg/ml and the suspension incubated for at least 3 hr at 37°C with occasional homogenization of the suspension. The tissue was then extracted three times with phenol and chloroform-isoamyl alcohol (24:1). The aqueous phase, containing RNA and DNA, was adjusted to 2% sodium acetate pH 5.0, two volumes ethanol added, and stored at -20°C for 16 hr. The precipitate was collected by centrifugation, the pellet resuspended in 0.01*M* Tris pH 7.2, 0.01*M* $MgCl_2$, RNAse-free DNAse I (Sigma Chemical) was added to a final concentration of 100 μg/ml, and the solution incubated 1 hr at 37°C. SDS was then added to a final concentration of 0.1%. The RNA solution was extracted with phenol and chloroform isoamylalcohol and the aqueous phase was dialyzed, lyophilized, and resuspended in distilled H_2O. RNA concentration was determined by optical density at 260 nm. DNA was extracted in a similar manner, except that after the initial ethanol precipitation, the pellet was resuspended in H_2O, adjusted to 0.5N NaOH for 3 hr at 37°C, dialyzed, and lyophilized. The DNA was then resuspended in H_2O, adjusted to a concentration of 1 mg/ml and sonically treated to an average size of 9 s prior to hybridization analysis (Marmur, 1961).

C. cDNA Preparation

^{3}H-cDNA specific for a replication-defective retrovirus of rats was prepared from two different sources:

^{3}H-cDNA$_{Ki-SV}$: The ^{3}H-cDNA utilized for most of the studies was obtained from the endogenous reverse transcriptase reaction of a feline leukemia virus (FeLV) pseudotype of Kirsten sarcoma virus (Ki-SV) grown in mink cells (Scolnick *et al.*, 1974). This pseudotype has been shown to produce a stable 20-fold excess of Ki-SV to FeLV or Ki-SV to endogenous mink viruses (Shih *et al.*, 1978). Virus preparations were banded one time in sucrose density gradients and the endogenous reaction was stimulated with calf thymus DNA fragments under conditions previously described (Taylor *et al.*, 1976). The ^{3}H-cDNA was then extracted twice with phenol and chloroform-isoamyl-alcohol and precipitated with ethanol overnight at -20°C. The precipitate was collected by centrifugation, resuspended in H_2O, and passed over a G-50 Sephadex column. The void volume, containing the ^{3}H-cDNA was then adjusted to 0.5*N* NaOH incubated 3 hr at 37°C, neutralized with glacial acetic acid, yeast RNA added to a final concentration of 25 µg/ml and precipitated with absolute ethanol at -20°C. The ^{3}H-cDNA was collected by centrifugation and resuspended in 0.01*M* Tris-HCl pH 7.2. To obtain the rat virus specific portions of Ki-SV in the ^{3}H-cDNA preparation, the ^{3}H-cDNA was hybridized to a 2000-fold excess of RNA extracted from a rat cell line, V-NRK (Benveniste and Todaro, 1973), which contains high levels of the endogenous replication-defective rat retrovirus RNA. Hybridization was performed under conditions described below. The hybridization mixture was then digested with S_1 nuclease (Leong *et al.*, 1972). After S_1 digestion, the reaction was phenol-chloroform extracted twice and precipitated with ethanol at -20°C. The ethanol precipitate was collected by centrifugation, resuspended in H_2O, and alkali-treated. The ^{3}H-cDNA$_{Ki-SV}$ obtained by this cycling procedure is specific for the rat portion of Ki-SV (i.e., the replication-defective endogenous retrovirus) (Scolnick *et al.*, 1978) and does not cross-hybridize with the genome of endogenous rat helper independent type-C retroviruses obtained from Osborne-Mendel (RT21C) Cremer *et al.*, 1970) or Wistar Furth (W/Fu) (Sarma *et al.*, 1973) or Sprague-Dawley rats (SD-1) (Rasheed *et al.*, 1976). In addition, no hybridization has been detected with the mink-endogenous virus (unpublished observations) or FeLV (Shih *et al.*, 1978).

(2) The second ^{3}H-cDNA specific for the replication-defective endogenous retrovirus was obtained from a DMBA-induced uterine adenocarcinoma cell line derived from a Sprague-Dawley rat (Sekiya *et al.*, 1972). This cell line, designated HTP, has been shown to contain high levels of the replication-defective retrovirus RNA (Scolnick *et al.*, 1976b). As previously described

(Scolnick *et al.*, 1974), the rat RNA was pseudotyped with a helper-independent virus obtained from a woolly monkey. The virus complex released from the cell contains approximately equal ratios of woolly virus RNA and rat RNA. The ^{3}H-cDNA was prepared from this virus complex and hybridized to a 2000-fold excess of RNA from the woolly leukemia virus alone. The hybridization reaction was then processed by hydroxyapatite chromatography to remove the hybridized cDNA (Benveniste and Scolnick, 1973). The remaining unhybridized ^{3}H-cDNA$_{HTP}$ obtained by this procedure is specific for the genome of the endogenous replication-defective type-C retrovirus found in HTP cells and has extensive homology to the rat portions of Ki-SV and Ha-SV (Scolnick *et al.*, 1974). Since the ^{3}H-cDNA$_{Ki-SV}$ and ^{3}H-cDNA$_{HTP}$ represent highly related, but not identical, copies of this class of replication-defective rat virus, both probes were used in the studies described below.

The ^{3}H-cDNA specific for the rat helper independent endogenous rat type-C retrovirus (^{3}H-cDNA$_{RaLV}$) was obtained from virus released by the RT21C Osborne-Mendel cell line (Cremer *et al.*, 1970). This cell line releases approximately a 50-fold excess of helper-independent virus to replication-defective rat virus (Scolnick *et al.*, 1976a,b). The ^{3}H-cDNA$_{RaLV}$ was prepared and processed, except that no additional hybridization cycling step was needed. The cDNA does not hybridize to the genome of the rat endogenous replication-defective retrovirus or to Kirsten sarcoma virus (Scolnick *et al.*, 1976a,b).

D. *Hybridization Analysis*

Hybridization of ^{3}H-cDNA to tissue RNA was performed in an 0.05 ml reaction mixture containing 0.01 Tris pH 7.2, 0.75*M* NaCl, 0.5% SDS, 0.1 mM EDTA, 2000-3000 tritiated cpm of the respective cDNA and various amount of RNA. The reaction mixture was incubated at 67°C for 20 or 40 hr. ^{3}H-cDNA·RNA hybrids were analyzed with S_1 nuclease (Leong *et al.*, 1972) and Crt values have been corrected for salt concentration (Scolnick *et al.*, 1976b).

E. *Cell Culture*

Fresh tumors were minced into small pieces with scissors, resuspended in 1% trypsin containing 0.001M EDTA, and the suspension was stirred at 37°C. Every 20 min free cells were poured off, fresh trypsin added, and this process was repeated three times. The cells were collected by centrifugation, washed with Dulbecco's medium containing 10% fetal calf serum and seeded at 1 x 10^{6} cells/100 mm Petri dish. Cells were maintained in

TABLE I. Summary of Tumors Obtained after DMBA Treatment

Treatment	No. animals[a]	No. tumors	Tumors/animal	Adenocarcinomas Total	Adenocarcinomas Analyzed[b]	Fibroadenomas total	Misc.[c] total
DMBA	17	50	1-7	35	21	5	10
Control	9	0	0	0	-	0	0
DMBA + Ovariectomy	9	20	1-4	14	8	5	1
Control (ovariectomy)	6	0	0	0	-	0	0
DMBA + ovariectomy + hormone replacement	11	40	1-5	25	12	4	11
Control (ovariectomy and hormone replacement)	7	0	0	0	-	0	0
DMBA Totals	37	110	1-7	74	41	14	30
Control Totals	22	0	0	0	-	0	0

[a]Only animals that developed tumors were included in this table. This represents 77% of DMBA-treated animals.

[b]Tumors less than 0.2 gm in weight were included in the total but were too small to be analyzed.

[c]This category included enlarged lymph nodes (7), epidermal cysts (4), basosquamous carcinomas (4), calcifying epitheliomas (3), trichoepitheliomas (2), and lymphomas (2).

Dulbecco's medium containing 10% fetal calf serum. 1 μg/ml protactin and $10^{-8}M$ 17 β-estradiol. However, subsequent studies revealed that prolactin and estradiol were not necessary for cell maintenance or growth and they were removed from the growth medium. After six passages, attempts were made to obtain cell clones from one tumor (1 gm wet weight) defined by histological examination of the tumor tissue as an adenocarcinoma. Cells were cloned by serial dilution in microtiter dishes (Falcon Plastics) as reported previously (Goldsby and Zipser, 1969). A number of isolates were obtained and one, B_8, was analyzed for endogenous retrovirus RNA expression.

III. RESULTS

A. *Classification of Tumors*

A total of 110 possible tumors from 37 DMBA-treated animals were obtained for histological and molecular analysis. Animals bearing tumors were divided into three categories: (1) DMBA treated at 50 days of age; (2) DMBA treated at 50 days of age and ovariectomized after tumor appearance; (3) DMBA treated at 50 days of age, ovariectomized after tumor appearance, and treated with estrogen after tumor regression was observed. Table I summarizes the number and type of tumors obtained in each of the three categories. A wide variety of tumor types was obtained by DMBA treatment, but as seen from this table, the majority of tumors obtained (67%) were mammary adenocarcinomas. These adenocarcinomas ranged in size from 0.08 to 10.8 gm.

As shown in Fig. 1, adenocarcinomas exhibited a variety of architectural patterns ranging from solid nests of sheets of epithelial cells, to variable-sized acini with piling up of the epithelium, to papillary cystic lesions with delicate stromal stalks covered with multiple layers of epithelial cells. The cells were oval to cuboidal with a moderate amount of slightly basophilic cytoplasm with round to oval vesicular nuclei. Nucleoli were prominent and usually single. The presence of mitotic figures was variable, being most frequent in the more solid epithelial areas. Most of the tumors were fairly well differentiated. In some cases, evidence of secretory activity was present as indicated by the presence of large vacuoles within tumor cells and/or the presence of a homogenous, eosinophilic, proteinaceous material within acinar or cyst lumens. The amount of stroma present was variable within tumors and especially between tumors of different sizes, and very little necrosis was observed in any of the tumors. In small tumors, the stroma was scant, and consisted of delicate bands

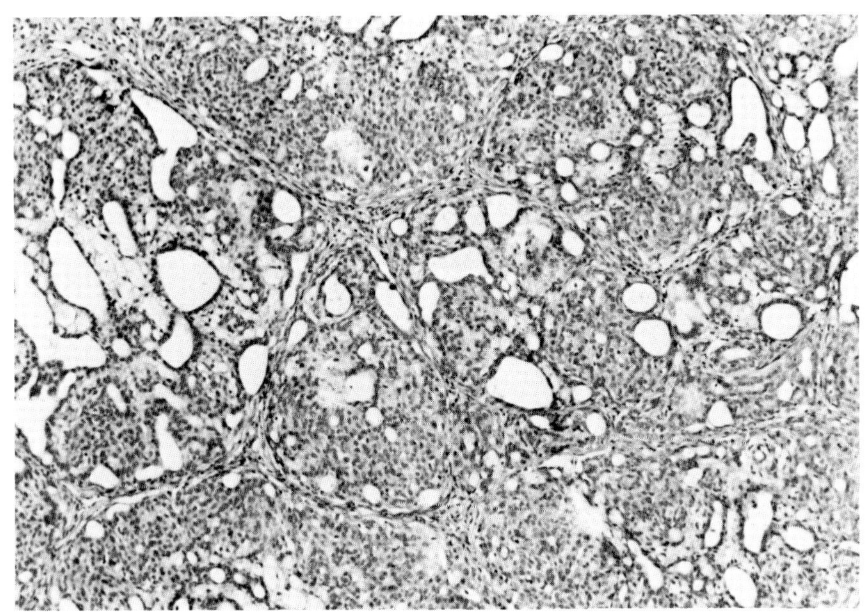

FIGURE 1. (a)

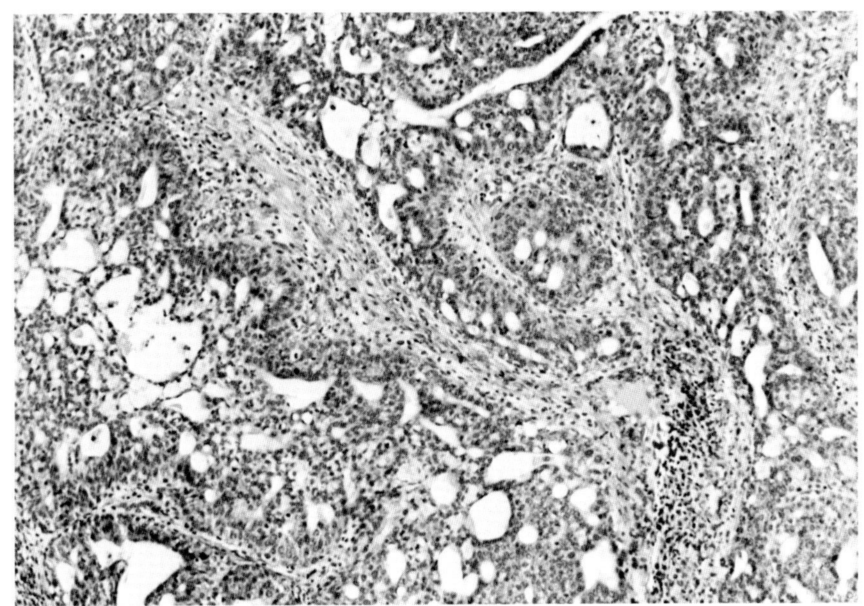

FIGURE 1. (b)

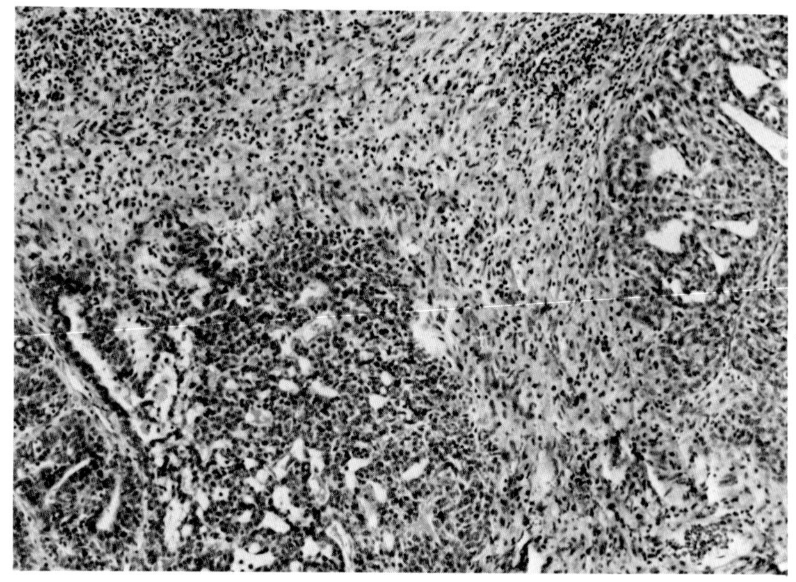

FIGURE 1. (c)

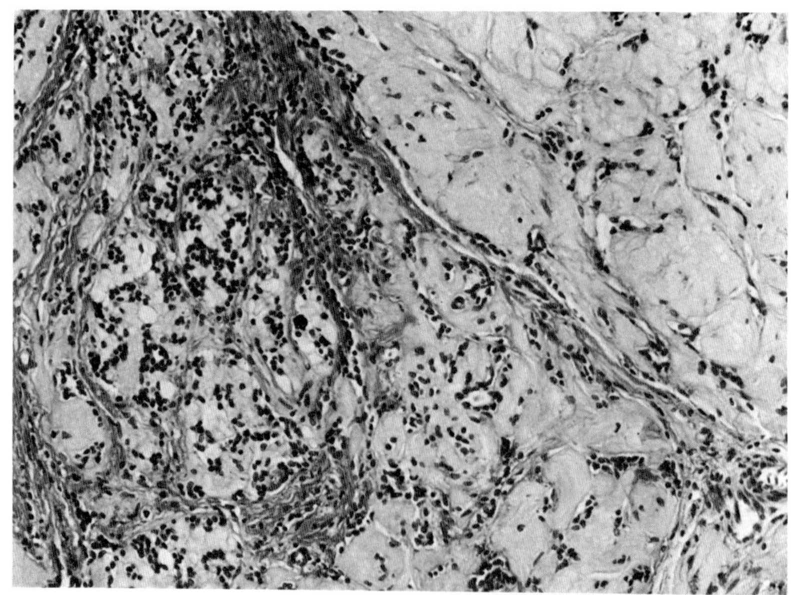

FIGURE 1. (d)

of connective tissue separating variable sized nests of epithelial cells (Fig. 1a). In larger tumors, the connective tissue bands were much more prominent (Fig. 1b,c). Lymphocytes were also frequently present in the stroma. Some tumors were fairly well encapsulated while others invaded the surrounding fat and muscle.

In ovariectomized animals, many of the tumors appeared to be involuting. The epithelial cells were small with scant cytoplasm and condensed nuclei. There was generally a single layer of epithelial cells lining cleftlike acini or tubules. In some cases, there was sloughing of degenerating epithelial cells into the lumens and in some tumors there were foci of viable neoplastic cells. The stroma between and surrounding the collapsed acini consisted of eosinophilic hyaline material (Fig. 1d). The tumors were separated into lobules by fibrous connective tissue bands and were generally surrounded by fibrous capsules.

A few fibroadenomas (13% of total) were detected in each category and a variety of other tumor types were also found. For this study, however, analysis was limited to mammary adenocarcinomas weighing more than 0.2 gm.

B. Hybridization of ^{3}H-cDNA Probes to Tumor RNA

RNA was extracted from adenocarcinomas and hybridized to cDNA specific for a replication-defective endogenous retrovirus (^{3}H-cDNA$_{KiSV}$) and to cDNA specific for the endogenous helper-independent type-C virus (^{3}H-cDNA$_{RaLV}$). Analysis of some tumor RNAs was limited, since the yield of RNA obtained from some small tumors was insufficient to fully saturate the ^{3}H-cDNA tested. Hybridization results on adenocarcinomas obtained from animals in the first category (i.e., those animals receiving only DMBA) was divided into four groups based on tumor size: 0.2-0.5 gm, 0.6-1.0 gm, 1.1-2 gh, and greater than 2 gm.

FIGURE 1. Histology of tumors of different sizes. (a) Adenocarcinoma with thin connective tissue septae dividing variable sized nests of epithelial cells. H & E, X80. (b) Adenocarcinoma with a moderate amount of connective tissue stroma dispersed throughout the tumor. Lymphocytes are scattered through the stroma. H & E, X80. (c) Adenocarcinoma with abundant connective tissue stroma separating island of epithelial structures. Lymphocytes are abundant in the stroma. H & E, X80. (d) Involuting adenocarcinoma in an ovariectomized rat. The epithelial cells lining cleftlike spaces are small with little cytoplasm and condensed nuclei. There is abundant hyalinized material separating the cells. H & E, X130.

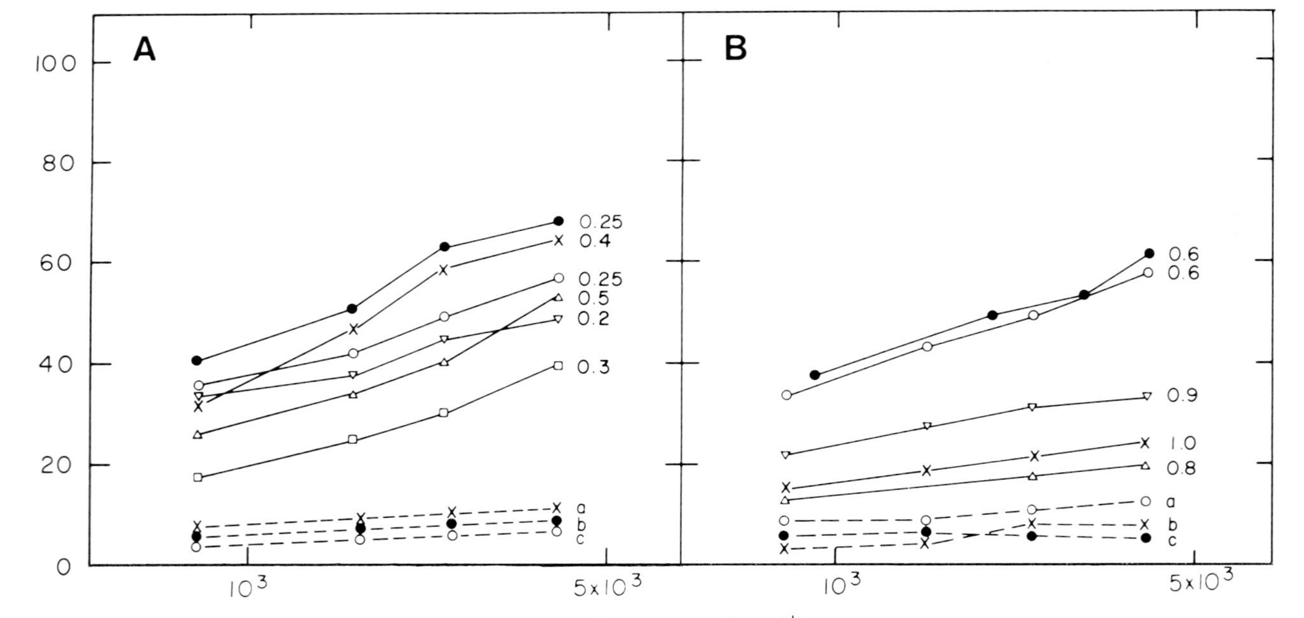

FIGURE 2. Viral RNA levels in tumors of different sizes. RNA was extracted from adenocarcinomas and hybridized to ^{3}H-cDNA$_{KiSV}$ as described in Materials and Methods. Approximately 2500-3000 TCA precipitable cpm of ^{3}H-cDNA were used in each reaction mixture. 100% hybridization represents hybridization of ^{3}H-cDNA$_{KiSV}$ to HTP RNA or ^{3}H-cDNA$_{RaLV}$ to RT21C RNA after subtraction of an S_1 nuclease background of 100 cpm (approximately 80% of input cpm hybridized). It was previously determined that ^{3}H-cDNA$_{RaLV}$ would hybridize to the RNA of the Sprague-Dawley helper-independent type-C virus (Rasheed et al., *1976) to the same extent as to RT21C RNA (unpublished observations).*

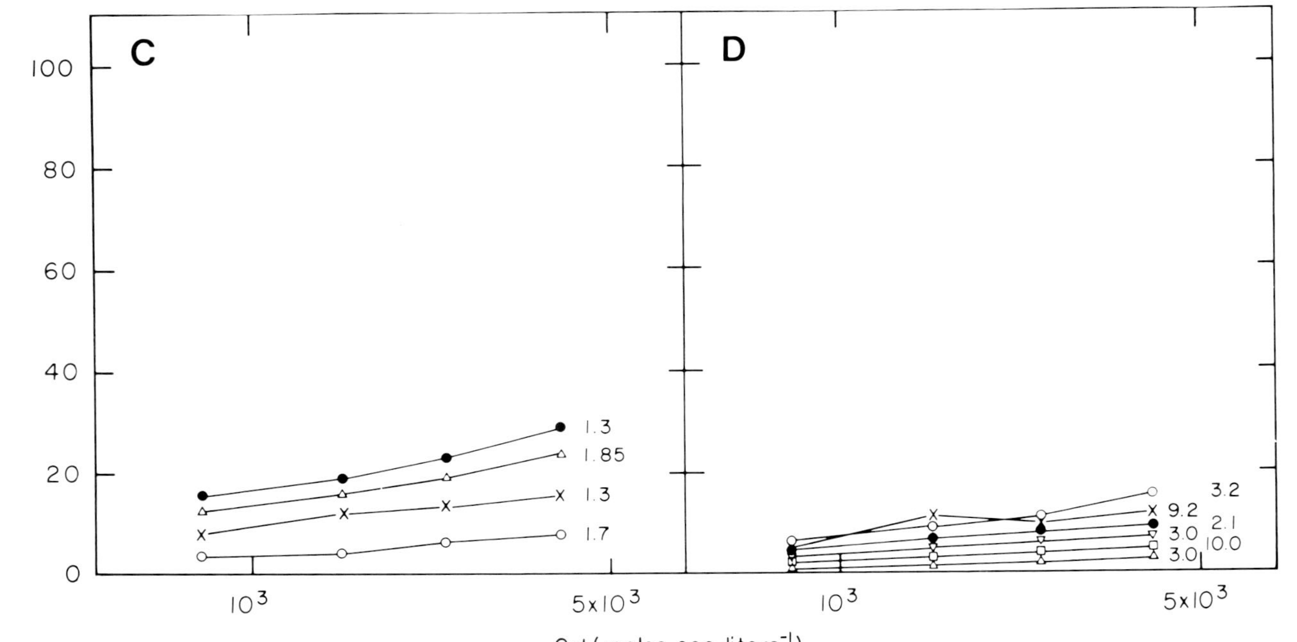

(Fig. 2. cont) (A) 0.2 - 0.5 gm tumors: dotted lines (a-c) represent hybridization of 0.4, 1.3, and 3.2 gm tumor RNA to ^{3}H-cDNA$_{KiSV}$. (B) 0.6 - 1.0 gm tumors: dotted line (a-c) represents ^{3}H-cDNA$_{KiSV}$ to mammary gland, normal spleen, and normal liver RNA. Liver and spleen RNA from DMBA-treated tumor-bearing animals gave essentially identical results. (C) 1-2 gm tumors. (D) >2 gm tumors. Data represent hybridization to tumors obtained from nine separate animals.

As seen in Fig. 2, division of tumors on the basis of weight produced an unexpected grouping of hybridization patterns. It is apparent from this figure that the smaller tumors (Fig. 2A,B) contained higher levels of RNA related to the replication-defective retrovirus than the larger tumors (Fig. 2C,D). RNA related to the helper-independent virus was not detected in any adenocarcinoma tested, regardless of size (Fig. 2A, a-c). In addition, no significant type-C virus RNA of either kind was detected in liver or spleen from control animal or in liver or spleen from the same DMBA treated rats, or in mammary gland from a retired breeder (Fig. 2B, a-c). As reported previously (Anderson and Robbins, 1976), RNA homologous to the replication-defective type-C retrovirus was detected in uteri (not shown), but the levels of the RNA appeared to vary from animal to animal without any as yet predictable pattern. Alkaline treatment of the tumor RNA abolished all hybridization, and RNA from large tumors did not inhibit the hybridization observed with the RNA from small tumors (not shown).

C. *Viral RNA Expression in Hormone-Dependent Tumors*

Expression of endogenous type-C retrovirus as RNA was also monitored in mammary adenocarcinomas that exhibited hormone responsiveness following ovariectomy. Those tumors that decreased in size for two consecutive weeks after ovariectomy were classified as hormone dependent and the results of RNA analysis of these tumors can be seen in Fig. 3. Based on the decrease in tumor volume, it is estimated that the size of these tumors at the time of ovariectomy was approximately 2-3 times that recorded when the animals were sacrificed, and thus these results should be compared to the data presented in Fig. 2 (B-D). When making this comparison, it appears that the steady-state level of the RNA of the endogenous replication-defective virus did not substantially change following ovariectomy although slightly less hybridization was observed. Similar comparisons were not possible with smaller tumors because their size after ovariectomy was too small to permit analysis. Though not shown in Fig. 3, no significant expression of RNA of helper-independent type-C virus was observed in these regressing tumors.

Tumors that decreased in size following ovariectomy and subsequently increased in size when animals were then treated with 17 β-estradiol were also classified as hormone dependent. However, the larger tumors did show a greater increase in size than the smaller tumors. Analysis of retrovirus RNA in these tumors can be seen in Fig. 4. Significant expression of RNA of the replication-defective virus was observed in both small

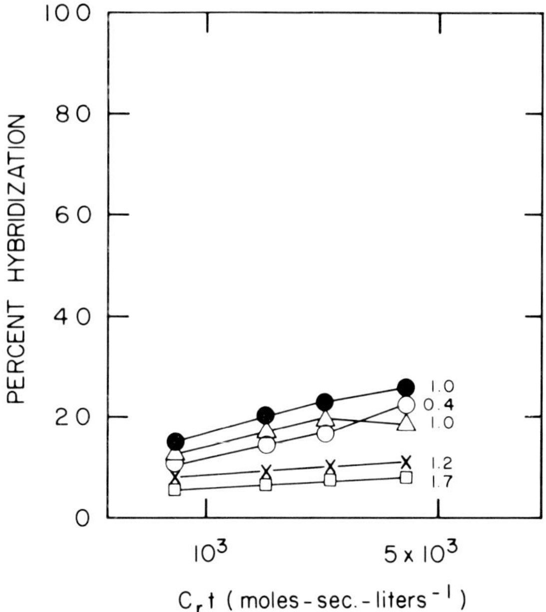

FIGURE 3. Viral RNA levels in hormone-dependent tumors following ovariectomy. RNA from adenocarcinomas that were removed after ovariectomy was analyzed by hybridization as described in Materials and Methods. 100% hybridization was determined as described in Fig. 2. Data represent tumors obtained from four separate animals.

(Fig. 4A) and, surprisingly, in large tumors (Fig. 4B). As with the other tumors, no significant expression of RNA of helper-independent retrovirus was observed in these tumors.

D. *Establishment of a Cell Line from a DMBA-Induced Mammary Tumor*

In order to further analyze the expression of RNA of endogenous type-C retroviruses in mammary adenocarcinomas, attempts were made to establish a cell line from these tumors. Three tumors (two adenocarcinomas, one fibroadenoma) from one animal were removed, trypsinized and the cells maintained in Dulbecco's medium containing $10^{-8}M$ 17 β-estradiol, 1 μg/ml prolactin, and 10% fetal bovine serum. A stable cell line (B_8) was obtained from one adenocarcinoma and analyzed for the RNA of both endogenous rat type-C retroviruses. As seen in Fig. 5, expression of RNA of the replication-defective retrovirus was readily de-

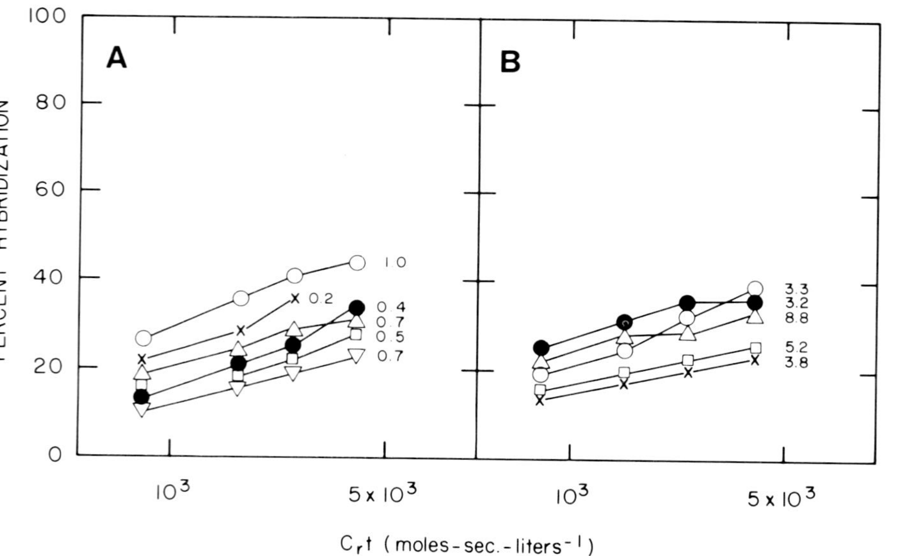

FIGURE 4. Viral RNA levels in hormone-dependent tumors following estrogen treatment. RNA from adenocarcinomas that regressed after ovariectomy and then increased in size following estrogen administration was analyzed by hybridization as described in Materials and Methods. 100% hybridization was determined as described in Fig. 2. (A) 0.2 - 1.0 gm tumors. (B) >1.0 gm tumors. Data represent tumors obtained from five separate animals.

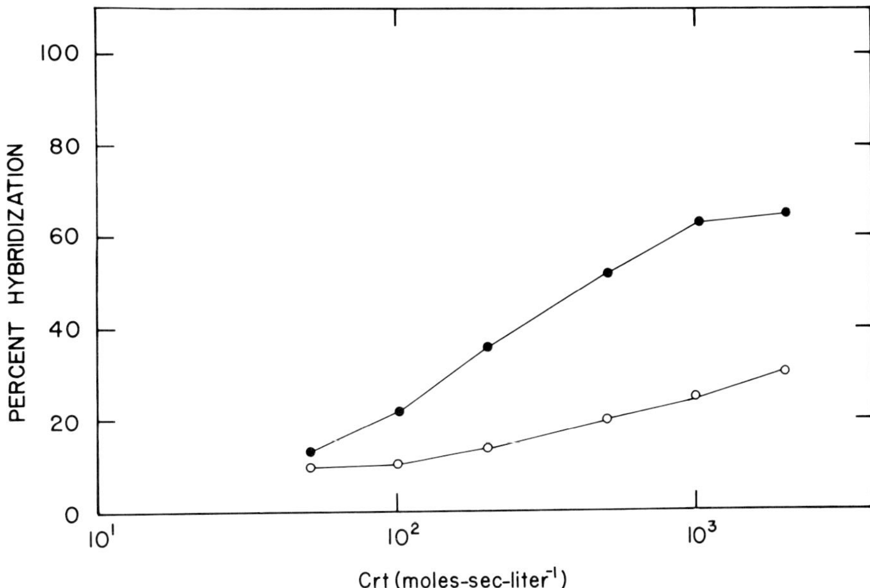

FIGURE 5. Hybridization to RNA of a cell line from a mammary adenocarcinoma. B_8 cells were grown in modified Dulbecco's medium containing 10% fetal calf serum. Cells were harvested, RNA was extracted, and this RNA analyzed as described in Materials and Methods. 100% hybridization was determined as described in Fig. 2 and represents 2000-25000 cpm. (●——●), ^3H-cDNA$_{KiSV}$; (○——○), ^3H-cDNA$_{RaLV}$.

tected and the 1/2 Crt (moles·secondxliters^{-1}) for this viral RNA was about 1-2 x 10^2, a value very similar to that observed in the small adenocarcinomas. A low level of endogenous helper-independent virus RNA was also detected in these cells but this RNA was at least 2 logarithim lower in concentration than the RNA for the replication-defective virus.

E. *Comparison of RNA in Cells of Mammary or Uterine Tumor Origin*

A second probe, ^{3}H-cDNA$_{HTP}$, specific for the replication-defective viral sequences in a uterine adenocarcinoma from another Sprague-Dawley rat was prepared as described in Materials and Methods. Hybridization of this probe to DNA and RNA from the uterine adenocarcinoma cell line (HTP), and to DNA and RNA from the mammary tumor cell line (B_8) was performed. As seen in Fig. 6A, the rate and extent of hybridization of ^{3}H-cDNA$_{HTP}$ to DNA$_{HTP}$ or DNA$_{B8}$ was identical. In contrast,

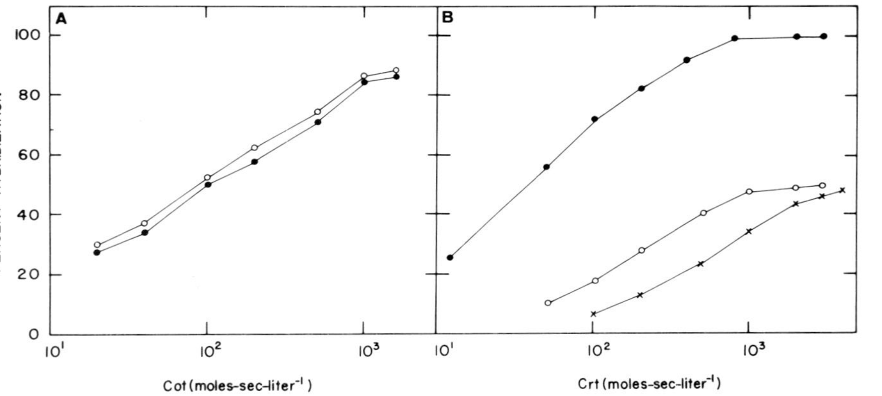

FIGURE 6. Hybridization to DNA or RNA of uterine and mammary tumor cell lines. Nucleic acids from the cell line HTP, the cell line B_8, and a primary mammary adenocarcinoma were prepared as described in Materials and Methods. Approximately 2500-3000 TCA precipitable cpm of ^3H-cDNA$_{HTP}$ were included in each hybridization reaction mixture. Analysis of DNA and RNA hybrids was done by S_1 nuclease (Leong et al., *1972). 100% hybridization represents final extent of hybridization of ^3H-cDNA$_{HTP}$ to excess HTP DNA or RNA after subtraction of an S_1 nuclease background of 100 cpm (2000-2500 cpm). The 1/2 Cot for rat unique sequence DNA has previously been determined to be 10^3 moles/sec/liter (Scolnick* et al., *1976a). (A) ●——● DNA$_{HTP}$; o——o DNA from mammary adenocarcinoma (0.4 gm tumor) or DNA$_{B8}$. (B) ●——● RNA$_{HTP}$ o——o RNA$_{B8}$; x——x mammary adenocarcinoma RNA (0.4 gm tumor).*

hybridization of this ^{3}H-cDNA$_{HTP}$ to RNA$_{B_8}$ or RNA from the parental mammary tumor (Fig. 6B) reached a plateau of 50% hybridization by S_1 nuclease analysis, as compared to hybridization of this ^{3}H-cDNA to RNA$_{HTP}$. A T_m analysis of the DNA-RNA hybrids was performed to further analyze the hybrids formed with these two cell RNAs.

In Fig. 7A, a similar T_m of 82.5°C was observed with the ^{3}H-cDNA$_{HTP}$·DNA$_{HTP}$ hybrids and the ^{3}H-cDNA$_{HTP}$·DNA$_{B_8}$ hybrids. However, the T_m of the ^{3}H-cDNA$_{HTP}$·RNA$_{HTP}$ hybrids was 83°C while the ^{3}H-cDNA$_{HTP}$·RNA$_{B_8}$ hybrids melted with a T_m of 77°C (7B). Thus, the expression of viral RNA in the B_8 mammary tumor from one Sprague-Dawley rat is distinguishable from the viral RNA in the DMBA-induced uterine tumor from another Sprague-Dawley rat.

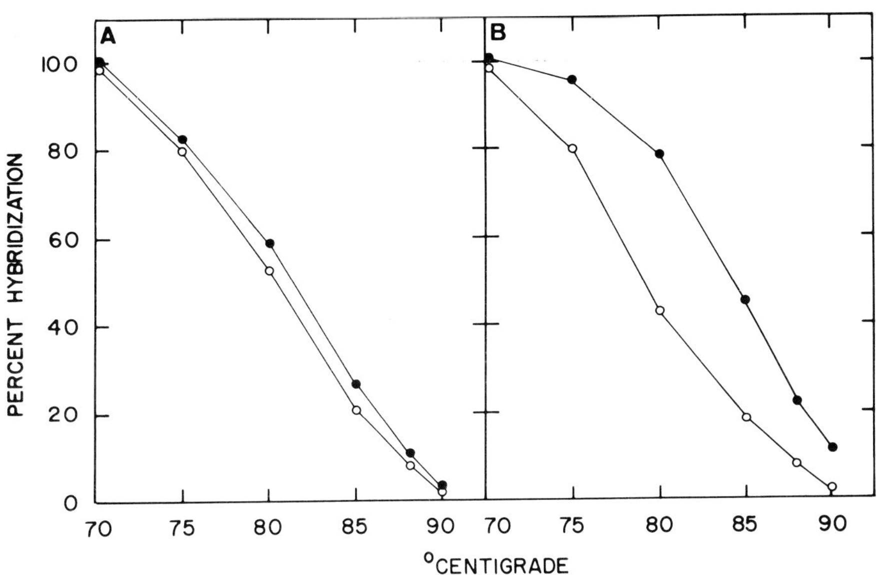

FIGURE 7. Thermal melting curves of hybrids. Hybridization of ^{3}H-cDNA$_{HTP}$ to HTP DNA or RNA, mammary tumor DNA or RNA, and B_8 DNA or RNA, was carried out to a Cot or CRT of 5 x 10^3 moles/sec/liters. At that time the hybridization reactions were frozen, duplicate tubes heated at various temperatures for 5 min and then immediately frozen in a dry ice-acetone bath. Analysis of hybrids was by S_1 nuclease as described previously (Leong et *al., 1972). 100% hybridization represents the hybridization of ^{3}H-cDNA$_{HTP}$ to HTP DNA or RNA after subtraction of an S_1 nuclease background of 100 cpm (2000-2500 cpm). (A) ●——● DNA$_{HTP}$; o——o mammary adenocarcinoma DNA (0.4 gm tumor) or DNA B_8; (B) ●——● RNA$_{HTP}$; o——o RNA$_{B_8}$ or mammary adenocarcinoma RNA (0.4 gm tumor).*

F. *Induction of Viral Sequences by Halogenated Pyrimidines*

When B_8 cells were treated with IUdR, a significant increase in both replication-defective retrovirus RNA and helper-independent type-C viral RNA was detected (Fig. 8). Interestingly, hybridization of ^{3}H-cDNA$_{HTP}$ to the B_8RNA now gave over 80% S_1 nuclease resistance indicating that additional related sequences of the replication-defective virus could be expressed as RNA in this cell line.

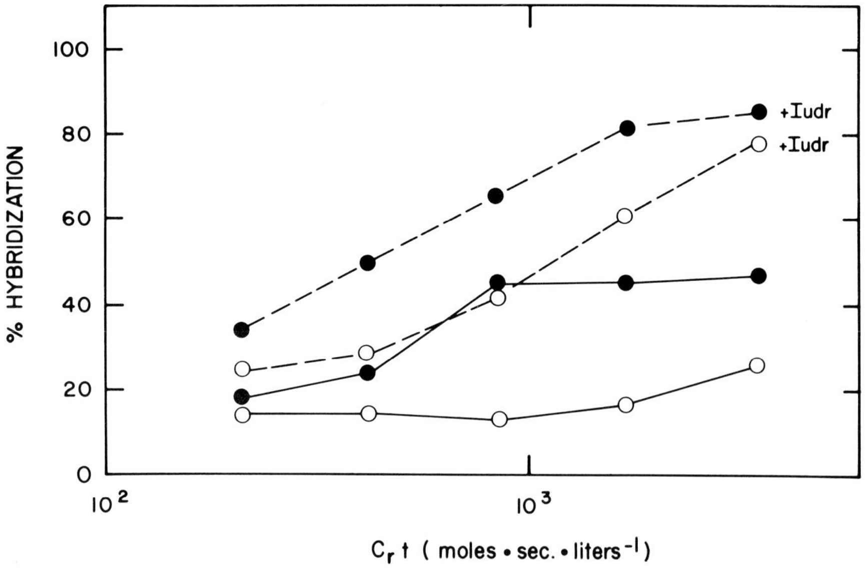

FIGURE 8. Hybridization to RNA obtained after 5-IUdR treatment of B8 cells. B8 cells were seeded in 150 cm² flasks and allowed to grow to 50-60% conflurncy. At that time 5-IUdR was added to a concentration of 20 μg/ml, the cultures incubated at 37°C for 48 hr and the RNA extracted as described in Materials and Methods. 100% hybridization represents hybridization of ^{3}H-cDNA$_{HTP}$ to RNA$_{HTP}$ or ^{3}H-cRNA$_{RaLV}$ to RT21C RNA after sub traction of an S_1 nuclease background of approximately 100 cpm (2000-2500 cpm). ●—● o---o ^{3}H-cDNA$_{HTP}$; o—o o---o ^{3}H-cDNA$_{RaLV}$.

IV. DISCUSSION

Dimethylbenz(a)anthracene-induced rat mammary tumors have proven to be an important experimental animal model in breast cancer research. The majority of mammary tumors induced by DMBA are adenocarcinomas which, like human mammary adenocarcinomas, are ductal in origin, do not appear to originate from hyperplastic alveolar nodules (Sinha and Dao, 1975; Russo *et al.*, 1977; Haslam and Bern, 1977), and are also highly responsive to hormonal manipulation. Ovariectomy of the animals causes most of the tumors to regress in size and this regression can be reversed by the administration of estrogen or prolactin (Dao, 1972; Meites, 1972; Leong and Sasaki, 1975: Weisch and Nagasawa, 1977). Individual mammary tumors can, however, vary greatly in such parameters as size, histology, enzyme content, latency, and response to hormonal manipulation (Stevens *et al.*, 1965; Archer and Orlando, 1968; Hilf *et al.*, 1969, 1970; McGuire and Julian, 1971; Boylan *et al.*, 1977; Hawkins *et al.*, 1977), thus making general conclusions about DMBA-induced tumors difficult. We have investigated another potential parameter for mammary tumor development by studying the expression of RNA of two endogenous rat type-C retroviruses. One virus is helper-independent, and is similar to other mammalian type-C viruses in its morphological and biochemical characteristics but appears to be ecotropic to the rat (Cremer *et al.*, 1970; Gazzolo *et al.*, 1971; Bergs *et al.*, 1972; Klement *et al.*, 1972, 1973; Sarma *et al.*, 1973; Benveniste and Todaro, 1973; Rasheed *et al.*, 1976). The other endogenous retrovirus is replication-defective and is of interest because a large portion of it is part of two known transforming viruses, the Kirsten and Harvey sarcoma viruses (Scolnick *et al.*, 1974; Roy-Burman and Klement, 1975; Scolnick *et al.*, 1976a; Shih *et al.*, 1978). From the current studies, several observations seem worthy of note.

(i) Most earlier studies involving chemical transformation of rat cells and chemically induced tumors were confined to analyses of markers of helper-independent rat viruses (Bergs *et al.*, 1970; Rhim *et al.*, 1973; Freeman *et al.*, 1973), and in contrast to these studies, we have detected significant expression of RNA of a replication-defective retrovirus but not RNA of a type-C helper-independent virus in DMBA-induced rat mammary adenocarcinomas. The highest levels of this RNA were observed in the smaller tumors (0.4 - 1.0 gm) which, in contrast to the larger tumors (>2.0 gm), had the highest proportion of tumor tissue to connective tissue. The molecular survey clearly does not allow us to indicate a causal relationship between expression of the rat viral RNA and tumor formation. However, the levels of this viral RNA in the small tumors are sufficient to potentially be etiological, as previous studies on Rous sarcoma virus transformation of mammalian cells have indicated that low levels (1/2 Crt 10^3 - 10^4) of sarcoma virus RNA are sufficient to maintain the transformed phenotype of the cell (Deng *et al.*, 1974).

(ii) The obvious hormonal control of tumor development has made a second observation in these studies of interest. Estrogen treatment following ovariectomy seems to increase the steady-state levels of the RNA of the replication-defective type-C virus in the larger tumors, in addition to increasing tumor size. Thus, it will be important in future studies to determine if estrogen is affecting at a transcriptional level the expression of RNA of the replication-defective type-C virus in specific cell populations of the hormone-responsive tumors.

(iii) It is important to consider in these studies the observation that all rats contain multiple copies of these retroviral genomes in their DNA (Scolnick *et al.*, 1976a). It is expected that there may be divergence among the 20-40 copies per genome of this defective rat virus. Thus, it is of interest that the expression of viral RNA in the HTP cell derived from a uterine adenocarcinoma is distinguishable from the RNA in the B_8 cell line derived from a mammary adenocarcinoma. Analysis of the T_m of the hybrids formed suggest that the expression of viral RNA in the B_8 cell is of a related but not identical copy of this defective endogenous virus. However, as seen in Fig. 8, it appears that the expression of RNA of additional related sequences in the B_8 cell can be detected under certain conditions. In future studies it will be important to determine if expression of RNA of different copies of this virus is random or has some specificity that correlates to the type of normal (e.g., uterus, testes) or transformed cell in which transcription of endogenous virus sequences occurs.

(iv) Up to now the only model of viral involvement in breast cancer development has been the mouse, in which the levels of expression of certain strains of type-B retroviruses are highly correlated to tumor formation (Bentvelzen and Daams, 1969; Nandi and McGrath, 1973; Bentvelzen, 1974; Heston and Parks, 1975). The observations on the DMBA-induced rat mammary tumors suggest an additional model system for viral involvement in breast cancer. As opposed to MMTV, the rat virus has RNA with many of the properties of type-C viral RNA, is replication-defective, does not form viral particles, and does not code for structural proteins immunoreactive with structural proteins of known type-B or type-C viruses (Scolnick *et al.*, 1976a,b). Thus, this type of retrovirus would not be detected in most conventional searches for expression of viral RNA or proteins in rat breast tumors or breast tumors in other species. Interestingly, we have also detected RNA related to the replication-defective virus in x-irradiation-induced and nitrosomethyl urea-induced breast tumors. Thus, these results, at minimum, indicate the necessity of considering the role or replication-defective endogenous retroviruses in carcinogen-induced, x-irradiation-induced, or naturally occurring tumors where viral particles have not been detected.

REFERENCES

Anderson, G. R., and Robbins, K. D. (1976). *J. Virol 17,* 335-351.

Archer, F. L., and Orlando, R. A. (1968). *Cancer Res. 28,* 217-224.

Bentvelzen, P. (1974). *Biochem. Biophys. Acta 355,* 136-259.

Bentvelzen, P., and Daams, J. H. (1969). *J. Natl. Cancer Inst. 43,* 1025-1035.

Benveniste, R. E., and Scolnick, E. M. (1973). *Virology 51,* 370-382.

Benveniste, R. E., and Todaro, G. J. (1973). *Proc. Natl. Acad. Sci. 70,* 3316-3320.

Bergs, V. V., Bergs, M., and Chopra, H. C. (1970). *J. Natl. Cancer Inst. 44,* 913-922.

Bergs, V. V., Pearson, G., Chopra, H. D., and Turner, W. (1972). *Int. J. Cancer 10,* 165-;73.

Boylan, E. S., Fowler, E. H., and Wittliff, J. L. (1977). *Brit. J. Cancer 35,* 602-609.

Chopra, H. C., Bogden, A. E., Zelljadt, I., and Jensen, E. M. (1970). *Europ. J. Cancer 6,* 287-290.

Cremer, N. E., Taylor, D. O., Oshiro, L. S., and Teitz, Y. (1970). *J. Natl. Cancer Inst. 45,* 37-48.

Dao, T. L. (ed). (1972). *In* "Estrogen Target Tissue and Neoplasia," pp. 257-353. University of Chicago Press, Chicago.

Deng, C. T., Boettiger, D., Macpherson, I., and Varmus, H. E. (1974). *Virology 62,* 512-521.

Engle, G. C., Shirahama, S., and Dutcher, R. M. (1969). *Cancer Res. 29,* 603-609.

Freeman, A. E., Gilden, R. V., Vernon, M. L., Wolford, R. G., Hugunin, P. E., and Heubner, R. J. (1973). *Proc. Natl. Acad. Sci. 70,* 2415-2419.

Gazzolo, L., Simkouic, D., and Martin-Berthelon, M. C. (1971). *J. Gen. Virol. 12,* 303-311.

Goldsby, R. A., and Zipser, E. (1969). *Exp. Cell Res. 54,* 271-275.

Harvey, J. J. (1964). *Nature 204,* 1104-1105.

Haslam, S. Z., and Bern, H. A. (1977). *Proc. Natl. Acad. Sci. 74,* 4020-4024.

Hawkins, R. A., Hill, A., Freedman, B., Killen, E., Buchan, P., Miller, W. R., and Forrest, A. P. M. (1977). *Europ. J. Cancer 13,* 223-228.

Heston, W. E., and Parks, W. P. (1975). *Can. J. Genet. Cytol. 17,* 493-502.

Hilf, R., Goldenberg, H., Michel, E., Carrington, M. J., Gruenstein, M., Meranze, D. R., and Shimkin, M. B. (1969). *Cancer Res. 29,* 977-988.

Hilf, R., Goldenberg, H., Gruenstein, M., Meranze, D. R. and Shimkin, M. B. (1970). *Cancer Res. 30,* 1223-1230.

Huggins, C., Briziarelli, G., and Sutton, H. (1959). *J. Exp. Med. 109,* 25-54.

Huggins, C., Grand, L. C., and Brillantes, F. P. (1961). *Nature 189,* 204-207.

Kirsten, W. H., and Mayer, L. A. (1967). *J. Natl. Cancer Inst. 39,* 311-335.

Klement, V., Nicolson, M. O., Gilden, R. V., Oroszlan, S., Sarma, P. S., Rongey, R. W., and Gardner, M. B. (1972). *Nature New. Biol. 238,* 234-237.

Klement, V., Nicolson, M. O., Nelson-Rees, W., Gilden, R. V., Oroszlan, S., Rongey, R. W., and Gardner, M. B. (1973). *Int. J. Cancer 12,* 654-666.

Leong, J., Garapin, A. C., Jackson, N., Fanshier, L., Levinson, W. E., and Bishop, J. M. (1972). *J. Virol. 9,* 891-902.

Leong, B. S., and Sasaki, G. H. (1975). *Endocrinology 97,* 564-572.

Marmur, J. (1961). *J. Mol. Biol. 3,* 208-218.

McGuire, W. L., and Julian, J. A. (1971). *Cancer Res. 31,* 1440-1445.

Meites, J. (1972). *J. Natl. Cancer Inst. 48,* 1217-1224.

Nandi, S., McGrath, C. M. (1973). *Adv. Cancer Res. 17,* 353-414.

Rasheed, S., Bruszewski, J., Rongey, R. W., Roy-Burman, P., Charman, H. R., and Gardner, M. B. (1976). *J. Virol. 18,* 799-803.

Rhim, J. S., Duh, R. G., Cho, H. Y., Elder, E., and Vernon, M. L. (1973). *J. Natl. Cancer Inst. 50,* 255-261.

Roy-Berman, P., and Klement, V. (1975). *J. Gen. Virol. 28,* 193-198.

Russo, J., Saby, J., Isenberg, W. M., and Russo, I. H. (1977). *J. Natl. Cancer Inst. 59,* 435-445.

Sarma, P. S., Kunchorn, P. D., Vernon, M. L., Gilden, R. V., and Berg, V. (1973). *Proc. Soc. Exp. Biol. 142,* 461-465.

Scolnick, E. M., Maryak, J. M., and Parks, W. P. (1974). *J. Virol. 14,* 1435-1444.

Scolnick, E. M., Goldberg, R. J., and Williams, D. (1976a). *J. Virol. 18,* 559-566.

Scolnick, E. M., Williams, D., Maryak, J., Vass, W., Goldberg, R. J., and Parks, W. P. (1976b). *J. Virol. 20,* 570-582.

Scolnick, E. M., Vass, W. C., Howk, R. S. and Duesberg, P. H. (1979). *J. Virol.* 964-972.

Sekiya, S., Takamizawa, H., Wang, F., Takane, T., and Kuwata, T. (1972). *Am. J. Obstet. Gynecol. 113*, 691-695.
Shih, T. Y., Young, H. A., Coffin, J. M., and Scolnick, E. M. (1978). *J. Virol. 25*, 238-252.
Sinha, D., and Dao, T. L. (1975). *J. Natl. Cancer Inst. 54*, 1007-1009.
Stevens, L., Stevens, E., and Currie, A. R. (1965). *J. Pathol. Bacteriol. 89*, 581-589.
Taylor, J. M., Illemensee, R., and Summers, J. (1976). *Biochim. Biophys. Acta 442*, 324-330.
Weinstein, I. B., Gerbert, R., Stadler, U. C., Orenstein, J. M., and Axel, R. (1972). *Science 178*, 1098-1100.
Weisch, C. W., and Nagasawa, H. (1977). Cancer Res. 37, 951-963.

IMMUNOLOGICAL ASPECTS OF BREAST CANCER

THE POTENTIAL OF VIRAL VACCINES FOR INTERVENTION IN MAMMARY NEOPLASIA: PRESENT STATUS AND A LOOK INTO THE FUTURE

Asher Frensdorff

Department of Microbiology,
The Dr. George S. Wise
Faculty of Life Sciences,
Tel Aviv University,
Tel Aviv, Israel

INTRODUCTION

In the past few years striking successes have been reported in preventing tumor-virus-induced neoplasias in animals by active or passive immunization with viral or subviral preparations, or with antisera directed against them. Suffice it to cite, in this context, the example of Marek's Disease which is today successfully controlled in fowl on an industrial scale by preventive vaccination.

The basic question becomes, therefore, not: "can virus-induced tumors be controlled by vaccination" but "what are the best and safest ways to achieve this purpose."

Much of the experimental work, which enables us to make this statement today, was done in C-type virus tumor models, and will be reviewed by J. N. Ihle elsewhere in this volume. It should, however, be emphasized that where B- and C-type viruses are concerned, host-virus interrelations may differ at crucial points. Extrapolation of conclusions from one model to another is therefore not only unwarranted, but may indeed be misleading. Viral vaccine studies in experimental mammary tumor models have so far been few and have progressed much more slowly in comparison. Two major difficulties have probably discouraged many investigators from engaging in this field. First, no practical methods to isolate MuMTV viral polypeptides,

ISBN 0-12-131150-3

acceptable *both* with respect to yield and to purity of the final product, were available. Methods which qualify to some extent for both these criteria have only very recently been published (Sarkar and Dion, 1975; Dion *et al.*, 1977; Ritzi *et al.*, 1976a,b; Frensdorff and Ben Yaakov, 1977; Creemers *et al.*, 1977). Second, the very model systems which, from the standpoint of similarity to human breast cancer, seem to be the most interesting and relevant ones, are characterized by the late age and low frequency at which spontaneous mammary tumors occur. Such model systems require, therefore, long-term studies and very large experimental groups if the effect of a given treatment on the incidence of spontaneous tumors is to be investigated. Not only is a great deal of patience required, but often existing animal facilities simply cannot accommodate this type of experiment.

Some investigators have attempted to circumvent the long observation period required to assess incidence of spontaneous tumors by studying instead the susceptibility of treated animals to a challenge with infective virus or with syngeneic viable tumor cells. Unfortunately, the susceptibility or resistance of an animal to such a challenge depends to a large extent on arbitrarily selected experimental conditions, and may therefore be a poor, or worse a misleading, parameter in assessing the efficacy of a vaccine (see also Section V).

One of the aims of these types of studies is to provide us with new insights about host-virus interrelationships and to provide additional proof, where required, that oncoviruses are indeed the causative agents of the tumor with which they are associated. Their real *raison d'être* is, however, the expectation that they will supply us with urgently needed information about the applicability of vaccination approaches to a few, selected, human cancers. Breast cancer, because of its high prevalence, its still very high mortality rate (Levine, 1977), and of course, because of its suspected association with a mammary tumor viruslike agent (discussed in Section VI) is one of the prime, if not *the* prime target for such studies. The importance of vaccination studies in experimental mammary tumor models can therefore, in spite of the cost and the effort involved, not be emphasized enough.

THE RATIONALE

Attempts to influence the host's susceptibility to naturally occurring, as well as to transplanted experimental tumors started early, on an entirely empirical basis. Experiments, in which the effect of immunizing mice with live or fixed mammary tumor cells, or with cell-free extracts prepared therefrom, were made at a time when it was still controversial as to whether mice are tolerant to murine mammary tumor virus (MuMTV) or not.

Recently, more and more emphasis has been put on studying the effect of immunogens ("vaccines"), which would be safe enough to be used in humans should results in experimental model systems warrant such a decision. This category comprises immunogens that are absolutely devoid of any potentially infective nucleic acid, viral or cellular. The two major groups of preparations that fulfill these criteria are purified structural components of MuMTV (mainly surface antigens) and tumor-specific nonviral antigens.

In retrospect the rationale for these experiements is perfectly sound; it is based on the following two arguments:

(a) MuMTV antigens are expressed in, but more importantly on, the surface of mammary tumor cells (Bentvelzen and Brinkhof, 1977; Yang, *et al.*, 1977. St. George *et al.*, 1978; Schochetman *et al.*, 1978). This has been particularly well documented for gp52, the major surface antigen of MuMTV. Tumor cells are thus a potential target for a recognition mechanism with specificity for these determinants:

(b) Mice are definitely not tolerant to their natural tumor virus antigens. A natural immune response (IR) to C- and D-type retroviruses has been detected in all species investigated so far in this respect; this has been particularly well documented in mice (for a recent review, see Ihle and Hanna, 1977), cats (Essex, 1977), and nonhuman primates (Fine *et al.*, 1978a). Similarly, mice do mount a natural immune response to MuMTV. This response is both humoral, as documented in immunodiffusion studies (Blair *et al.*, 1966; Bentvelzen *et al.*, 1970; Blair, 1971; Müller and Zotter, 1973), by immunofluorescence using tumor cells as targets (Bentvelzen and Creemers, 1977), and more recently, by radioimmunoassay (Ihle *et al.*, 1976; Fine *et al.*, 1978b; Wald, *et al.*), as well as cell mediated (Heppner, 1969; Blair *et al.*, 1974; Bentvelzen and Creemers, 1977; Tagliabue *et al.*, 1978).

Both forms of reactivity are detectable early in life. Even in mouse strains in which mammary tumors appear (i.e., become palpable) as early as six or seven months of age antibodies, as well as cytotoxic lymphocytes, are probably present long before the first tumor cells have started to divide. The driving force of this IR must therefore be virus load or virus expression, and not the growing tumor itself. In other words, the virus-induced tumor develops on the background of a preexisting immune response directed against antigenic determinants expressed on the tumor cells.

This type of natural, or autogenous, IR is also regularly present in strains of mice genetically selected by inbreeding for very high tumor incidence, such as the RII/Imr strain maintained by us, in which all female breeders develop early tumors (average age 189 days, range 145-275 days) (Frensdorff and Wald, 1978). It must therefore be concluded that this form of natural IR provides very little, if any, protective effect against the tumor. This may be due to a multitude of reasons, such as a quantitative insufficiency; a balance between humoral and cell/mediated immunity that is unfavorable for tumor cell destruction; a fine specificity of the recognition mechanism of the IR, directed against an antigenic determinant on tumor cell membrane-associated gp^{52}, which is sterically inaccessible or protected. Alternatively, active mechanisms emanating from the tumor cell, which inactivate the effector mechanisms of the IR, such as a constant shedding of surface antigen molecules from the cell, secretion of proteolytic enzymes, or of immunosuppressive substance, to name only a few, must also be considered. It may be assumed that more than one mechanism is operative. At present, however, our knowledge does not permit us to go beyond simply listing some of the possibilities.

Much more germane to the present problem is the notion that vaccination, at least that form induced by active immunization, is thur not a *de novo* immunization of an animal with a hitherto unknown antigen, but must be seen as an attempt to manipulate an existing natural IR in such a way as to elicit a better result, i.e., achieve a tumor protective effect.

It is noteworthy that the rationale of the vaccination approach as presented here is entirely independent of the etiological involvement of MuMTV in murine mammary tumors.

DESIGN OF A GENERAL VACCINATION STRATEGY

At present we have not yet reached the stage where we can design a strategy, let alone a generally applicable one, to be followed in vaccination experiments, and which would ensure some measure of success. At best, we can define the major risks and conclude there-from a few criteria to be observed.

A. *Introduction, Via the Inoculum, of Potentially Oncogenic Genetic Material of Viral or Cellular Origin*

Clearly, we do not want to expose the individual we wish to protect by vaccination to an agent known to induce neoplasia, even if we were certain that the host range of the virus does not permit replication in that particular species. MuMTV was thought for many years to be restricted to mouse cells and some investigators have indeed contemplated using an inactivated MuMTV vaccine in humans (J. Charney, personal communication). Only very recently Lasfargues, after laborious efforts, has shown that this is not so; MuMTV can be grown in cat, mink (Lasfargues and Sheffield, 1976; Howard *et al.*, 1977), and human cells (Lasfargues and Coutinho, 1978).

Inactivation of the virus, like any chemical reaction, cannot be expected to achieve absolute completion and is therefore not to be relied on. In addition, isolates of one virus may be expected to be contaminated with small amounts of other viruses endogenous to the host from which they are isolated, and which may be hazardous to the vaccinated organism (Zuckerman, 1978). Tumor cells cannot be used for vaccination for precisely the same reasons.

A safe vaccine for the future would therefore have to be entirely free from genetic information in any form, such as purified viral polypeptides or nonvirus associated tumor cell-membrane antigens. This intends, in no way, to belittle the extremely valuable information that vaccination studies with structurally intact viruses have yielded.

B. *Induction of Autoimmune Disease*

It is mainly a matter of semantics whether antigens of endogenous (i.e., germ-line transmitted) viruses expressed on normal or on tumor cells represent "self" or "non-self" constituents. The natural IR, which exists normally against these antigens, although it may be considered an autoimmune reaction, and in spite of the fact that it leads to deposition of antibody-viral antigen complexes in the kidneys (Yoshiki *et al.*, 1974; Slovin *et al.*, 1977), obviously does not lead to autoimmune disease. The only well/documented exception to this seems to be in NZB mice (for recent review, see Levy, 1977). Deliberate immunization against such an antigen could of course change the picture entirely, and damage or destroy vital normal cells in which the virus, or closely related and cross/reactive endogenous viruses, are propagated. Interestingly, this does not seem to be the case. To the best of our knowledge, no case of autoimmune disease resulting from vaccination with purified viral antigens has been reported to date.

Since, however, most virus preparations, which serve as starting material for the preparation of vaccines, are contaminated with host/cell antigens, it is felt that every possible precaution should be taken to remove these contaminants.

Purification of disrupted MuMTV preparations over a solid immunoadsorbent consisting of goat-anti-mouse normal mammary gland tissue antibodies (Creemers *et al.*, 1977) or an immune precipitation of gp^{52} from lectin-sepharose-purified glycoproteins of MuMTV by a goat antiserum monospecific to gp^{52} (Frensdorff and Ben-Yaakov, 1977; Ben-Yaakov and Frensdorff, 1977) are examples in point. By the same token vaccines should be, as far as possible, free from structural antigens of other C-type tumor viruses.

C. *Tumor Enhancement Resulting from Vaccination*

Tumor enhancement, i.e., accelerated appearance and/or increased incidence of tumors is by far the most real danger inherent in vaccination procedures as demonstrated by recent observations in our own lab (Burowski, *et al.*, 1979; as well as reports by Jones *et al.*, 1977; Creemers *et al.*, 1977, 1978). It is probably our most urgent task to clarify the precise immune mechanisms that are induced by immunization and that lead to enhancement of an oncorna-virus-induced tumor, so that it will be possible to avoid inducing these in designing vaccination protocols. Before this goal is satisfactorily achieved, no extension of experimental vaccinations to human cancer can be safely envisaged.

It is beyond the scope of this presentation to review in detail all the possible mechanisms that have been evoked to explain enhancement. The most commonly held concept concerning enhancement was introduced to vaccination studies by tumor immunologists and implied, in a much oversimplified way, that protection against tumors is provided solely by the cell-mediated IR. In contrast, antibodies to tumor antigens are assumed to facilitate tumor growth in all cases, either by combining with tumor cell surface antigens, thus shielding them from recognition by effector cells of CM immunity, or by combining with soluble tumor antigens with the resulting formation of immune complexes, with either inactivate effector cells or stimulate the proliferation of suppressor T cells. (Creemers and Bentvelzen 1977).

In mouse leukemias, lymphomas (Ihle and Hanna, 1977), and also in murine mammary tumors, high titers of autogenous antibodies directed against the causative virus were regularly detected (Ihle *et al.*, 1976; Wald, *et al.*, in preparation). Free (i.e., not in antigen-antibody complex form) gp^{52} was detected in the plasma of mammary-tumor-bearing mice (Ritzi *et al.*, 1976a,b 1977), which supposedly also had antibodies against the same antigen. These observations reinforced the view that antibodies represent no essential part of tumor immunity. It should be borne in mind, however, that many of the experimental data on which this concept is based were obtained in systems substantially different from the set-up of a virus-induced tumor growing on the background of a preexisting IR.

This concept of tumor enhancement by antibodies may apply to the situation which prevails when a non-virus-induced tumor (e.g., chemical carcinogen induced) develops; indeed, many of the observations which led to its formulation were made in carcinogen-induced, or in serially transplanted tumors. It must be borne in mind that in such models the host is exposed to the tumor specific antigens (TSAs) for the first time at the moment the first tumor cell makes its appearance; when transplantation is practiced, the organism is suddenly confronted with a considerable antigen load. In naturally occurring virus-induced tumors, such as the murine mammary tumors, the organism is exposed to the TSAa according to an entirely different time course. In the tumors which are induced by endogenous germ/line transmitted MuMTVs and which occur late and in low frequency (in C_3Hf, RIIIf, BALB/c and related mouse strains), there is no "infection." The organism is exposed from the moment that virus expression starts to the same TSAs (the virus surface antigens) that are ultimately also expressed on the surface of the tumor cells when the tumor eventually develops. In the early, high frequency, tumors induced by exogenous (horizontally transmitted) MuMTVs (those arising in the C_3H, RIII, BALB/cfC_3H and related mouse strains) there is an initial, sudden exposure to massive doses of infective virus. It may be very important that this exposure occur in the neonatal period, when the organism is immunologically not fully competent. However, no tolerance is induced. This initial exposure is followed by progressively increasing expression of *de novo* synthesized virus on normal cells, which proceeds uninterrupted until the first neoplastic cell arises. Thus, the common donominator of virus-induced tumors, endogenous as well as exogenous, is the prolonged exposure to TSAs, which precedes tumor development, whereas in the other tumors this first exposure is simultaneous with tumor development. Moreover, the prolonged progressively increasing virus expression by host cells (in the case of exogenous tumor virus this stage probably represents the infection, by virus, of more and more target cells) seems to be a necessary prelude to tumorigenesis.

The difference in the time course of events between virus/ induced and other tumors, as well as a growing body of reports describing successful tumor control using antisera directed against virus-associated tumor cell surface antigens (Hunsmann *et al.*, 1975; Huebner *et al.*, 1976; Gardner *et al.*, 1977; De Norhona *et al.*, 1978; Collins *et al.*, 1978a,b; Haagensen *et al.*, 1978) led us to reexamine the concept that antibodies to viral antigens have no effect, or even an enchancing effect on tumorigenesis, and to consider whether it seemed warranted to arrtibute the same enhancing effect to an immune-effector mechanism during the pretumor, as well as the tumor phase. These two phases should be clearly distinguished, and the possibility of different effects of the humoral IR on the course of events in each one should be considered.

THE EFFECT OF PASSIVE IMMUNIZATION WITH ANTISERUM TO MuMTV ON MuMTV EXPRESSION AND ON MAMMARY TUNORIGENESIS

To test this hypothesis we have studied the effect of an antiserum to MuMTV, administered to newborn female RIII/Imr mice during the period in which infection with exogenous MuMTV takes place (i.e., the suckling period), on the regulation of MuMTV expression in the stages that precede tumorigensis and its effect on tumor igenesis (Frensdorff and Wald, 1978; Wald and Frensdorff, 1979; Wald, *et al.*, in preparation).

The RIII strain carries both an exogenous (milk transmitted) and an endogenous (germline transmitted) MuMTV (Moore *et al.*, 1976; Michalides and Schlom, 1975). Tumor incidence in multiparous females in our RIII colony is 100% at an average age of occurrence of 189 days (range: 4.5-9 months). The antiserum used in these experiments (αMuMTV) was a high titered precipitating goat antiserum (50% endpoint in double antibody RIA: $7 \chi 10^{-5}$), produced in our laboratory against MuMTV-S grown in tissue culture (Fine *et al.*, 1974). It reacted with MuMTV-S as well as with MuMTV-P. The bulk of antibody in this serum was directed against the major surface antigen of MuMTV, gp52, and, recognized in addition to gs determinants on this glycoprotein also ts determinants, present only in gp52 of MuMTV-S (Sidransky *et al.*, 1979).

Antiserum was administered in 10 i.m. injections, equally spaced over the first 21 days of life; before receiving the last injection, the newborns were separated from their mothers. One group received increasing amounts of whole antiserum (50 μl/injection), a total of 3.75 ml/mouse. A second group received 50 μl of a 10 χ concentrated globulin fraction of the antiserum at each injection, totaling 5.0 ml of antiserum equivalent per mouse. Controls consisted of untreated mice and of mice treated with normal goat serum (NGS) or the globulin fraction thereof.

At the age of four weeks all females, including controls, were force bred; this regimen [which considerably enhances mammary tumor development (Boot, 1969)] was maintained until each surviving female had terminated the ninth pregnancy.

The most striking observations made in the course of this study were the following:

a) MuMTV expression (assessed by the concentration of MuMTV antigens in the milk of treated and untreated mice) was completely supressed or at least sharply reduced and delayed in most of the αMuMTV-treated animals, whereas NGS had no effect whatsoever; 14 out of a total of 44 αMuMTV-treated mice had no detectable virus antigen in their milk of third lactation, whereas all untreated and NGS/treated mice had high concentrations. MuMTV expression was more strongly suppressed in those animals receiving the globulin fraction of αMuMTV (equivalent to 5 ml of antiserum/mouse); 10 out of a total of 20 animals in this group were negative. Seven out of the negative mice remained negative throughout the milk of ninth lactation.

b) The effect of treatment on the appearance of mammary tumors was even more dramatic. Only five of the mice (25%) treated with the globulin fraction of αMuMTV developed tumors before the age of nine months as opposed to 100% in the control groups. Ten of the remaining mice are still tumor free at more than 19 months of age, whereas four died at 18-19 months without tumors. Here, too, the effect of treatment was much more marked in the mice which had been treated with the globulin fraction (75% tumor-free animals) than in the group treated with whole antiserum (17% tumor free). Animals which had no, or very low, MuMTV antigen in the milk of third lactation remained tumor free throughout their life. However, no regression curve could be fitted for the plot of antigen concentration in milk vs. the age of appearance of the tumors.

It is of interest to note that none of the mice treated with αMuMTV or with NGS showed any gross signs of autoimmune disease, in spie of the fact that the antiserum slightly reacted with various mouse serum proteins.

MuMTV concentration in mouse milk increases with parity (Moore *et al.*, 1976; Frensdorff and Wald, unpublished data). This suggests that the initial virus load, which each suckling newborn mouse receives, also increases with parity of the mother. It was therefore of interest to investigate the age of spontaneous tumor occurrences in females originating from different parities of their respective mothers. Surprisingly, descendants from late (>5) parities, developed tumors which occurred later (range: 145-275 days) than descendants from early (first and second) parities (range: 145-212 days). The difference between the two cumulative tumor incidence curves was statistically significant ($p < 0.01$). This could result from the higher efficiency of infection of MuMTV (when injected parenterally) at low concentrations, reported by Charney and Moore (1972), or alternatively, by another factor, which in addition to initial virus load, plays a regulatory role in virus expression. Passively transferred maternal antibody to MuMTV could be such a factor. The titer of this antibody in female MuMTV-carrying mice increases with age (Ihle *et al.*, 1976; Wald, *et al.*, in preparation). Whether an intricate interplay between these two factors is indeed operative is at present under investigation.

In any case, this study has clearly demonstrated that antibodies to MuMTV do have a profound effect on exogenous MuMTV expression and on tumorigenesis when administered during the period of massive infection with the exogenous tumor virus, and that this effect is quite the opposite from enhancement.

An extremely important question is whether this type of immune intervention, i. e., administration of antibodies to a heterologous cross-reacting exogenous virus, affects the expression of only exogenous MuMTV, or whether that of the germ-line transmitted MuMTV is also suppressed. It is possible that the passively administered antibody simply resulted in the elimination of most, or all, of the exogenous virus introduced via milk in some of the animals. However, the fact that seven tumor-free mice did not express MuMTV antigens in the milk at the ninth lactation, an age at which most exogenous virus-free RIIIf mice express endogenous MuMTV in their milk (D. H. Moore, personal communication), raises the possibility that expression of endogenous MuMTV has also been affected by the administration of αMuMTV. Kende *et al.* (1978) have recently shown that active immunization of BALB/c, C57Bl, and NIH/Swiss mice with a formalin-inactivated exogenous virus (MuLV-R) leads to suppression of expression of endogenous C-type virus in these mice. Whether a similar suppression of endogenous MuMTV has occurred in our mice is presently being investigated in our laboratory. In any case, in designing future vaccination experiments these effects will have to be considered.

THE EFFECT OF ACTIVE IMMUNICATION WITH VIRAL OR SUBVIRAL VACCINES ON SUSCEPTIBILITY TO CHALLENGE WITH INFECTIOUS VIRUS AND ON SPONTANEOUS TUMORIGENESIS

A. Vaccination With Structurally Intact but Inactivated MuMTV

1. Effect on Susceptibility to Challenge with Infective Exogenous Virus. The foundations for systematic studies in active immunization against MuMTV were laid in Charney's and Moore's (1972) experiments. The protocol, which was also essentially followed in experiments reported later (Charney *et al.*, 1976), consisted for a single intramuscular injection of formalin-inactivated MuMTV (purified from RIII milk), given with complete Freund's adjuvant to 4-6 week old mice. Animals were challenged by injection of 30 ng of infective RIII virus. Absence of MuMTV antigens in milk obtained from vaccinated mice after their third pregnancy, tested in agar-gel immunodiffusion (Charney *et al.*, 1969), was taken as an indication that animals were protected.

The basic experiment in this series was performed in C57Bl/Haag mice. Mice of this subline (Charney *et al.*, 1969) normally neither express MuMTV nor develop mammary tumors, but are susceptible to infection with infective RIII MuMTV at 8-10 weeks of age (55% of mice became positive after inoculation with 30 ng of virus in the infectivity assay used by the authors). In these experiments it was established that by the criteria used C57Bl mice can be completely protected against subsequent challenge with infective virus with inactivated MuMTV by a single vaccination. In subsequent studies (Charney *et al.*, 1976; Sarkar and Moore, 1978) the dose dependency of the protective effect was established; 10 and 1 μg of vaccine proveded complete protection; at lower doses the effect decreased rapidly. Interestingly, low doses (10^{-3} and 10^{-4}μg) of vaccine, especially when given with incomplete Freund's adjuvant, seemed to enhance MuMTV expression under the experimental conditions.

2. *Effect on Incidence of Spontaneous Mammary Tumors in Mouse Strains which Naturally Develop Such Tumors.* In RIII mice (95% of the females in the colony studied were positive in the infectivity assay at third lactation and 85% of multiparous females developed early tumors) the effect of this vaccination protocol was only marginal. Tumor incidence was not decreased, but development was consistently delayed (27 days at 50% endpoint).

In similar experiments involving mouse strains which express endogenous MuMTV (RIIIf and Af) (Charney *et al.*, 1976) a very substantial protective effect was achieved: Only 9.2% of vacinated RIIIf females had tumors at 23 months of age, as compared to 25% in untreated animals. If Af mice the tumor incidence at this age was similar to control groups, but there was a very substantial delay in their appearance.

The authors concluded from these observations that by their criteria a high degree of protective immunity could be achieved in mice expressing endogenous MuMTV only, whereas mice expressing endogenous and exogenous MuMTV could not be protected at all.

In retrospect, these conclusions may have been overcautious. One is tempted to assume that a suboptimal immunization protocol may have adversely influenced the results in these studies. A recent study involving murine C-type retrovirus

(Kende *et al.*, 1978) indicates that using large and repeated doses of similarly inactivated MuLV-R (a total of 1,150 μg given in 12 injections spaced over a few months) almost completely suppressed expression of endogenous ecotropic C-type viruses in immunized mice, thus establishing that a vaccine prepared from exogenous tumor virus can indeed suppress expression of endogenous virus. It is also possible that better results could have been achieved in the RIII strain had a heterologous vaccine (e.g., one prepared from C_3H virus) rather than a homologous one, been used, as earlier observations made in the GR strain would suggest (Bentvelzen, 1972).

B. Vaccination With Subviral Vaccines (Partially Purified Polypeptides of MuMTV Devoid of Nucleic Acid)

1. Effect on Susceptibility of Mice, Which Do Not Express MuMTV, to Challenge with Exogenous MuMTV. The effect of vaccination with the major surface antigen of MuMTV,(gp^{52}), on the susceptibility of C57Bl mice to challenge with RIII virus was studied by Sarkar and Moore (1978) using a vaccination protocol essentially similar to that of Charney and Moore, (1972) (see Section V. A.1). Two preparations of gp^{52} were tested; in one, the glycoprotein was released from the virions by repeated sonication in the presence of detergent, followed by two-step chromatographic purification (Sarkar and Dion, 1975); in the other, gp^{52} was released from virions by acid treatment (Sarkar *et al.*, 1976). Vaccination with 10 μg (but not with 1 μg) of purified gp^{52} conferred complete protection (no MuMTV antigen in milk of the third lactation and no mammary tumors at the end of a two-year observation period, as opposed to 50% and 56%, respectively, in unvaccinated control mice). The acid-solubilized gp^{52} was ineffective, suggesting that it had been too denatured to retain immunogenicity. The fact that more of the purified protein was required to confer protection than when inactivated but structurally intact virus was used probably reflects the generally decreased immunogenicity of antigenic determinants presented on soluble molecules as opposed to the same determinant on a carrier particle.

2. The Effect on Susceptibility to Tumor Challenge of Mice Which Do Express Endogenous MuMTV (BALB/c and DBAF). The gp^{52} enriched fraction used in experiments of Creemers *et al.*, 1977) was prepared from virus purified from BALB/cfC_3H tumors and disrupted by sonication. MuMTV-unrelated host proteins were removed by sepharose-coupled goat antiserum to normal mouse mammary gland tissue. Glycoproteins were separated from nonglycosylated polypeptides with Con-A-Sepharose.

According to the authors, about 60% of the protein in the preparation is gp52, whereas the rest is mostly Con A. Substantial "leakage" of lectin, coupled to CNBr-activated Sepharose 4B and contaminating eluates has also been our own experience (Ben-Yaakov and Frensdorff, unplublished), and has led us since to abandon CNBr-activated Sepharose as a matrix for lectins. This contamination of the vaccine with Con A may be of considerable importance in assessing the effects of the vaccine, especially those elicited by large doses, since there are numerous reports on the immunosuppressive effect of Con A (activation of suppressor T cells) when injected together with antigen into mice (Markowitz *et al.*, 1968; Markham *et al.*, 1977; Ekstedt *et al.*, 1977; Machida *et al.*, 1977; to cite only a few examples).

The vaccination protocol consisted of an, i.p., injection of vaccine (different doses were used) in PSB, as alum precipitate or with a fraction isolated from Mycobacterium smegmatis. Both adjuvants have been shown to exert a nonspecific antitumor activity of their own. Twenty days later animals were challenged with cells from a serially subcutaneous transplanted BALB/c mammary tumor originally induced by MuMTV-O or alternatively with L 1210 leukemia cells (which also express MuMTV antigens), which were alternatively passaged in (DBAf x BALB/c) F_1 mice and *in vitro*.

In BALB/c mice challenged with BALB/c tumor cells, 1 μg of vaccine administered with 5 μg of alum led to a 10-week delay in appearance of the tumors as compared to controls, but all animals finally succumbed. 100 μg of vaccine given with 500 μg of alum markedly accelerated tumor development. Booster injections were found to be without significant effect.

3. *The Effect on the Incidence of Spontaneous Tumors.* The same authors (Creemers *et al.*, 1978) have also now reported their first observations on the effect of different doses of their vaccine (see above, Section V. B.2), as well as the effect of combinations of the vaccine with different adjuvants, on spontaneous tumors. Mice of the high tumor incidence GR and BALB/cfC3H strains, as well as of the low tumor incidence strains, BALB/c and C3Hf, were included in this study. One of the most striking findings was that the administration of 10 μg of the vaccine significantly delayed tumors in the two high-tumor strains, whereas the same treatment accelerated their appearance in BALB/c and C3Hf mice. The effect of a vaccine prepared from MuMTV-O on tumors in BALB/cfC3H mice was also studied. When 10 μg of this vaccine were injected in alum precipitated form, a 61% decrease in tumor incidence occurred. Again, it was observed that booster injections, (two or five injections of one tenth of the initial

vaccine dose) did not further increase the effect on tumor development achieved by the first immunization, although they induced an increase in antibody titer.

Another important finding was the poor correlation between the effect of the vaccine on the susceptibility of BALB/c mice to a tumor challenge and its effect on primary tumorigenesis in mice of the same strain. This observation will have to be considered when designing further experiments.

In several respects (e.g., dose dependence of the effect of the vaccine and occurrence of enhancement) the results reported by these investigators with the subviral vaccine differ from those reported by groups who have used structurally intact, but inactivated, virus. Such differences have not been observed with different types of C-type virus vaccines.

Whether these differences are really related to the use of solubilized virus proteins, rather than particles, for immunization, or whether they are due to contaminating components present in the vaccine awaits further clarification.

CONCLUSIONS AND A LOOK INTO THE FUTURE

The picture that emerges from the studies reviewed in Sections IV and V is a rather complex one. There are, however, two basic conclusions to be drawn.:

(a) Manipulation of the natural immune response of mice against MuMTV by either passive or active vaccination with viral, subviral, or antiviral vaccines *can* lead to a state where substantially fewer and/or later tumors develop in a treated population, than would normally occur.

(b) Such manipulation can induce, under certain circumstances, the very opposite effect. Thus, in the murine mammary tumor model, enhancement of tumors is not only a potential risk but a very real danger.

Though immunity can prevent tumors, clearly not all effector mechanisms of immunity positively contribute to their control; moreover; the same effector mechanism, may, in different stages of the host-virus interrelation behave differently, and thus the timing of vaccination with respect to tumor appearance will probably become a very important consideration.

We are still mostly in the dark as to what triggers, or what specifically stimulates, those effector mechanisms which negatively affect tumor control, such as suppressor T cells, so that the balance may ultimately be tipped in favor of tumor development. Many factors have been implicated: the dose of immunogen and the extent of antigenic difference between it and the virus naturally expressed in the host; the type and amount of adjuvant used; timing of the immune manipulation; and the genetic background of the host. Doubtless this list will still grow before we start to see some light.

Clearly, getting to understand which effector mechanisms favor tumorigenesis and learning how to control them is now the central issue if we want to make use of the great tumor-preventive potential of vaccines without running the danger of inducing tumor enhancement. To achieve this goal more studies, in which all measurable parameters of the IR are constantly and longitudinally monitored in individual untreated, as well as in vaccinated, animals will be necessary. It has been shown that the susceptibility to tumor challenge, shortly after vaccination, is not a reliable parameter of protective immunity against spontaneous tumors; long-term studies, which last until all animals have a chance to develop spontaneous tumors will therefore be necessary to gain a better understanding of this problem. Mouse strains which display an intermediate tumor incidence, and in which the immune status of surviving animals that ultimately did develop tumors can be compared, retrospectively, with those that did not develop them will probably prove to be the most valuable models in this respect. Such studies are already under way in several laboratories including those in Rijswijk, the Netherlands, and our own.

Will attempts to control neoplasia by vaccination ever be applicable to breast cancer? There is definitely a rationale for such a hope. Since the first reports in the early 1970s, that a MuMTV-like particle could be demonstrated in, an isolated from, human breast cancer (Spiegelman *et al.*, 1972, Schlom *et al.*, 1972), there has been a growing body of evidence indicating that breast cancer tissues contain an antigen which cross-reacts with MuMTV, and which has not been detected in normal breast tissue or in benign mastopathies. This antigen was most often demonstrated by its reaction with antisera to MuMTV (Müller and Grossman, 1972, Seman and Dmochowski, 1973, Moore, 1974, Black *et al.*, 1975). Recently, the methods and reagents used to detect and localize this antigen have become better and better controlled with respect to specificity (Newgard *et al.*, 1976, Keydar *et al.*, 1978, Mesa-Tejada *et al.*, 1978, Black *et al.*, 1978, Wanebo *et al.*, 1978). The cross reaction could be specifically blocked by purified gp52 of MuMTV or elicited with a monospecific antiserum to gp52 (Keydar *et al.*, 1978).

If this antigen is also expressed *on* the membrane of tumor cells, the host's immune system could be trained by prior vaccination to recognize and attack selectively tumor cells as they arise. In view of the cross reactivity of this antigen with gp52 of MuMTV such vaccination could conceivably be performed with purified gp52 of MuMTV, or with antibodies against it. This would bring such a project to the realm of the logistically feasible.

The basis for this concept is the existence, in human breast cancer tissue, of an antigen which cross reacts with murine gp52. It is important to note that it does not imply that the cross-reacting antigen is somehow involved in the etiology of human breast cancer, nor does the validity of this concept require this. However, before we proceed to apply this idea to immunoprevention of human breast cancer we must learn to prevent tumor enhancement lest immunoprevention turn accidentally into immunoinduction.

ACKNOWLEDGMENTS

The experimental work performed in the author's laboratory and described in this publication was funded in part by Public Health Service Contracts NO1 CP 53517 and NCI-CP-VO-71011-63 from the Virus Cancer Program within the Division of Cancer Cause and Prevention, National Cancer Institute. Some of the materials used in these studies were obtained through the Office of Program Resources and Logistics, Virus Cancer Program.

REFERENCES

Bentvelzen, P.,(1972). *In* "Fundamental Research on Mammary Tumors" (J. Mouriquand, ed.). p 129. Inserm, Paris.

Bentvelzen, P., and Brinkhof, J. (1977). *Eur. J. Cancer 13,* 241-245.

Bentvelzen, P., and Creemers, P. C. (1977). *In* "Contemporary Topics in Immunobiology" (M. G. Hanna Jr. and F. Rapp. eds.) Vol. 6, pp. 229-238. Plenum Press, New York.

Bentvelzen, P., Van Der Gugten, A., Hilgers, J., and Daams J. H. (1970). *In* "Immunity and Tolerance in Oncogenesis" (L. Severi, ed.), pp. 525-539. Perugia, Italy, Division of Cancer Research.

Ben-Yaakov, M., and Frensdorff, A. (1977). *Israel. J. Med. Sci. 13,* 1034-1035.

Black, M. M. (1977). *In* "Contemporary Topics in Immunobiology" (M. G. Hanna Jr. and F. Rapp, eds.) Vol. 6, pp. 239-262. Plenum Press, New York.

Black, M. M., Zachrau, R. E., Shore, B., Moore, D. H., and Leis, H. P. (1975). *Cancer 35,* 121-128.

Black, M. M., Zachrau, R. E., Shore, B., and Leis, H. P. (1978). *Proc. Am. Assoc. Cancer Res. 19,* 15.

Blair, P. B. (1971). *Israel J. Med. Sci. 7,* 161-186.

Blair, P. B., and Lane, M. A. (1978). *Internat. J. Cancer, 21,* 476-481.

Blair, P. B., Lavrin, D. H., Dezfulian, M., and Weiss, D. W. (1966). *Cancer Res. 26,* 647-652.

Blair, P. B., Lane, M. A., and Yagi M. J. (1974). *J. Immunol. 112,* 693-705.

Boot, L. M. (1969). Ph. D. thesis, Induction by prolactin of Mammary tumors in mice. University of Amsterdam; Amsterdam, The Netherlands.

Burowski, Witz, and Frensdorff, A. (1979). *Israel J. Med. Sci.,* (in press).

Charney, J., and Moore, D. H. (1972). *J. Natl. Cancer Inst. 48,* 1125-1129.

Charney, J., Pullinger B. D., and Moore, D. H. (1969). *J. Natl. Cancer Inst. 43,* 1289-1296.

Charney, J., Holben J. A., Cody, C. M. and Moore, D. H. (1976). *Cancer Res. 36,* 777-780.

Collins, J. J., Sanfilippo, F., Tsong-Chou, L., Ishizaki, R., and Metzgar, R. S. (1978a). *Internat. J. Cancer Inst. 21,* 51-61.

Collins, J. J. Roloson, G., Haagensen, D. E., Fischinger, P. J., Wells, S. A., Holder, W., and Bolognesi, D. P. (1978b). *J. Natl. Cancer Inst. 60,* 141-152.

Creemers, P., and Bentvelzen, P. (1977). *Eur. J. Cancer 13,* 261-267.

Creemers, P., Ouwehand, J., and Bentvelzen, P. (1977). *J. Natl. Cancer Inst. 59,* 895-903.

Creemers, P., Ouwehand, J., and Bentvelzen, P. (1978). *J. Natl. Cancer Inst. 60,* 1461-1466.

De Norhona, F., Schäfer, W., Essex, M., and Bolognesi D. P. (1978). *Virology 85,* 617-621.

Dion, A. S., Williams, C. J., and Pomenti, A. A. (1977). *Anal. Biochem. 82,* 18-28.

Ekstedt, R. D., Waterfield, J. D., Nespoli, L., and Möller, G. (1977). *Scand. J. Immunol. 6,* 247-253

Essex, M. (1977). *In* "Contemporary Topics in Immunobiology" (M. G. Hanna Jr. and F. Rapp, eds.) Vol. 6, pp. 71-106. Plenum Press, New York.

Fine, D. L., Arthur, L. O., and Plowman, J. K. *et al.* (1974). *Appl. Microbiol. 28,* 1040-1046.

Fine, D. L. Arthur, L. O., and Smith, G. H. (1978a). *Proc. Am. Assoc. Cancer Res. 19,* 111.

Fine, D. L., Devare, S. G., Arthur, L. O., Charman, H. P., and Stephenson, J. R. (1978b). *Virology 86,* 567-571.

Frensdorff, A., and Ben-Yaakov, M. (1977). *Israel. J. Med. Sci. 13,* 967.

Frensdorff, A., and Wald, A. (1978). *J. Natl. Cancer Inst. 61,* 437-439.

Gardner, M. B., Klement, V., Estes, J. D., Gilden, R. V., Toni, R., and Huebner, R. J. (1977). *J. Natl. Cancer Inst. 58*, 1855-1857.

Haagensen, D. E., Roloson, G., Collins, J. J., Wells, S. A., Bolognesi, D. P., and Hansen, H. J. (1978). *J. Natl. Cancer Inst. 60*, 131-139.

Heppner, G. H. (1969). *J. Natl. Cancer Inst. 4*, 608-615.

Howard, D. K., Colcher, D., Teramoto, Y. A., Yound, J. M., and Schlom, J., (1977). *Cancer Res. 37*, 2696-2704.

Huebner, R. J. Raymond, V. G., Toni, R., Hill, R. W., Trimmer, R. W., Fish D. C., and Sass, B. (1976). *Proc. Natl. Acad. Sci. 73*, 4633-4635.

Hunsmann, G., Moennig, V., and Schafer, W. (1975). *Virology 66*, 327-329.

Ihle, J. N., and Hanna, M. G., Jr., (1977). *In* "Contemporary Topics in Immunobiology" (M. G. Hanna Jr. and F. Rapp, eds.) Vol. 6, pp. 169-194, Plenum Press, New York.

Ihle, J. N., Arthur, L. O., and Fine, D. L. (1976). *Cancer Res. 36*, 2840-2844.

Jones, J. M., Kennel, S. J., and Feldman, J. D. (1977). *J. Immunol. 118*, 371-373.

Kende, M., Stephenson, J. R., Kelloff, G. J., Al Ghazzouli I. K., and Dinowitz M. (1978). *Nature (London) 273*, 383-385.

Keydar, I., Mesa-Tejada, R., Ramanarayanan M., Ohno, T., Fenoglio, C, Hu, R., and Spiegelman, S. (1978). *Proc. Natl. Acad. Sci. 75*, 1524-1528.

Lasfargues, E. Y., and Sheffield, J. B. (1976). *J. Microsc. Biol. Cell. 26*, 29-34.

Lasfargues, E. Y., and Coutinho, W. G. (1978). *Proc. Am. Assoc. Cancer Res. 19*, 188.

Levine, P. H. (1977). *In* "Contemporary Topics in Immunobiology" (M. G. Hanna Jr. and F. Rapp, eds.), Vol 6, pp. 263-286, Plenum Press, New York.

Levy, J. A. (1977). *In* "Autoimmunity Genetic, Immunologic, Virologic and Clinical Aspects" (N. Talal, ed.), pp. 404-453, Academic Press, New York.

Machida, A., Yasuda, S., Kumazawa, Y. and Mizunde, K. (1977). *Appl. Immunol. 54*, 158-164.

Markham, R. B., Stashak, P. W., Prescott, B., Amsbaugh, D. F., and Baker, P. J. (1977). *J. Immunol. 118*, 952-956.

Markowitz, H., Person, D. A., Gitnick, G. L., and Ritts R. E., Jr. (1968). *Science 163*, 476-478.

Mesa-Tejada, R., Keydar, I., Ramanarayanan, M., Ohno, T., Fenoglio, C., and Spiegelman, S. (1978). *Proc. Natl. Acad. Sci. 75*, 1529-1533.

Michalides, R., and Schlom, J. (1975). *Proc. Natl. Acad. Sci. 72*, 4635-4639.

Moore, D. H. (1974). *Cancer Res. 34*, 2322.

Moore, D. H. (1978). Personal Communication.
Moore, D. H. Holben, J. A., and Charney, J. (1976). *J. Natl. Cancer Inst. 57,* 889-896.
Müller, M., and Grossman, H. (1972). *Nature, New Biol. 237,* 116-117.
Müller, M., and Zotter, S. (1973). *J. Natl. Cancer Inst. 50,* 713-717.
Newgard, K. W., Cardiff, R. D., and Blair, P. B. (1976). *Cancer Res. 36,* 765-768.
Ritzi, E., Baldi, A., and Spiegelman, S. (1976a). *Virology 75,* 188-197.
Ritzi, E., Martin, D. S. Stolfi, R. L., and Spiegelman, S. (1976b). *Proc. Natl. Acad. Sci. 73,* 4190-4194.
Ritzi, E. Martin, D. S., Stolfi, R. L., and Spiegelman, S. (1977). *J. Exp. Med. 145,* 999-1013.
St. George, J. A. Cardiff, R. D., and Young, L.I.T. (1978). *Proc. Am. Assoc. Cancer Res. 19,* 51.
Sarkar, N. H., and Dion, A. S. (1975). *Virology 64,* 471-491.
Sarkar, N., and Moore, D. H. (1978). *Cancer Res. 38,* 1468-1472.
Sarkar, N. H., Taraschi, N. E., Pomenti, A. A., and Dion, A. S. (1976). *Virology 69,* 677-690.
Schlom, J., Spiegelman, S., and Moore, D. H. (1972). *J. Natl. Cancer Inst. 48,* 1197.
Schochetman, G., Fine, D. L., and Massey, R. (1978). *Proc. Am. Assoc. Cancer Res. 19,* 110.
Seman, G., and Dmochowski, L. (1973). *Cancer 32,* 148.
Sidransky, Y., Ben-Yaakov, M., and Frensdorff, A. (1979). *Israel. J. Med. Sci. 15,* 192.
Slovin, S. F., Bennet, S. J., and Pascal, R. R. (1977). *J. Natl. Cancer Inst. 59,* 1499-1501.
Spiegelman, S., Axel, R., and Schlom, J. (1972). *J. Natl. Cancer Inst. 48,* 1205.
Tagliabue, A., Herberman, R., and Mc Coy, J. (1978). *Proc. Am. Assoc. Cancer Res. 19,* 55.
Wald, A., Ben-Yaakov, M., and Frensdorff, A. (1979). in preparation.
Wald, A., and Frensdorff, A. (1979). *Israel J. Med. Sci. 15,* 194-195.
Wanebo, H. J., Tukuda M., Tsuei, L., Sarkar, N. H., and Modak, M. J. (1978). *Proc. Am. Assoc. Cancer Res. 19,* 146.
Yang, Y., Tang, R., and Nandi, S. (1977). *Biochem. Biophys. Res. Commun. 76,* 1044-1050.
Yoshiki, T., Mellors, R. C., Strand, M., and August, J. T., (1974). *J. Exp. Med. 140,* 1011-1027.
Zuckerman, A. (1978). *Nature (London) 272,* 579-580.

CELL-MEDIATED IMMUNITY TO MAMMARY TUMORS: SO WHAT?*

G. H. Heppner
and
F. R. Miller

Department of Medicine
Roger Williams General Hospital
Division of Biology and Medicine
Brown University
Providence, Rhode Island

I. INTRODUCTION

That tumor-associated immune responses can be detected in mice sensitized to or bearing syngeneic mammary tumors has been known since the pioneering work of Weiss and co-workers (1966). The antigens responsible for the immunity have been found to be of both viral (Weiss *et al.*, 1966; Morton, 1969) and nonviral (Vaage, 1968; Morton, 1969; Heppner and Pierce, 1969) origin. Both spontaneously arising MMTV (murine mammary tumor virus) associated (Weiss *et al.*, 1966; Morton, 1969) and chemically induced (Lopez and Sigel, 1975; Ruppert *et al.*, in press) breast tumors have been found to be immunogenic. The immune effector mechanisms have been shown to be of both the humoral and cell-mediated type and include cytotoxic T- and non-T-cells (Lane *et al.*, 1975), cytotoxic antibodies (Stolfi *et al.*, 1975), serum-blocking factors (SBF) (Heppner, 1969; Blair *et al.*, 1976a), and lymphocyte-dependent antibodies (LDA) (Pollack *et al.*, 1972; Blair *et al.*, 1976b). Similar results have been obtained with human breast cancers (Black *et al.*, 1974; Hollinshead *et al.*, 1974; McCoy *et al.*, 1976; Heppner 1976),

**Supported by USPHS Grants CA 23390 and CA 17074. Dr. Miller is the recipient of USPHS Research Fellowship Award CA 05845.*

ISBN 0-12-131150-3

although the technical difficulties inherent in tumor immunological studies with an outbred, variable population make these studies much more difficult to perform or interpret. Finally, evidence has been presented from animal work indicating that immunotherapy may influence mammary tumor growth (Martin *et al.*, 1964; Rios and Simmons, 1973; Fisher *et al.*, 1975). Thus, a wealth of evidence exists for the presence of active immunity in breast cancer hosts, at least at some times and under some circumstances. Nevertheless, it appears to us that a major question about this immunity, and cell-mediated immunity in particular, remains to be answered. Briefly stated, that question is "So what?" What role does immunity play in the clinical course of breast neoplasia? In order to begin to answer this question, it is necessary to understand some of the basic biological and clinical features of breast cancer so that one may have an idea of where immunity could play a role. It is also necessary to know what the various types of assays for cell-mediated immunity measure *in regard to clinical tumor behavior.* The extensive heterogeneity of breast cancer must be realized and investigated from an immunological standpoint. In addition, the presence of immune reactions *in situ,* within the neoplasm itself, must be known. Over the past two years we, and our colleagues, Dr. Jean Hager, Dr. Beverly Blazar, and Dr. Dan Dexter, have been attempting to resolve these problems and, although we cannot yet definitively do so, we have come to know some of their complexities.

II. CLINICAL CORRELATIONS OF ASSAYS FOR CELL-MEDIATED IMMUNITY

A. *Clinical Behavior of Mouse Mammary Tumors*

The most fundamental characteristic of the clinical behavior of mouse mammary tumors, either autochthonous or early transplants, is variability. This variability is seen not only between tumors of similar origin but even within the same tumor over the course of time. A second fundamental characteristic is the lack of relationship among the various parameters of clinical behavior. This independent assortment of clinical characteristics has been amply documented by Foulds (1969, 1975) for a large number of animal and human cancers. We (Hager *et al.*, 1978) recently analyzed a series of 60 strain BALB/cfC3H mammary tumor populations implanted in syngeneic hosts. For each population we measured the latency period (time to produce a palpable outgrowth from 10^5 cells injected subcutaneously) and the growth rate. We also determined by autopsy and histology the extent of local invasion of the primary implant and the presence of metastases in lungs and visceral organs. These four behavioral parameters were found to be independently assortable. That is, the latency period of a tumor was not related to how fast it grew after it became palpable. Neither of these characteristics were related to invasion or metastasis. Finally, invasion and metastasis, the two hallmarks of malignancy, were themselves unrelated. This last point is illustrated in Fig. 1.

It seems obvious that if the various characteristics of a tumor that contribute to its clinical course are themselves independent variables, it will be impossible for any immune response to be interacting uniformly to influence all of them or to have a clear-cut relationship with some general characteristic, such as survival. Failure to appreciate this may be contributing to the poor success rate of attempts to "monitor" immune reactivity in terms of clinical course in human cancer patients. In any event we have tried to see whether immune reactivity is related to any behavioral characteristic by doing

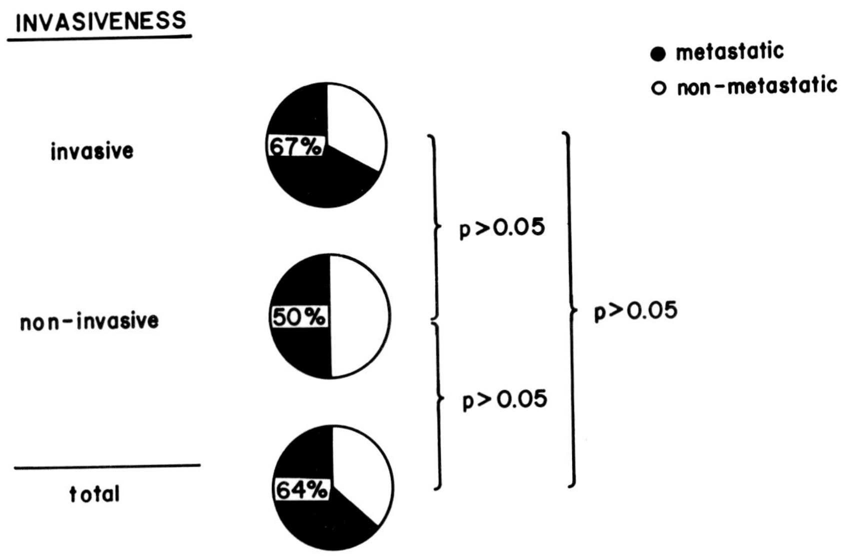

FIGURE 1. The relationship between the presence of local invasion by subcutaneous implants of strain BALB/cfC$_3$H mammary tumors and the presence of metastases in lungs or visceral organs. The upper circle represents the tumors which were invasive; the middle circle represents those which were noninvasive. The bottom circle represents all tumors. The shaded areas are for metastatic, the open areas nonmetastatic tumors. Invasion and metastases are shown to be independent.

a multivariate analysis of the four characteristics and the ability of the same 60 BALB/cfC3H mammary tumors to induce CMI, SBF, and LDA.

B. *Clinical-Immunological Correlates of Mouse Mammary Tumors as Measured by Microcytotoxicity Assay*

Strain BALB/cfC3H male mice were sensitized to the mammary tumors by subcutaneous injection of 10^5 tumor cells followed by surgical removal of the resulting tumor. At 10-14 days after surgery, their lymph node cells (LNC) were tested for CMI against the sensitizing and other tumor cells. Sera taken at the time and 10-14 days after surgery were tested for their ability to both block CMI and to arm LNC in an antibody-dependent cellular cytotoxicity assay. Thus, both SBF and LDA were assessed. The data were analyzed to see which immune parameters correlated with which behavioral characteristics. As shown in Table I, the relationships were sharply defined. CMI was more frequently detected with slower growing or metastatic tumors. SBF were more frequent in mice sensitized to nonmetastatic, or faster growing tumors, or to those with shorter latency periods. LDA were more frequent with slower growing or noninvasive tumors. CMI was not associated in either direction with length of latency period or invasiveness. SBF were not associated with invasiveness. LDA were independent of latency period and metastasis. Thus, each immune parameter was associated with a unique set of behavioral characteristics. Further, the association of immunity with behavior did not always suggest an interaction beneficial to the host. A positive association between CMI and metastasis has been also seen by Fidler (1974) and others (Fisher *et al.*, 1965).

Our results were obtained using one particular immune assay, the microcytotoxicity test. Recently we have completed a similar study using two other tests for CMI, the chromium-release and Winn assays.

C. *Clinical-Immunological Correlates of Mouse Mammary Tumors as Measured by Chromium-Release and Winn Assays*

The literature on assessment of CMI to tumors is a confusing one. Various assays are available, and although they differ in many technical details, it is unclear whether or not they are of equal value in measuring clinically relevant reactivity. In order to see whether results with the MCT assay were comparable to those obtained with other assays of CMI, we (Miller *et al.*, 1978) recently carried out a large number of experiments in which we simultaneously assayed CMI by the MCT, a long term ^{51}Cr

cytotoxicity test (CRT), and the Winn Assay. The latter is an *in vivo* test in which tumor and either sensitized or control lymphoid cells are mixed together and then injected into non-sensitized hosts. CMI is indicated by a decrease in tumor growth in the presence of sensitized cells. For this study both MMTV-associated BALB/cfC3H tumors and BALB/c tumors developing spontaneously from hyperplastic alveolar nodule lines induced by either hormones or chemicals (Medina, 1976) were used. The mice were sensitized by a variety of protocols. Regardless, however, of protocol or tumor type, the results showed that the three assays are not equivalent. Thus, results with the MCT tests were unrelated to those obtained by the other two. Detection of CMI by the CRT was strongly associated with detection by Winn assay, although a negative CRT did not necessarily predict a negative Winn test, suggesting that CRT is a less sensitive assay. The reason for the discrepancy between MCT and CRT-Winn assays may be a difference in the type of effector cells active in the three assays, although this will have to be further investigated. Regardless, it seems likely that the detection of CMI by CRT and Winn assays will not show the same correlation with tumor behavior as does detection by MCT. To test this hypothesis we analyzed latency period and growth rate data from a series of mammary tumors for correlation with detection of CMI by CRT and Winn tests. With these assays detection of CMI was independent of growth rate but was more frequent with tumors of longer latency period (Table I). For example, the average latency period for tumors inducing CMI detectable by Winn assay was 35 days, as opposed to 21 days for the CMI negative tumors ($P<0.05$).

In summary, the relationship of cell-mediated, and other types of, immunity to the clinical behavior of a mammary tumor is complex. Each type of immunity, if it plays a role at all, only interacts with certain aspects of the disease. Further, different assays, which overall measure similar types of immunity, reveal different points of host-tumor interaction. Of course, our studies deal with correlations, which may or may not indicate causal relationships. It is clear, however, that CMI is not involved in all phases of neoplastic disease and, where it may be involved, is schizophrenic - in some ways favoring the host, in some ways the tumor.

III. IMMUNOLOGICAL HETEROGENEITY OF MOUSE MAMMARY TUMORS

Another complexity to be considered when trying to assess the role of CMI in growth of mammary tumors is the extensive heterogeneity within these neoplasms. This heterogeneity has been especially noted by Dunn (1959) and both Henderson and

TABLE I. Clinical-Immunological Correlates of Mouse Mammary Tumors

Assay[a] (type of immunity)	Relationship of clinical characteristic to presence of immunity			
	Latency period	Growth rate	Invasiveness	Metastasis
MCT (CMI)	independent	slower	independent	increased
MCT (SBF)	shorter	faster	independent	decreased
MCT (LDA)	independent	slower	decreased	independent
CRT (CMI)	longer	independent	NT	NT
WINN (CMI)	longer	independent	NT	NT

[a]MCT, microcytotoxicity test; CRT, chromium release test; Winn, Winn assay; CMI, cell-mediated immunity; SBF, serum blocking factors; LDA, lymphocyte dependent antibodies; NT, not tested.

Rous (1962) and Sluyser and Van Nie (1974) have presented experimental evidence for it. Recently, Dexter and others (1977) isolated four subpopulations, lines 66, 67, 68H, and 168, of tumor cells from a single, autochthonous, strain BALB/cfC3H mammary tumor. These subpopulations were obtained by a variety of cell culture and separation methods. A fifth subpopulation, 4.10LM, was obtained by culturing a single lung metastatic nodule from a subcutaneous implant of the tenth *in vivo* passage generation of the same tumor which yielded the other four lines. All five of these cell populations have been characterized extensively for *in vitro* and *in vivo* growth properties, as well as for expression of MMTV surface antigen and karyotype. They differ markedly in all properties except one: they all produce tumors when injected subcutaneously into syngeneic mice. We have maintained these lines for almost two years. They are quite stable *in vitro*. When passaged *in vivo*, and then returned to culture, they also generally "breed true," except for 68H which exhibits a remarkable ability to differentiate into several morphologically distinct variants after either *in vivo* passage or exposure to chemical inducers *in vitro* (Hager *et al.*, unpublished observations). Thus, we have five distinct subpopulations of mammary tumor cells all derived from a single tumor. The most likely explanation, given the extensive morphologic and karyotype heterogeneity present in the parent tumor, is that these subpopulations were present in the original tumor cell population. We have recently been exploring the immunological characteristics of the five subpopulations and of the parent tumor in terms of expression of MMTV antigens and also the ability to induce CMI in strain BALB/c (MMTV-free) and BALB/cfC3H (MMTV-positive) hosts. Our assays for MMTV antigens include membrane immunofluorescence with rabbit C3H MMTV antiserum and intracellular immunoperoxidase to (primarily) gp52 (this assay has been graciously performed by Spiegelman and coworkers). Our CMI assays are MCT, CRT, and Winn assays. These studies are still in progress, but the data to date are summarized in Table II.

As can be seen, the immune characteristics of the subpopulations are heterogeneous. Thus, only one line, 68H, strongly expresses membrane MMTV antigens. Indeed, >90% of the cells are routinely positive. [Dr. Hager in our laboratory has recently shown (data presented at this meeting) that the other four lines will also express this reactivity when exposed to 5-iodo-2'-deoxyuridine.] Different assays with the parent tumor showed 2-17% of the cells express MMTV membrane antigen. Intracellular gp52 can be detected in 66, 68H, and 4.10LM, but not in 67. Lines 67, 168, 68H, and 4.10LM have all induced CMI effective against themselves in BALB/c hosts, whereas line 66 has not.

TABLE II. *Immune Reactivity of Subpopulations of a Single BALB/cfC3H Mouse Mammary Tumor*

Subpopulation	Membrane MMTV antigen	Intracellular gp52	Induction of self CMI in	
			BALB/c	BALB/cfC3H
66	0*	+, focal	0	+
67	0	0	+	+
168	0	NT	+	0
63H	+++	+++	+	0
4.10LM	±	++	+	0
Parent tumor	+	NT	+	+

*+, Detection of indicated reactivity; 0, reactivity not detected; NT, not tested.

In BALB/cfC3H hosts lines 66 and 67 are immunogenic, whereas 168, 68H, and 4.10LM so far are not. The parent tumor induces detectable CMI in both types of host.

The failure of 66 to induce self-CMI in BALB/c hosts is interesting. The fact that it can do so in BALB/cfC3H mice shows that it is not simply immunoinsensitive to killing by cytotoxic lymphocytes. Furthermore, its failure to induce self-CMI in BALB/c hosts is not due to a defect in immunogenicity since it can induce lymphocytes reactive against lines 67 and 68H (Table III).

The induction of cross-reactive CMI by the subpopulations in both BALB/c and BALB/cfC3H mice further reveals immunologic heterogeneity. Table III summarizes the results obtained in BALB/c mice. Mice have been sensitized as described above to each of the subpopulations. Their LNC were then tested against the sensitizing and the other four tumor cell populations. The cross-reactive relationships so far revealed by these, and by similar experiments in BALB/cfC3H hosts, are diagrammed in Fig. 2. Interestingly, in BALB/c hosts the cross-reactive patterns are less complete than in BALB/cfC3H hosts. Thus, in BALB/c's, depending upon the assay (see above discussion) the five populations can be linked but certain of them do not induce cross-reactive immunity. In BALB/cfC3H hosts, lines 66 and 67, 168, and 4.10LM all mutually cross-react, whereas 68H neither induces nor is affected by CMI to the other lines. Clearly interpretation of these results will require further data. From the point of view of this presentation, however, it is clear that there can be nonimmunogenic subpopulations within a tumor that is itself immunogenic. It is also clear that the type and distribution of the relevant antigens can be different on the different subpopulations within that tumor. Whether these antigens are viral, organ, or tumor-specific will require further analysis. However, one's view of the role CMI, and its manipulation by immunotherapy, could play in a tumor that is made up of such immunologically heterogeneous subpopulations is certainly different from that predicated on a belief in the essential homogeneity of tumors. It need hardly be pointed out that that belief is the dominant one in experimental cancer research today.

IV. *IN SITU* CELL-MEDIATED IMMUNITY TO MOUSE MAMMARY TUMORS

Most of our knowledge about CMI to breast cancer comes from studies using peripheral lymphoid cells - in blood, spleen, or lymph nodes. Haskill and associates (1975) described the lymphoid cells infiltrating implants of the mouse mammary tumor line T1699 and found them to be predominantly T cells, Fc-re-

TABLE III. CMI-Induced in Strain BALB/c Mice to Subpopulations of a Single BALB/cfC3H Mouse Mammary Tumor

Target cell subpopulation	Assay	LNC[a] Donor sensitized to 66	67	168	68H	4.10LM
66	MCT	0	0	0	0	0
	CRT	0	0	0	0	+
	Winn	0	0	0	NT	+
67	MCT	+	+	+	NT	+
	CRT	+	+	+	NT	0
	Winn	+	+	+	NT	0
168	MCT	0	0	0	NT	0
	CRT	0	0	0	NT	0
	Winn	0	+	+	NT	0
68H	MCT	+	0	0	+	0
	CRT	0	0	0	+	+
	Winn	NT	0	NT	NT	NT
4.10LM	MCT	0	+	0	0	+
	CRT	0	0	0	+	0
	Winn	0	+	0	NT	0

[a]LNC, lymph node cells; +, detection of CMI; 0, CMI never detected; NT, not tested.

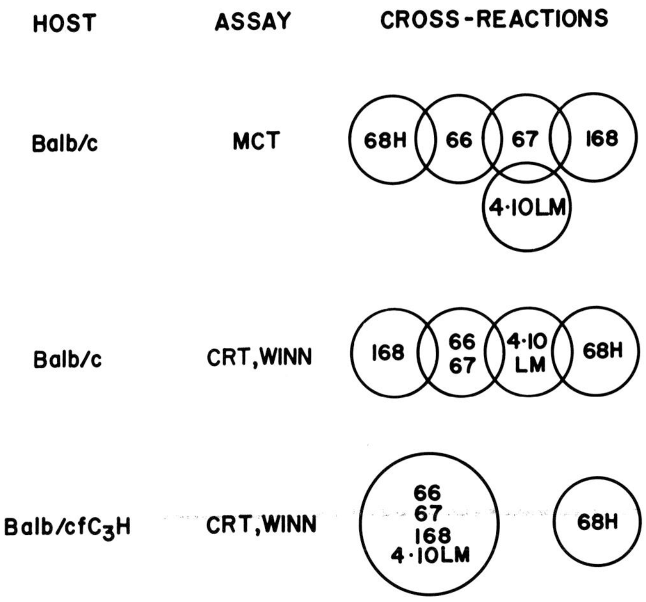

FIGURE 2. Immunological cross-relationships of five subpopulations of a single strain BALB/cfC3H mammary tumor. MCT, microcytotoxicity test; CRT, chromium release test; Winn, Winn Assay. Interlocking circles denote cross-reactivity. When the assay did not detect immunological differences, the subpopulations are enclosed within a single circle.

ceptor bearing cells, and eosinophils. More recently, in our laboratory Blazar (1978a,b) has defined the lymphoid populations of a series of autochthonous and first generation transplants of strain BALB/cfC3H mammary tumors and of tumors arising in Medina's (1976) hyperplastic alveolar nodule lines. She found that T cells and cells sensitive to lysis by antilymphocyte serum and complement were always the largest subpopulations, but that there were enormous differences between different tumors in the percentage of these cells. Fc receptor cells and phagocytic cells were also present. Interestingly, although there was great variability between tumors in the relative proportion of the different lymphoid cell types, tarnsplants of given tumors contained the same relative proportions of the infiltrating cells as were found in the autochthonous tumors. Thus, the type of infiltrate is a tumor, not host, characteristic.

Assay by MCT of the functional capacity of the lymphoid cells isolated from the tumors showed them to be, not cytotoxic, but markedly stimulatory to tumor cell growth and survival (Blazar *et al.*, 1978). This stimulation was seen even when the lymph node cells of the tumor donor were cytotoxic. Ruppert *et al.* (1979) have shown that 4-7 days after removal of the tumor, the lymph node and spleen cells are then also stimulatory to tumor cells, but by day 10 cytotoxicity is regained. These results show that assessment of CMI with peripheral cells can be a misleading guide to the status of immunity within a tumor. They further point up the dual nature (Prehn, 1976) of CMI in regard to its ability to influence mammary tumor growth.

V. CONCLUSION

It should by now be obvious that the question presented in the title of this paper cannot yet be answered. It is certain, however, that CMI does not play a role in all phases of cancer growth, nor is its presence consistently favorable to the host. It is also apparent that different assays can reveal different relationships between CMI and tumor growth. The choice of assay, therefore, should depend on the clinical features of the particular neoplastic disease, or stage of disease, being studied. Understanding of the role of CMI in neoplasia must also take into account the heterogeneity of tumors. All tumor cells within a tumor are not immunologically equivalent. Isolation of a single tumor cell line cannot begin to reveal the complexities of a "real" neoplasm. Finally, it will be increasingly necessary to learn about CMI *in situ*, within primary tumors, metastatic lesions, and, undoubtedly, in the natural site of tumor growth, such as the mammary fat pads. Efforts to simplify experimental systems by eliminating the complexities present in spontaneous neoplasia may result in ultimate failure to understand, and hence control, CMI to tumors.

REFERENCES

Black, M. M., Moore, D. H., Shore, B., Zachrau, R. E., and Leis, H. P. (1974). *Cancer Res. 34*, 1054-1060.

Blair, P. B., Lane, M. A., and Mar, P. (1976a). *J. Immunol. 116*, 606-609.

Blair, P. B., Lane, M. A., and Mar, P. (1976b). *J. Immunol. 116*, 610-614.

Blazar, B. A., and Heppner, G. H. (1978a). *J. Immunol. 120*, 1876-1880.

Blazar, B. A., and Heppner, G. H. (1978b). *J. Immunol. 120*, 1881-1886.

Blazar, B. A., Miller, F. R., and Heppner, G. H. (1978). *J. Immunol. 120,* 1887-1891.

Dexter, D. L., Kowalski, H. M., Fligiel, Z., and Heppner, G. H. (1977). *Proc. Am. Assoc. Cancer Res. 18,* 45.

Dunn, T. (1959). *In* "Physiopathology of Cancer" 2nd Ed. (F. Homburger and N. H. Fishman, eds.), pp. 38-84. P. H. Hoeber, Inc., New York.

Fidler, I. J. (1974). *Cancer Res. 34,* 481-488.

Fisher, B., Fisher, E. R., and Sakai, A. (1965). *Cancer Res. 25,* 993-996.

Fisher, B., Wolmark, N., Rubin, H., and Saffer, E. (1975). *J. Natl. Cancer Inst. 55,* 1147-1153.

Foulds, L. (1969, 1975). "Neoplastic Development," Vols. I, II. Academic Press, New York.

Hager, J. C., Miller, F. R., and Heppner, G. H. (1978). *Cancer Res.* in press.

Haskill, J. S., Yamamura, Y., and Radov, L. (1975). *Int. J. Cancer 16,* 798-809.

Henderson, J. S., and Rous, P. (1962). *J. Exp. Med. 115,* 1211-1229.

Heppner, G. H. (1969). *Int. J. Cancer 4,* 608-615.

Heppner, G. H. (1976). *In* "Breast Cancer: A Multidisciplinary Approach" (G. St. -Arneault, P. Band, and L. Israel, eds.), pp. 95-108. Springer-Verlag, Berlin.

Heppner, G. H., and Pierce, G. (1969). *Int. J. Cancer 4,* 212-218.

Hollinshead, A. C., Jaffurs, W. T., Alpert, L. K., Harris, J. E., and Herberman, R. B. (1974). *Cancer Res. 34,* 2961-2968.

Lane, M. A., Roubinian, J., Slomich, M., Trefts, P., and Blair, P. B. (1975). *J. Immunol. 114,* 24-29.

Lopez, D. M., and Sigel, M. M. (1975). *J. Reticuloendothelial Soc. 18,* 305-312.

McCoy, J. L., Jerome, L. F., anderson, C., Cannon, G. B., Alford, T. C. Connor, R. J., Oldham, R. K., and Herberman, R. B. (1976). *J. Natl. Cancer Inst. 57,* 1045-1049.

Martin, D. S., Hayworth, P., Fugmann, R. A., English, R., and McNeill, H. W. (1964). *Cancer Res. 24,* 652-654.

Medina, D. (1976). *Cancer Res. 36,* 2589-2595.

Miller, F. R., Dexter, D. L., and Heppner, G. H. (1978). *Proc. Am. Assoc. Cancer Res. 19,* 38.

Morton, D. L. (1969). *J. Natl. Cancer Inst. 42,* 311-330.

Pollack, S., Heppner, G. H., Brawn, R. J., and Nelson, K. (1972). *Int. J. Cancer 9,* 316-323.

Prehn, R. T. (1976). *Transplant. Rev. 28,* 34-42.

Rios, A., and Simmons, R. L. (1973). *J. Natl. Cancer Inst. 51,* 637-644.

Ruppert, B., Blazar, B., Medina, D., and Heppner, G. H. (1979). *J. Immunology,* in press.

Ruppert, B., Wei, W., Medina, D., and Heppner, G. H. (1978). *J. Natl. Cancer Inst. 61.* 1165-1169.

Sluyser, M., and Van Nie, R. (1974). *Cancer Res. 34,* 3253-3257.

Stolfi, R. L., Fugmann, R. A., Stolfi, L. M., and Martin, D. S. (1975). *J. Immunol. 114,* 1824-1830.

Vaage, J. (1968). *Cancer Res. 28,* 2477-2483.

Weiss, D. W., Lavrin, D. H., Dezfulian, M., Vaage, J., and Blair, P. B. (1966). *In* "Viruses Inducing Cancer" (W. J. Burdette, ed.), pp. 138-168. Univ. of Utah Press, Salt Lake City.

MURINE LEUKEMIA: APPROACHES TO IMMUNOPREVENTION*

James N. Ihle

Cancer Biology Program
NCI Frederick Cancer Research Center
Frederick, Maryland

Werner Schäfer

Max-Planck-Institut für Virusforschung
D-7400 Tübingen
Germany

I. INTRODUCTION

Murine leukemias encompass a number of pathological disorders induced by a diversity of agents. The predominant type of leukemia is a lymphosarcoma of thymic origin, although a variety of leukemias or lymphomas have been found including reticulum cell sarcomas, myeloid leukemias, myelomas, and plasmacytomas. Perhaps the most intriguing aspect of murine leukemia, however, is the number of factors that induce it. The best known examples are the spontaneous leukemias that occur at high frequencies in strains of mice such as AKR, C58, and C3H/figgy. In addition, however, radiation, chemical carcinogens, and estrogen can readily induce leukemia in appropriate strains of mice. An essential, but yet unanswered, question is whether all these leukemia-inducing agents have a common etiological denominator or even a common mechanism of transformation.

The most provocative observation noted in studies of the biology of murine leukemias was that of a C-type viral etiology

Research sponsored in part by the National Cancer Institute under Contract No. NO1-CO-75380 with Litton Bionetics, Inc.

ISBN 0-12-131150-3

of AKR leukemias (Gross, 1951). Since this initial observation, considerable information has been acquired concerning the structure and regulation of C-type viruses (for review see Vogt and Hu, 1977). C-type viruses serologically indistinguishable from the AKR-type of MuLV have been shown to be associated with a variety of inbred strains of mice, although in most cases they are not associated with leukemia. In general, the transmission of C-type viruses is genetic (Rowe *et al.*, 1971; Lowy *et al.*, 1971, 1974), although cases of maternal transmission of C-type viruses have been demonstrated (Melief *et al.*, 1975). In the results presented here we have extended some of these observations and have specifically addressed the questions of the etiological relationship of the virus to leukemia, the characteristics of virus expression associated with induction of leukemia, and the possibility of immunoprevention to modify these events.

II. BIOLOGICAL AND GENETIC CHARACTERISTICS OF THE VIRUSES ASSOCIATED WITH LEUKEMIA

C-type viruses structurally and functionally similar to the virus associated with AKR leukemias are found in a variety of inbred strains of mice. The genetic transmission of these viruses has been assessed by DNA-DNA hybridization, serological and virological assays, and by the observation that halogenated pyrimidines can induce expression of the virus in cultured fibroblasts from backcrossed mice. The results of several such experiments are summarized in Table I. The genetics of the AKR C-type viruses has been the most extensively studied. Rowe *et al.* (1972) have determined the linkage of one of the AKR viral loci to be near Gpi-1 on chromosome 7. In studies employing a combination of serological and virological approaches, it appears that the AKR harbors a total of three such endogenous viral genomes (Ihle and Joseph, 1978a). Each of the viral loci has an early phenotype *in vivo,* in that it is expressed early in life (see below). Comparable to the AKR, C3H/figgy mice, a high spontaneous leukemia strain, have multiple loci for an AKR-type virus. One of the viral loci has been tentatively mapped on chromosome 7 near the hemoglobin B gene (Rowe, 1973).

In addition to the high leukemia strains, a number of additional strains have been examined for viral loci. Several strains such as the NIH Swiss and 129/J shown in Table I lack the AKR-type proviral sequences (Lowy *et al.*, 1974). However, several low leukemia strains such as C3H, BALB/c, and C57BL/6 have a single viral locus. The gene for the BALB/c viral locus appears to be allelic with the C3H locus, while the viral locus of C57BL/6 mice appears to be at a different site as shown by the experiments summarized in Fig. 1. In these studies the

TABLE I. *Distribution of AKR MuLV-Type Viruses Among Inbred Strains of Mice*

Strain	No. viral loci	Phenotype[a]	Locus	Chromosome	Linkage
AKR	3	Early	Akv-1	7[b]	Gpi-1 (12)[c]
			Akv-2, Akv-3	Unknown	
C3H/figgy	>3	Early	Cfv-1	7[d]	Hbb
			Additional	Unknown	
C3H/HeJ	1	Early	C3v-1	5[e]	Pgm-1 (24)
BALB/c	1	Late	Bv-1	5	Pgm-1
C57BL/6	1	Intermediate		Unknown	
NIH Swiss	0	---		---	
129/J	0	---		---	

[a]Phenotypes of virus expression were determined by serological assays as described in the text.
[b]Rowe et al., 1972.
[c]Map units (recombination frequencies) from the marker locus.
[d]Rowe, 1973.
[e]Gene linkage was determined by serological assays in backcrossed mice for virus expression (Ihle and Joseph, 1978) and isoenzyme differences in phosphoglucomutase-1 (Ihle and Domotor, unpublished data).

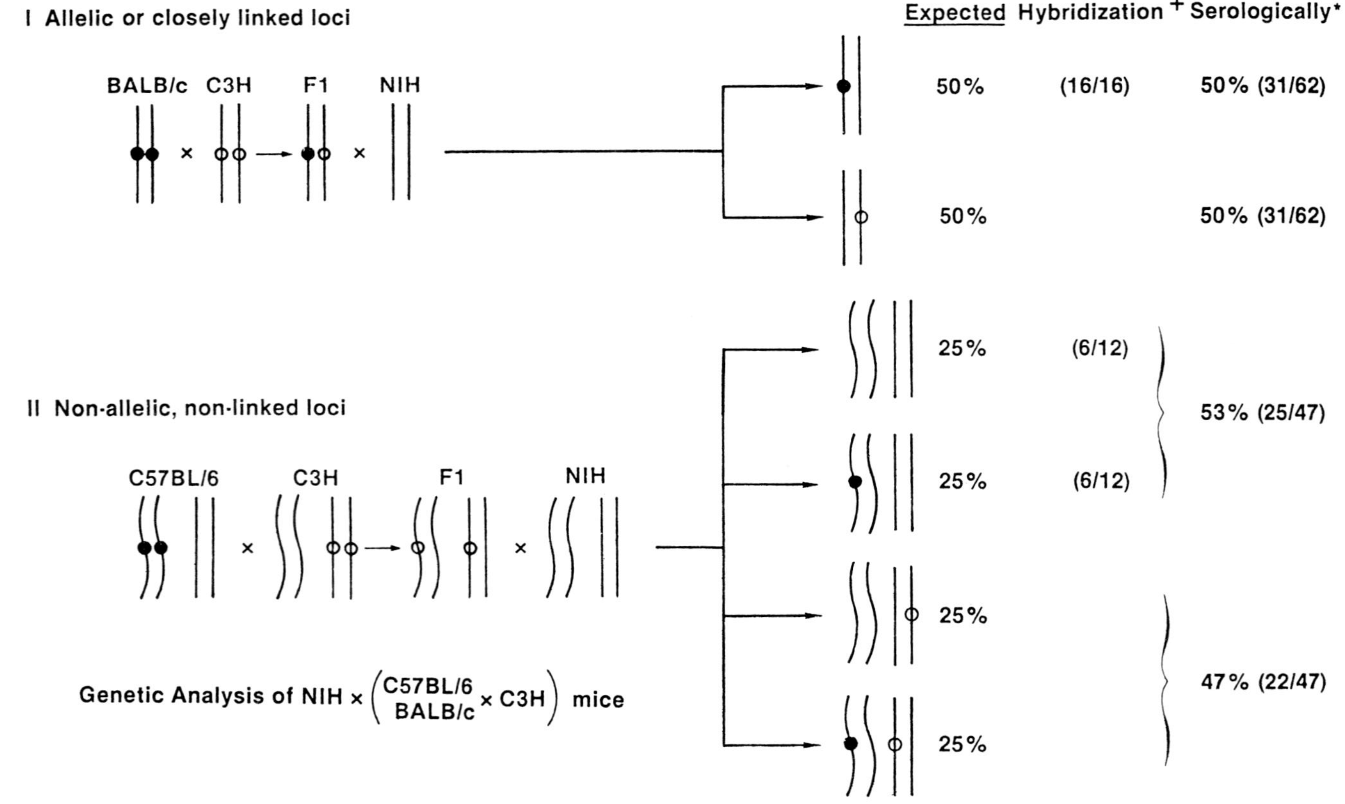

FIGURE 1. +, *The C57BL/6 or BALB/c viral locus was detected by DNA-DNA hybridization;* *, *the C3H phenotype was detected serologically.*

linkage of viral loci was determined by a combination of serological and hybridization experiments as previously described (Ihle and Joseph, 1978b). For example, the C3H and BALB/c viral loci can be distinguished serologically, while both loci can be detected by hybridization. Assuming the viral loci are allelic, the cross BALB/c ⊗ C3H gives an F_1 homozygous for the presence of a viral locus with one allele of the BALB/c and one of the C3H. The cross to the virus-negative NIH Swiss would then give offspring, *all* of which have either the BALB/c or C3H locus. As determined by serological assays, this was exactly the situation observed in that 50% of the mice examined had the C3H locus, while the other 50% had the proviral sequences of the BALB/c locus. Preliminary evidence suggests that the BALB/c-C3H viral locus is on chromosome 5 linked to the gene phosphoglucomutase-1. The converse situation, nonlinked viral loci, was seen when C3H and C57BL/6 mice were examined. For two nonlinked viral loci, the F_1 is heterozygous for viral loci and the two loci segregate independently in the F_1 x NIH Swiss cross. In this case, again approximately 50% of the population had the C3H locus, but of the non-C3H-type mice only 50% had the C57BL/6 locus, demonstrating independent segregation of the viral loci. Thus, the site of virus integration in various inbred strains is variable.

As illustrated in Table I, each of the viral loci has a characteristic phenotype of expression *in vivo*. These phenotypes are best determined by serological assays (Ihle *et al.*, 1976c; Ihle and Joseph, 1978a,b) and have been arbitrarily grouped in early, intermediate, and late phenotypes. The early phenotype is one in which endogenous virus expression is detected in 50% of the mice within 2 months of age, whereas the 50% point for the intermediate phenotype is 6-8 months of age, and for the late phenotype is greater than 12 months of age. Interestingly, although the phenotype of virus expression has been shown to segregate with the structural genes for the virus, no structural differences in the viruses have been observed to account for the differences in the expression *in vivo*. Initially it was thought that the site of integration might determine the phenotypic differences, although the observation that the BALB/c and C3H viruses are allelic and have quite distinct phenotypes of expression seems to exclude this possibility. Nevertheless, as experiments begin, which study the physical structure of integrated viruses, it may be possible to identify regulatory sequences that control these phenotypic differences.

In terms of the biology of ecotropic C-type viruses and their relationship to leukemia, these types of studies have defined several important principles. First, integrated C-type viruses display quite unique phenotypes of expression *in vivo* and this property appears to be associated with the provirus itself and is not a host function. Second, the site of integration is highly variable. This observation argues against an evolutionary derivation of endogenous ecotropic viruses and suggests that horizontal transmission and germ-line integration may have occurred independently in the parental mice from which our inbred strains were derived. Third, the number of viral loci is highly variable, ranging from none to greater than three loci. Last, of the high spontaneous leukemia strains of mice examined, all are characterized by multiple viral loci, all of which appear to have the early phenotype of expression.

III. CHARACTERISTICS OF VIRUS EXPRESSION ASSOCIATED WITH LEUKEMIA

Although AKR-type ecotropic viruses are widespread among various inbred strains of mice, the high incidence of spontaneous leukemias is limited to relatively few strains. This is not because of inherent differences in pathogenicity of the viruses, since ecotropic viruses from low leukemia strains under appropriate conditions can be shown to be pathogenic (Greenberger *et al.*, 1975; Jolicoeur *et al.*, 1978). As discussed above, one important difference between leukemia-prone strains and "normal" strains is the number of integrated virus genomes. In addition, however, a variety of genetic factors have been shown to influence pathogenesis, the most striking of which is the Fv-1 gene that affects the *infectious* replication of the virus in the host (Rowe and Hartley, 1972) without affecting the primary expression of integrated provirus (Ihle and Joseph, 1978b). The results from these and other experimental approaches have demonstrated that with few exceptions there is a compelling correlation between the levels of infectious virus replication (viral burden, extent of viremia) and the induction of leukemia.

The correlation between virus burden and leukemia has been illustrated by several experimental approaches. One approach has utilized the Fv-1 gene to restrict virus expression (Lilly *et al.*, 1975). For example, AKR mice lack free antibody against the virus and have high levels of infectious virus and have the Fv-$1^{n/n}$allele, the permissive allele for AKR virus replication. When AKR mice are crossed with Fv-$1^{b/b}$ mice, such as BALB/c mice, which restrict virus expression, the F_1 is phenotypically antibody-positive and has low levels of infectious virus. If the F_1 mice are then backcrossed to AKR mice, all the progeny have a complete genetic dowry of virus, but segregate with respect to the gene-controlling restriction of virus replication.

When these mice are then examined for the extent of viremia at six weeks and this is correlated with the induction of leukemia, there is a direct correlation. Thus, the higher the level of viremia, the more likely the probability of leukemia.

A second approach involves "spreading out" the AKR viral loci on a strain lacking an AKR-type virus but which is permissive ($Fv\text{-}1^{n/n}$) for virus replication. In this case the appropriate backcross is NIH ⓧ NIH x AKR) and several aspects of such crosses have been examined including the presence of proviral DNA, free antibody against the virus, viral antigen levels, and infectious virus (Ihle and Joseph, 1978a). As shown in Table II this backcross generates several phenotypes and several observations relevant to the AKR virus. First, the only phenotype that lacks proviral DNA is a nonviremic, antibody-free mouse (data not shown). These mice represent 12-13% of the population, illustrating the existence of three viral loci in the AKR. A second phenotype includes mice that lack detectable infectious virus but that are antibody-positive. This population is relatively leukemia-free and in most respects is similar to strains such as the C3H. Lastly, a phenotype comparable to the AKR itself is observed that are viremic without evidence of free antibody. Like the AKR, these mice have a high probability of leukemia. In these results it is also important to note the contrasting phenotypes of viremia and antibody. The above experiments have illustrated an impressive requirement for the genetic presence of the virus for leukemia and, more importantly, the requirement of expression at viremic levels throughout life.

In spite of years of research, the mechanisms involved in leukemogenesis by the AKR-type viruses are not known. The lack of information is due to the properties of the disease including the viremia that precludes precisely defining activation of virus expression and "transformation," the long latencies involved in the disease, and the lack of appropriate *in vitro* transformation systems. The observation, however, that chronic life-long viremia is required for leukemia argues against a direct "transformation" event and suggests that induction of leukemia may be by an indirect mechanism. A variety of such mechanisms have been proposed, including generation, by recombination of altered viruses, alteration of thymic environments, induction of virus-mediated somatic mutations, etc. Our current hypothesis is that the induction of leukemia is associated with and dependent upon a chronic cellular immune response of the host against the virus. This hypothesis was suggested by the observation that in contrast to the transient T-cell blastogenic response of normal mice to the viral envelope glycoprotein (Lee and Ihle, 1977), *viremic* AKR mice or NIH backcrossed mice display a chronic 4-5 month blastogenic response that precedes the onset of leukemias (Lee and Ihle, in preparation). It is conceivable that this chronic im-

TABLE II. Phenotypes of Virus Expression at 6 Months in AKR, (NIH x AKR) and NIH x (NIH x AKR) Mice

Strain	Antibody	p30[a]	p12[a]	Infectious virus[b]	Percent of population	Leukemia incidence at 9 months
AKR	<1:10	800-1000	50-100	>1000	100	82%
NIH x AKR	<1:10	600-900	40-75	>1000	100	72%
NIH x (NIH x AKR)	<1:10	200-1000	10-100	100->1000	64	68%
NIH x (NIH x AKR)	1:10-1:320	70-100	5-15	5-70	3.5	
NIH (NIH x AKR)	1:80-1:640	20-100	5-10	0	19.8	5%
NIH (NIH x AKR)	<1:10	10-20	<0.1	0	12.8	0%

[a]Ngm/mg protein in spleen extracts determined by radioimmune competition assays.
[b]FFU of virus from 1-cm sections of tail tissue.

mune stimulation is required to establish a rapidly dividing population of cells in which spontaneous transformation is highly likely.

IV. APPROACHES TO IMMUNOPREVENTION

Various immunological approaches to regulating virus expression in AKR mice are possible, including active immunization with virus or viral components, passive immunotherapy with antisera either xenogeneic, allogeneic, or syngeneic against the virus or viral antigens, or a combination of these approaches. Presumably the success or failure of these approaches will rely heavily on the ability to reduce the high viral burdens to a level that host immunity can cope with residual virus. Active immunization using viral gp71 has been shown to be effective against Friend virus disease (Hunsmann *et al.*, 1975). In this case immunization was prior to virus challenge and was not complicated by the expression of an endogenous virus. Nevertheless, based on the success of this approach in Friend disease, attempts were made to protect AKR mice by active immunization with FLV gp71. In contrast to the expected result, active immunization with FLV gp71 accelerated the mortality due to leukemia in AKR mice (Ihle *et al.*, 1976e). This acceleration occurred in spite of (or perhaps because of) a vigorous response against gp71 detectable by antibody and cellular reactivity such as blastogenesis. The response was type-specific in that it was specific for FLV gp71 and did not cross-react with the AKR-type virus. The lack of cross-reactivity did not appear to be due to the absorption of the cross-reactive population of antibodies by endogenous viruses because in other strains having little or no expression of the endogenous virus, the response to FLV gp71 immunization was similarly type-specific (Ihle *et al.*, 1976a,b).

Active immunization using formalized AKR virus has also been examined in low leukemia, low virus strains. In such strains, formalized viral vaccines induce a vigorous humoral immune response that is capable of mediating virus neutralization (Lee *et al.*, 1977). As above, the immune response against gp71 was primarily type-specific and in this case was type-specific for the AKR-type virus gp71. In addition to a gp71 response, antibodies were also detectable with specificity for p15(E). This response was group-specific in that it cross-reacted with several murine virus serotypes but was nonneutralizing. In spite of these reports, however, the ability of active immunization of AKR mice to reduce leukemia has not been reported. It appears that inducing an immune response by active immunization in naive animals might be quite distinct from trying to immmunize mice already suffering from a state of viremia.

In contrast to the lack of apparent efficacy of active immunization, passive immunotherapy in AKR mice appears to have a beneficial effect. Schäfer *et al.* (1977a,b) have demonstrated that passive immunotherapy utilizing a high-titered goat anti-FLV gp71 is effective in treatment of both FLV disease as well as AKR mice. It should be noted in this case that the xenogeneic antiserum used was group-specific and reacted equally well with either FLV or the AKR virus. Results of treatment of AKR mice, however, were somewhat complex in that little effect was seen when 2- or 6-month-old mice were treated, whereas treatment of newborn mice or, even better, treatment of the mother and newborns prolonged their life significantly. These results were interpreted to suggest that the essential component of treatment is the reduction of virus burdens *early* in life. Interestingly, this conclusion was also predicted by the genetic experiments correlating virus expression with leukemia (Lilly *et al.*, 1975). The additional requirement for treatment of the mothers was interpreted to suggest that one component establishing a high viral burden early in life was maternal transmission of the virus. This is interesting in view of previous results that demonstrated a maternal effect on AKR leukemias in that foster nursing could reduce the incidences and onset of leukemias (Miller, 1961). Neverthless, in terms of leukemia, the net effect of passive immunotherapy was the reduction of the incidence of leukemia at 12 months of age from 60% to approximately 10%. In terms of various parameters of virus expression *in vivo*, the effects shown in Table III were observed, which illustrate the differences between a treated and untreated family of mice. As shown, passive immunotherapy significantly reduced virus expression as measured by infectious plasma virus or serum levels of the viral antigen p12. More importantly, detectable antibodies against the virus were found among the treated mice but were not detectable in untreated mice. Thus, passive immunotherapy can reduce virus burdens, allow recovery of host immune functions in some cases, but more importantly prolong life.

Effects comparable to the above have also been obtained using xenogenic antisera against whole virus alone or in combination with vaccines of inactivated virus (Huebner *et al.*, 1976). As above, passive immunotherapy early in life of AKR mice significantly reduced the levels of infectious virus and concomitantly reduced the incidence of leukemias at 1 year of age. Unfortunately the immune status of the protected mice was not assessed. Nevertheless, the above results taken together indicate that spontaneous leukemias in high frequency strains are associated with active replication of high levels of virus expression. The

TABLE III. *Virus and Antibodies in Untreated and IgG-Treated AKR Mice*

Mouse			Virus						Antibody					
Family	Sex	No.	FIU/ml plasma at months of age			AKR-p12 ng/ml serum at months of age			AKR-neutral. (Vn/Vo) at months of age			AKR-precip. RIP titer at months of age		
			7	11½	16	7	11½	16	7	11½	16	7	11½	16
Ig-treated 54/8	M	1	NT	0[a]		0[b]	0		0[c]	0		0[d]	0	
		2	NT	0	0	0	0	0	0	0	0	0	0	0
		3	NT	0	0	0	0	0	0	0	0	0	0	0
		4	NT	0	0	0	0	0	0	0	0	0	0	0
		5	NT	0	0	0	0	0	0	0	0	0	100	100
		6	NT	0	0	0	0	0	0	0	0	0	0	0
		7	NT	0		0	0		0	0		0	300	
		8	NT	0		0	0		0	0		0	0	
	F	1	NT	0	0	NT	NT	0	0	0	0	100	300	100
		2	NT	0	0	NT	NT	0	0	0	0	0	100	0
		3	NT	0	0	NT	NT	0	.04	.08	.05	300	1000	1000
Control	M	1	NT			300			0			0		
		2	NT	350	3500	100	NT	2000	0	NT	0	0	NT	0
		3	NT	100		100	600		0	0		0	0	
		4	NT			0			0			0		
		5	NT			0			0			0		

NT = not tested. [a]<50 FIU/ml. [b]<50 ng p12/ml. [c]≥0.15 Vn/Vo. [d]<40.

essential goal in immunoprevention is therefore to reduce or eliminate this burden early in life. The most effective and perhaps only way to achieve this goal in AKR mice is by passive immunotherapy early in life with high-titered antiviral reagents.

V. IS THERE A COMMON VIRAL ETIOLOGY FOR MURINE LEUKEMIAS?

As shown above, immunological techniques appear quite promising as a preventive approach for controlling the types of leukemias found in strains of mice such as the AKR. The next question is whether these approaches are generally applicable to other murine leukemias such as those induced by radiation or carcinogens. Implicit in generalizing the techniques of virus-specific immunoprevention is the concept that there exists a common viral etiology of all forms of murine leukemia. Although such a concept has been widely accepted, it now appears that perhaps *only* the type of leukemias found in strains such as the AKR have a viral etiology.

Perhaps second to AKR leukemias, the most studied leukemia is that induced by irradiation. Initially it was hypothesized that radiation-induced leukemias had a viral etiology based on the observation that leukemogenic virus could occasionally be isolated from radiation-induced lymphomas (Gross, 1959; Lieberman and Kaplan, 1959). However, a number of recent studies have demonstrated that the virological pattern in radiation-induced leukemias is quite distinct from that found in AKR mice (Ihle *et al.*, 1976d,f). In particular, in none of the cases examined has the induction of leukemia following irradiation been associated with viremic levels of virus expression such as those that are essential for leukemia induction in AKR mice. Secondly, in terms of either overt virus expression or seroepidemiological studies, the expression of the endogenous ecotropic virus does not correlate with leukemia induction. Lastly, leukemia can be readily induced in strains of mice lacking the proviral sequences of the ecotropic virus (Ihle, 1978; Arnstein *et al.*, 1976). These observations strongly imply that there probably is not a viral etiology for radiation-induced leukemias, or if there is, the virological patterns are quite distinct from that observed in AKR mice and may not be amenable to comparable immunoprevention.

As previously shown, however, occasionally viruses can be isolated from radiation-induced leukemias that are weakly oncogenic. Continued *in vivo* passage of such viruses can give rise to highly leukemogenic viruses (Lieberman and Kaplan, 1959). Recently, one such virus preparation has been extensively studied biologically and biochemically (Decleve *et al.*, 1976, 1978). The results demonstrate that the majority of virion proteins are serologically identical to the B-tropic, ecotropic virus commonly found in old C57BL mice. The envelope glycoprotein, gp71, however is serologically unique and appears to have arisen by recombination between the endogenous ecotropic and xenotropic viruses. Nevertheless, we could find neither seroepidemiological evidence for the existence of this virus in primary radiation-induced leukemias using serological assays, nor could we find this unique glycoprotein in primary radiation-induced lymphomas using competition radioimmunoassays (Ihle and Lieberman, in preparation). Therefore, it appears that the most likely origin of radiation leukemia virus is the occasional isolation of a lymphoma, which fortuitously expresses the endogenous ecotropic virus, which is weakly leukemogenic, and the subsequent selection during continued *in vivo* passage of recombinant viruses with greatly enhanced leukemogenic potential.

Irrespective of the lack of consistent ecotropic virus expression in primary radiation-induced lymphomas, attempts have been made to intervene in radiation leukemias by passive and active immunotherapy. Initial experiments involved passive immunotherapy, utilizing a rat antiserum against radiation leukemia virus (Ferrer *et al.*, 1973). The results were equivocal, however, since both immune and normal sera gave the same degree of protection. More recently attempts were made to immunize C57BL/6 mice with Friend leukemia virus gp71 and although immunity was established, no protection was seen against radiation-induced lymphomas (Ihle *et al.*, 1976b). In another study (Peters *et al.*, 1977) active and passive immunoprevention were attempted. Immunization with either inactivated Gross MuLV (an AKR-type virus) or simian sarcoma virus had no effect on development of leukemia, whereas immunization with inactivated Rauscher MuLV reduced the incidence of lymphomas by approximately 50%. The effect of passive immunotherapy with a goat anti-Gross MuLV was also examined. As in previous experiments, control IgG treatment gave approximately a 25% protective effect compared to that of untreated mice. The specific IgG treatment gave approximately a 40% reduction in lymphomas compared to that of the controls. Because of the marginal effects seen thus far, it has been difficult to assess the feasibility of immunoprevention in radiation-induced leukemia. It should also be noted that these effects cannot be equated with causation since the fortuitous expression of endogenous viruses in lymphomas, although providing an immunological target for protection, need not imply direct etiology. In fact, the partial protection seen may be due to exactly this relationship.

Similar to the virus-induced leukemias, little is known concerning the mechanisms in radiation-induced leukemias. Recent experiments have demonstrated very distinct alterations in the normal differentiation of early thymocytes in the bone marrow that are correlated with leukemia induction (Pazmiño *et al.*, 1978). These results have suggested that intervention in the leukemic process might best be effected by treatment with specific polypeptide hormones that control the early stages of thymocyte differentiation. Moreover, these results have suggested that the mechanism of radiation-induced leukemia may be quite distinct from that of the virus-induced diseases since none of the specific alterations induced by radiation are seen in virus-induced leukemias. Nevertheless, it appears that it may be extremely difficult to generalize as to either etiology *or* treatment of the various murine leukemias.

VI. SUMMARY AND FUTURE PROSPECTS

The results to date demonstrate a compelling relationship between endogenous, ecotropic C-type viruses and the spontaneous leukemias found in strains of mice such as the AKR. Equally compelling are the virological patterns associated with the induction of leukemia. Clearly the lack of a direct correlation between the presence of the virus and leukemia, and the requirement for a chronic life-long state of viremia will be significant in determining the mechanisms involved in the induction of leukemia. With regard to immunotherapy, however, the spontaneous leukemias have presented a number of challenges not previously encountered in infectious diseases. The most obvious difference is that unlike most infectious diseases, the etiological agent is an endogenous, genetically transmitted virus. Associated with this observation are a number of theories that could have had a significant impact on immune intervention, including the concepts that mice were immunologically tolerant to endogenous viruses, C-type virus expression was involved in normal differentiation, and that because of apparent widespread viral antigen expression any immune intervention would lead to a devastating autoimmune disease. In fact, however, to date, none of these effects has been seen. In contrast, observations such as the variable number and site of viral loci and the existence of immune responses against the virus strongly suggest that the AKR-type virus is a classical infectious agent that fortuitously, because of its replicative mechanism, can and has become integrated in certain strains of mice. In this regard, it is interesting to note that in other species, the C-type viruses associated with leukemia are exogenous viruses, suggesting that inbred strains of mice may be unique in this regard.

The successful immunoprevention of leukemias in AKR mice has been dependent upon understanding the unusual characteristics of the relationship of the virus to the disease. Unlike the majority of infectious diseases in which immunization is utilized to effectively deal with the *possible* encounter with an infectious agent, the AKR disease is characterized by an established viral infection from birth. This infectious process is in full swing prior to the development of the host immunological functions. This situation is analogous to infecting newborn mice with an exogenous leukemia virus such as Moloney leukemia virus that rapidly induces leukemia. If, however, the virus is given after maturation of immune functions, the host is resistant to both the viremia and leukemia. In the AKR mouse the infectious spread of the virus is essential as illustrated by the lack of viremia and leukemia in the Fv-1-resistant crosses. By the leukemic phase at 8-12 months, the virus can represent approximately 0.01% of the mouse. Clearly, this type of infectious process would tax the best efforts for immune intervention. As expected, therefore, passive immunotherapy of leukemic mice results in lethal passive anaphylaxis (Ihle, unpublished observation). For these reasons, retrospectively, it appears that passive immunotherapy early in life, prior to the establishment of chronic viremia, is perhaps the only effective treatment.

The next obvious question is whether the viral leukemias of AKR mice or the treatment has any broader implication in terms of leukemias. In terms of other known viral leukemias in other species, the results may be directly applicable since similar virological patterns are often encountered. In terms of human leukemia, it appears that at least the therapeutic approaches may have limited, if any, significance. This is primarily because of the lack of a comparable virological pattern. However, if AKR leukemias are mechanistically related to chronic cellular immune reactivity as suggested above, this disease may be extremely significant with regard to the mechanisms of induction of leukemia. In particular it is known that certain leukemias are regularly associated with immune deficiencies (Louie and Schwartz, 1978), which could result in comparable chronic cellular immune reactivities against a variety of environmental agents. Thus, in the AKR mouse the immune deficiency is the inability to mount an immune response that can cope with the viremia. Nevertheless, any direct applicable consequences of curing AKR mice are not readily obvious at this time.

Perhaps the most applicable concept emerging from studies on leukemia in mice is one of variable etiology. It has been assumed that because viruses are associated with leukemias in several species, there must be a common viral etiology in all cases. Actually quite the contrast appears to be true in that within one species it appears that the etiology need not always be viral. In particular, in mice the radiation-induced leukemias clearly illustrate a distinctly different virological pattern from AKR leukemias and in fact are probably not virus-induced. Irrespective of the underlying etiological arguments, these observations have profound significance for immunotherapy.

For example, as mentioned above, passive immunotherapy of leukemic AKR mice results in acute passive anaphylaxis; however, comparable treatment of mice suffering from radiation-induced leukemia has no effect either in terms of anaphylaxis or death due to ultimate growth of the tumor. In addition to this aspect, the mechanism of leukemia-induction may be quite distinct and undoubtedly will have a direct impact on human leukemia since it is now clear that radiation is an important leukemogenic factor for humans. Nevertheless, in summary, it is appropriate to state that at this time it is difficult to generalize with respect to either etiology or immunotherapy of leukemia.

REFERENCES

Arnstein, P., Riggs, J. L., Oshiro, L. S., Huebner, R. J., and Lewette, F. H. (1976). *J. Natl. Cancer Inst. 57,* 1085-1089.

Decleve, A., Lieberman, M., Ihle, J. N., and Kaplan, H. S. (1976). *Proc. Natl. Acad. Sci. 73,* 4675-4679.

Decleve, A., Lieberman, M., Ihle, J. N., Rosenthal, P. N., Lung, M. L., and Kaplan, H. S. (1978). *Virology 90,* 23-35.

Ferrer, J. F., Lieberman, M., and Kaplan, H. S. (1973). *Cancer Res. 33,* 1339-1343.

Greenberger, J. S., Stephenson, J. R., Moloney, W. C., and Aaronson, S. A. (1975). *Cancer Res. 35,* 245-252.

Gross, L. (1951). *Proc. Soc. Exp. Biol. Med. 78,* 342-348.

Gross, L. (1959). *Proc. Soc. Exp. Biol. Med. 100,* 102-105.

Huebner, R. J., Gilden, R. V., Toni, R., Hill, R. W., Trimmer, R. W., Fish, D. C., and Sass, B. (1976). *Proc. Natl. Acad. Sci. 73,* 4633-4635.

Hunsmann, G., Moennig, V., and Schäfer, W. (1975). *Virology 66,* 327-329.

Ihle, J. N. (1978). *Sem. Hematol. 15,* 95-115.

Ihle, J. N., and Joseph, D. R. (1978a). *Virology 87,* 287-297.

Ihle, J. N., and Joseph, D. R. (1978b). *Virology 87,* 298-306.

Ihle, J. N., Collins, J. J., Lee, J. C., Fischinger, P. J., Moennig, V., Schäfer, W., Hanna, M. G., Jr., and Bolognesi, D. P. (1976a). *Virology 75,* 74-87.

Ihle, J. N., Collins, J. J., Lee, J. C., Fischinger, P. J., Pazmiño, N., Moennig, V., Schäfer, W., Hanna, M. G., Jr., and Bolognesi, D. P. (1976b). *Virology 75,* 102-112.

Ihle, J. N., Domotor, J. J., Jr., and Bengali, K. M. (1976c). *Bibl. Haematol. 43,* 177-179.

Ihle, J. N., Joseph, D. R., and Pazmiño, N. H. (1976d). *J. Exp. Med. 144,* 1406-1423.

Ihle, J. N., Lee, J. C., Collins, J. J., Fischinger, P. J., Pazmiño, N. H., Moennig, V., Schäfer, W., Hanna, M. G., Jr., and Bolognesi, D. P. (1976e). *Virology 75,* 88-101.

Ihle, J. N., McEwan, R., and Bengali, K. (1976f). *J. Exp. Med. 144,* 1391-1405.

Jolicoeur, P., Rosenberg, N., Cotellessa, A., and Baltimore, D. (1978). *J. Natl. Cancer Inst. 60,* 1473-1476.

Lee, J. C., and Ihle, J. N. (1977). *J. Immunol. 118,* 928-934.

Lee, J. C., Ihle, J. N., and Huebner, R. (1977). *Proc. Natl. Cancer Inst. 74,* 343-347.

Lieberman, M., and Kaplan, H. S. (1959). *Science 130,* 387-388.

Lilly, F., Duran-Reynals, M. L., and Rowe, W. P. (1975). *J. Exp. Med. 141,* 882-889.

Louie, S., and Schwartz, R. S. (1978). *Sem. Hematol. 15,* 117-138.

Lowy, D. R., Rowe, W. P., Teich, N. M., and Hartley, J. W. (1971). *Science 174,* 155-156.

Lowy, D. R., Chattopadhyay, S. K., Teich, N. M., Rowe, W. P., and Levine, A. S. (1974). *Proc. Natl. Acad. Sci. 71,* 3555-3559.

Melief, C. J. M., Louie, S., and Schwartz, R. S. (1975). *J. Natl. Cancer Inst. 55,* 691-698.

Miller, J. F. A. P. (1961). *Adv. Cancer Res. 6,* 291-368.

Pazmiño, N. H., McEwan, R., and Ihle, J. N. (1978). *J. Exp. Med. 147,* 708-718.

Peters, R. L., Sass, B., Stephenson, J. R., Al-Ghazzouli, I. K., Hino, S., Donahoe, R. M., Kende, M., Aaronson, S. A., and Kelloff, G. J. (1977). *Proc. Natl. Acad. Sci. 74,* 1697-1701.

Rowe, W. P. (1973). *Cancer Res. 33,* 3061-3068.

Rowe, W. P., and Hartley, J. W. (1972). *J. Exp. Med. 136,* 1286-1301.

Rowe, W. P., Hartley, J. W., Lander, M. R., Pugh, W. E., and Teich, N. (1971). *Virology 46,* 866-876.

Rowe, W. P., Hartley, J. W., and Bremner, T. (1972). *Science 178,* 860-862.

Schäfer, W., Bolognesi, D. P., de Noronha, F., Fischinger, P. J., Hunsmann, G., Ihle, J. N., Moennig, V., Schwarz, H., and Thiel, H.-J. (1977a). *Med. Microbiol. Immunol. 164,* 217-229.

Schäfer, W., Schwarz, H., Thiel, H.-J., Fischinger, P. J., and Bolognesi, D. P. (1977b). *Virology 83,* 207-210.

Vogt, P. K., and Hu, S. S. F. (1977). *Ann. Rev. Genet. 11,* 203-238.

IDENTIFICATION OF VIRAL GENE PRODUCTS WHICH INDUCE IMMUNE RESPONSES IN NORMAL AND MAMMARY TUMOR-BEARING MICE

D. L. Fine
L. O. Arthur
R. J. Massey
and
G. Schochetman

Viral Onocology Program
Frederick Cancer Research Center
Frederick, Maryland

I. INTRODUCTION

Development of neoplasia in animals basically results from two processes. The first consists of transformation of normal cells to neoplastic cells with altered phenotypic properties. The second is the failure of the host's immune response to recognize or cope with the transformed cells. Cell transformation by viruses or chemicals results in altered phenotypic expression which includes the synthesis of specific classes of antigens not normally present on nontransformed cells. These antigens and the host immune responses directed against them thus represent markers which can serve (1) diagnostically in detecting tumor presence, (2) prognostically in predicting clinical status, and (3) prophylactically in preventing tumor development.

Important models for developing the use of such biological markers to monitor tumor development would be antigens specifically associated with or induced by oncogenic viruses, such as those of the mouse mammary tumor virus (MMTV). This virus has well-characterized structural proteins and is unique because it represents the only mammalian RNA tumor virus known to induce carcinomas in its host of origin (Bittner, 1936). Highly specific antisera to the MMTV structural components provide immunological probes which can be used to monitor specific

ISBN 0-12-131150-3

viral gene expression. Despite the presence of MMTV as a genetic factor in all mice (Varmus *et al.*, 1972; Scolnick *et al.*, 1974), only those strains which express the virus have a high incidence of mammary cancer (Parks *et al.*, 1974; Noon *et al.*, 1975). In the studies described here, we identify those MMTV-specific antigens which are expressed in normal and tumor-bearing mice from moderate and high mammary tumor strains and which are present on cell membranes of target tissues as true cell-surface antigens recognizable by host immune responses. Furthermore, we demonstrate that mice which express MMTV antigens develop specific humoral and cell-mediated immune responses which recognize these virus-coded and mammary tumor cell surface-associated antigens.

II. OVERVIEW OF HIGH AND MODERATE MAMMARY TUMOR MOUSE STRAINS AND MAMMARY TUMOR CELL SYSTEMS

High-incidence mammary cancer strains, such as C3H, RIII, and GR, develop mammary tumors early in life (6-12 months). In these strains, MMTV is expressed in an exogenous (particulate) form in milk, mammary tumors, and male reproductive organs (Bernard *et al.*, 1956; Bittner, 1940; Smith, 1966). Subsequent horizontal transmission of this virus through milk and/or seminal fluid (Andervont and Dunn, 1948; Strong, 1943) from the parent results in tumor development in recipient offspring. Consequently, horizontal transmission of exogenous MMTV is responsible for maintenance of high mammary cancer incidences. High mammary tumor strains can be freed of the exogenous MMTV (but not proviral MMTV) by foster nursing on low tumor incidence strains (Heston *et al.*, 1950). These foster-nursed or *f* strains exhibit a greatly reduced mammary tumor incidence as well as a significant delay (12-20 months) in the onset of tumor occurrence (Heston *et al.*, 1950). Despite removal of the highly oncogenic exogenous MMTV, strains such as C3Hf continue to express MMTV antigens and MMTV virus particles in their milk (Verstraeten and Van Nie, 1974) and mammary tumors (Dmochowski *et al.*, 1954). The virus expressed in these tissues represents an extrachromosomal form of the proviral or endogenous MMTV and induces a high frequency of late-arising tumors after inoculation into susceptible recipient animals (Hageman *et al.*, 1968). The availability of MMTV-expressor strains of mice, such as C3H and C3Hf, and the feasibility of developing continuous cultures of MMTV-producing mammary tumor cells (Fine *et al.*, 1974) have provided homologous *in vivo* and *in vitro* MMTV sources (both exogenous and endogenous) as well as systems for studying expression of MMTV antigens. Although our predominant *in vivo* source of MMTV has been the

Mm5mt/c_1 cell line originally derived from a mammary tumor of a C3H/Cgrl mouse (Owens and Hackett, 1972), we have recently established two mammary tumor cell lines from C3H/HeNf mice. Virus from these cell lines possess proteins similar to those of MMTV of other mouse strains. These proteins have molecular weights of 10,000 (p10), 14,000 (p14), 20,000 (p20), 27,000 (p27), 30,000 (p30), 36,000 (gp36), and 52,000 (gp52) (Fig. 1). Monospecific antisera have been prepared (Arthur *et al.*, 1978a,c; Schochetman *et al.*, 1977) against most of the proteins from MMTV derived from the Mm5mt/c_1 cell line and sensitive radioimmunoassays for several proteins have been developed (Arthur *et al.*, 1978a,c). The development of highly specific competition radio-

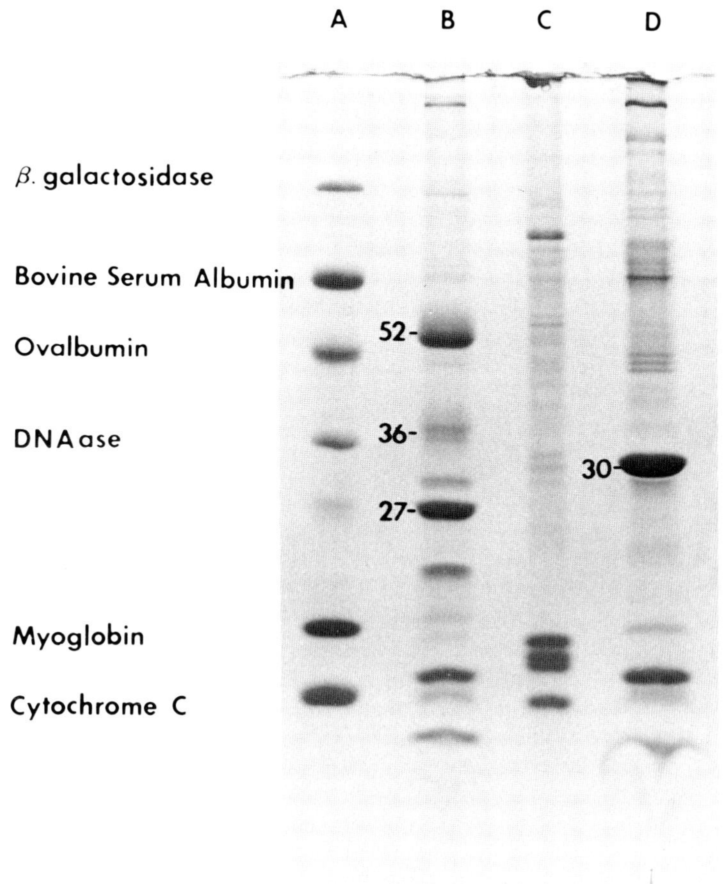

FIGURE 1. SDS-PAGE analysis of MMTV proteins (column B) from purified MMTV derived from Mm5mt/c_1 cells. Major envelope polypeptides gp52, gp36, and major internal polypeptide p27 are designated. Comparison with purified intracytoplasmic particles (column C), and purified Rauscher MuLV (column D). Molecular weight standards are shown in column A.

immunoassays for antigens such as the major MMTV envelope glycoprotein gp52 provides a means for detecting the expression of this antigen in specific tissues of normal and tumor-bearing mice.

III. *IN VIVO* DISTRIBUTION OF MMTV ENVELOPE GLYCOPROTEIN GP52

Previously we have demonstrated (Arthur *et al.*, 1978a; Fine *et al.*, 1978) strains with a high incidence of mammary cancer, such as C3H and GR/N, express MMTV gp52, primarily in mammary tumors, normal mammary glands, and lymph nodes of female mice. While no gp52 was detected in lymph nodes of male C3H/HeN mice, appreciable quantities were found in the vas deferens and the vesicular, coagulating, and prostate glands. No antigen was detected in either the testes or epididymis. The male C3H/HeN submaxillary gland also contained low levels of gp52. In addition, MMTV gp52 is expressed in the sera of mammary tumor bearing mice (Arthur *et al.*, 1978a; Ritzi *et al.*, 1976; Zangerle *et al.*, 1977), where it coexists with precipitating antibodies to MMTV (Arthur *et al.*, 1978a). These latter findings, in conjunction with the fact that MMTV gp52 is the major external MMTV protein (Schloemer *et al.*, 1976; Witte *et al.*, 1973; Cardiff *et al.*, 1974), may indicate that this protein represents an important antigen involved in immune responses to MMTV expression. Therefore, it is important to understand the distribution of MMTV gp52 in various organs of normal mice from moderate and low mammary tumor strains in order to correlate MMTV expression and immune responses to the virus. Tissue extracts and sera from age-matched C3H, GR/N, C3Hf, and BALB/c male and female mice were examined (Table I). Tissue distribution of MMTV gp52 in the moderate mammary tumor strain C3Hf was similar to that found in both high mammary tumor strains, C3H and GR/N. Tissues including liver, spleen, kidney, brain, heart, bone marrow, and preputial glands were routinely negative for all strains of mice.

Concentration of MMTV gp52 antigen in organs of C3H and GR/N mice was consistently higher (as much as 20-fold) than that found in C3Hf mice, whereas corresponding tissues of BALB/c mice were negative. The presence of MMTV gp52 in mammary tumors of C3Hf mice indicates that endogenous MMTV is expressed at relatively high levels in this mouse strain. Similarly, the presence of MMTV gp52 in the sera of C3Hf mice demonstrates that the major glycoprotein of endogenous MMTV is released into the sera, presumably as a result of disruption of the barrier between the mammary gland and the circulatory system. The presence of this antigen in the sera of tumor-bearing C3Hf mice is analogous to its presence in the sera of mice which harbor and transmit exo-

TABLE I. Distribution of MMTV gp52 in Tissues of Inbred Mice[a]

Strain	Sex	Tumor status	MMTV gp52[b]						
			Serum	Tumor	Mammary tissue	Submaxillary gland	Coagulating gland	Vesicular gland	Vas deferens
C3Hf	F	-	9(5)		31(15)	3(10)			
C3Hf	F	+	500(2)	410(2)	N.T.[c]	N.T.			
C3Hf	M	-	2(5)			2(10)	1(10)	2(10)	5(10)
C3H	F	-	4(15)		279(6)	21(6)			
C3H	F	+	775(9)	1286(8)	N.T.	N.T.			
C3H	M	-	3(4)			2(10)	29(9)	5(9)	100(10)
GR	F	-	12(4)		809(15)	8(10)			
GR	F	+	120(4)	270(3)	N.T.	N.T.			
GR	M	-	N.T.			11(10)	43(9)	29(10)	57(10)
BALB/c	F	-	3(12)		N.A.[d]	N.T.			
BALB/c	M	-	2(5)			N.A.	N.A.	N.A.	N.A.

[a]MMTV gp52 was measured in tissue extracts of retired breeders by competition radioimmunoassays as described in Materials and Methods.

[b]Average concentration of gp52 is expressed as ng MMTV gp52/mg protein in tissue extracts and as ng MMTV gp52/ml in the sera samples. Number of animals tested is given in parenthesis.

[c]Not tested.

[d]No antigen detected within limits of assay.

genous MMTV. Based on the results of the moderate and low-cancer strains, the C3Hf strain appears to be an MMTV-expressor like C3H, whereas BALB/c is a low or nonexpressor of the virus. A similar tissue distribution of MMTV gp52 was observed in groups of normal and tumor-bearing feral mice trapped in Southern California. However, in contrast to the finding that MMTV gp52 is expressed in all C3H, C3Hf, and GR mammary tumors, we were able to detect MMTV gp52 in only three of seven mammary tumors from feral mice. In addition, levels of MMTV gp52 antigen in the mammary tumors of the feral mice were low in comparison to mammary tumors of the inbred mice. Normal organs (e.g., lymph nodes, submaxillary, and vesicular glands) contained levels of gp52 equivalent to those levels detected in the same organs of inbred mice (Fine *et al.*, 1978). We can conclude from these data that although feral mice have a low incidence of spontaneous mammary tumors (Gardner *et al.*, 1976) they are low expressors of MMTV.

Expression of MMTV antigens in tumor-bearing mice is not restricted to MMTV gp52. This conclusion is based on our observations that MMTV p14 (Arthur *et al.*, 1978c) is expressed in mammary tumors. Furthermore, using a competitive radioimmunoassay for MMTV p10, we have recently found that MMTV p10 is expressed in the sera of mammary tumor bearing mice. Levels of p10 are higher in sera of mammary tumor bearing mice than in sera of non-tumor-bearing animals. Levels of p10 ranged from 45 to 300 ng/ml in the sera of tumor-bearing C3H/HeN and GR/N mice, whereas p10 was not detected (<2 ng p10/ml serum) in the sera of tumor-free C3H/HeN and GR/N female mice.

IV. DISTRIBUTION OF PRECIPITATING ANTIBODIES TO MMTV

Radioimmunoprecipitation assays using radiolabeled virus or viral antigens have provided a highly sensitive tool for detecting antiviral immune responses (Ihle *et al.*, 1974, 1976). We have used radioimmunoprecipitation of ^{125}I-MMTV as an indicator of humoral immunity in attempting to correlate immune responses to MMTV with MMTV antigen expression. MMTV precipitating antibody was detected in all high and low mammary tumor strains as well as in a group of feral mice trapped in several geographic locations in Southern California (Table II). However, significant differences were noted between the high and low tumor strains with regard to titer and frequency of antibody-positive animals. Sera from the two high mammary tumor strains, C3H and GR/N, had the highest titers (1:3,200) and frequency of antibody to MMTV (60-90%). Approximately 50% of the sera from the C3Hf strain contained the antibody and these sera also had high titers (maximum 1:3,200). In contrast, mice

TABLE II. *Distribution of Precipitating Antibodies to MMTV in Mice of High, Moderate, and Low Mammary Tumor Incidence*

Strain[a]	Sex	Tumor	Incidence[b] (months)	Anti-MMTV Antibody: Number positive[c] / Number tested	Anti-MMTV Antibody: Maximum titer
C3H/HeN	F	99	7	32/36 (89%)	1:3200
C3H/HeN	M			21/28 (75%)	1:3200
C3H/HeNf	F	40	16	17/30 (57%)	1:3200
C3H/HeNf	M			14/36 (38%)	1:3200
GR/N	F	85	9	11/16 (69%)	1:2560
GR/N	M			6/10 (60%)	1:2560
BALB/c (NIV)[d]	F	32	16	3/3 (100%)	1:1280
BALB/c (NIV)	M			1/1 (100%)	1:640
BALB/c	F	5	16	1/25 (4%)	1:20
BALB/c	M			0/15 –	–
C57BL/6	F	1	18	3/57 (5%)	1:320
C57BL/6	M			0/9 –	–
Feral Mice	F	3	>18	6/49 (12%)	1:400
Feral Mice	M			4/43 (9%)	1:400

[a] All mice were non-tumor bearing animals greater than six months of age.

[b] Percent of forced breeders which develop mammary tumors. Average age of tumor appearance is given in parenthesis. Tumors arising after nine months of age are considered late arising.

[c] Sera which precipitated greater than 20% of the ^{125}I-MMTV at a 1:20 dilution were considered positive.

[d] All BALB/c (NIV) mice were greater than 14 months of age.

with low incidences of mammary tumors (1-5%), such as BALB/c, C57BL/6, and feral mice, had low-titered (1:20) low-frequency (4-12%) antibody-positive sera. Interestingly, BALB/c mice infected with the nodule-inducing variant (NIV) of MMTV (Deome *et al.*, 1967), had high-titered antibodies to MMTV and a higher incidence of spontaneous mammary tumors than did uninfected BALB/c mice. As such, NIV-infected BALB/c mice exhibited immune responses and tumor development characteristics similar to those of the C3Hf strain. The presence of antibody in these two strains is indicative of both expression and immune recognition of endogenous MMTV. In correlating the distribution of antibody to MMTV with the previous data on MMTV gp52 expression (Table I), it appears that strains of mice (both male and female) which express MMTV antigens similarly develop precipitating antibodies to MMTV, whereas MMTV nonexpressing strains (e.g., BALB/c and C57BL6) do not develop MMTV-precipitating antibodies at high frequency. Although antibody was detected in one of 25 BALB/c mice, the antibody titer in this serum was too low (1:20) to demonstrate specificity. Three of 57 C57BL/6 mice developed antibodies which were specific for MMTV by competition assays; however, these mice had been housed in the same room with C3H and GR/N mice. Therefore, it is possible that the immune responses in these mice were due to exposure to MMTV expressed by these other strains.

V. AGE-DEPENDENT DEVELOPMENT OF PRECIPITATING ANTIBODIES TO MMTV IN C3H AND C3HF MICE

Because exposure to MMTV antigens may be instrumental in stimulating antibody production, we examined the effect of age on the development of MMTV precipitating antibodies. Groups of five virgin female C3H and C3Hf mice were bled beginning at six weeks of age and then at three-week intervals and their sera examined for MMTV precipitating antibody. Antibodies were detected in the sera of six-week-old C3H mice (Fig. 2). Antibody titers in this group of mice increased with age and by 15 weeks of age ranged from 1:1,600 to 1:3,200. The early immune responses in C3H mice may result from infection with the milk-borne MMTV transmitted by nursing on C3H females. This hypothesis is supported by the lack of development of MMTV antibodies in six-week-old C3Hf mice. MMTV antibodies were detected in this group, but not until the mice were 15 weeks of age. These antibodies were presumably directed at endogenous MMTV antigens, which are expressed at a relatively early age. The development of antibodies in virgin C3Hf would exclude the possibility that the immune response is directed at MMTV antigens transmitted by male mice during breeding.

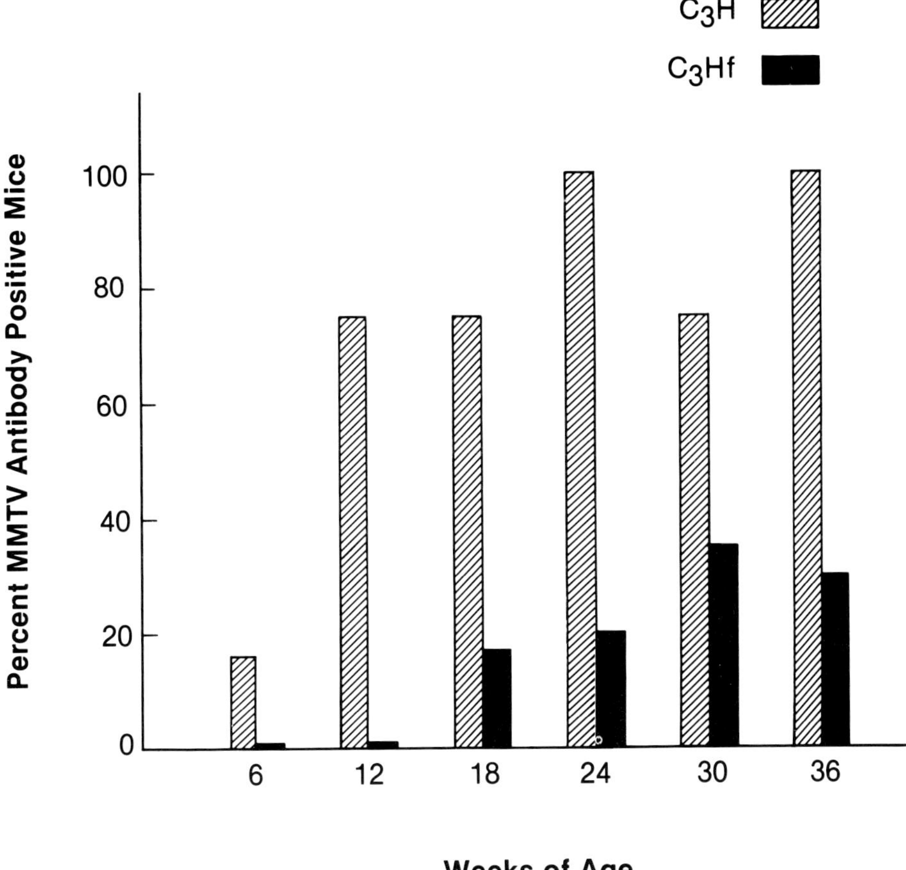

FIGURE 2. Age-dependent development of MMTV precipitating antibody in virgin female C3H and C3Hf mice.

VI. SPECIFICITY OF NATURALLY OCCURRING ANTIBODIES TO MMTV

It is consistent with the tissue-specific expression of gp52 in high and moderate tumor incidence strains to predict that the natural antibodies which develop in these same mouse strains are directed against gp52. One method for demonstrating specificity of the natural sera is to compete the binding of ^{125}I-MMTV with unlabeled virus and/or virus antigens. In this test binding of the natural sera for ^{125}I-MMTV was displaced by either unlabeled MMTV or purified MMTV gp52, but not by A-MuLV (Fig. 3). In addition, neither G-MuLV, MPMV, nor SMRV competed (data not shown), indicating the specificity of

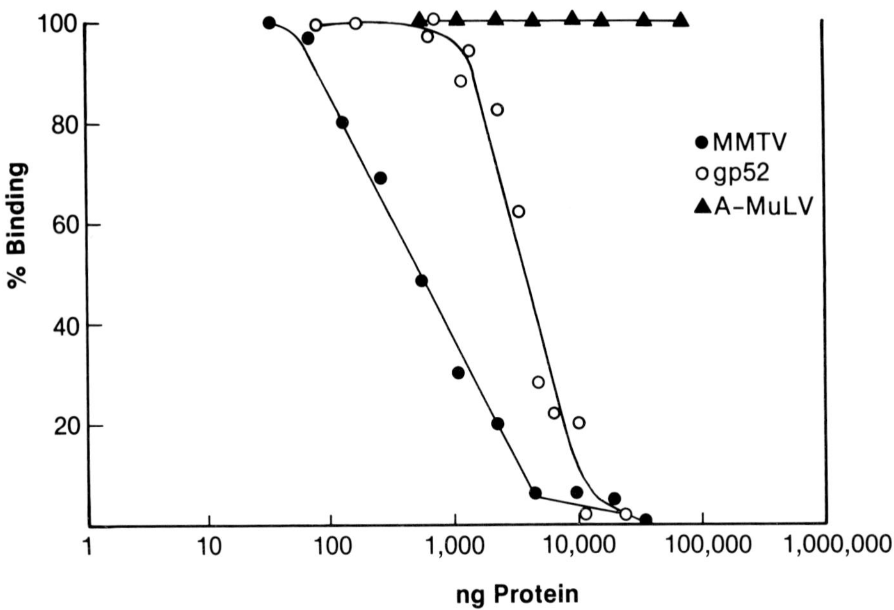

FIGURE 3. Demonstration of specificity for binding of natural mouse serum to ^{125}*I-MMTV. Binding was displaced by unlabeled MMTV (●——●), and purified MMTV gp52 (O——O) but not by amphotrophic MuLV (A-MuLV) (▲——▲).*

the serum reactivity for MMTV. The ability of purified MMTV gp52 to compete in this assay indicates that at least part of the naturally occurring humoral immune response is directed against this antigen. 550 ng of MMTV were required to displace 50% binding of the ^{125}I-MMTV. Since gp52 represents approximately 15% of the virion proteins, it is estimated that 82.5 ng of this protein associated with the intact MMTV were present at 50% displacement. In contrast, 4,500 ng (or nearly 50-fold more) purified MMTV gp52 was required to give equivalent displacement of the ^{125}I-MMTV. This difference might be due to the alterations which occur in the three-dimensional configuration of the glycoprotein during purification and which render it less antigenic for binding to the natural sera.

In a corollary experiment we examined mouse sera for antibodies to purified MMTV gp52. Sera from 22 MMTV antibody-positive C3H and C3Hf mice were assayed for precipitating antibodies to MMTV gp52 and no precipitation of gp52 was found. In contrast, high-titered sera from 4 of 11 MMTV antibody-positive x-irradiated feral mice and one BALB/c NIV-infected mouse were found to precipitate ^{125}I-MMTV gp52. Precipitations of ^{125}I-MMTV gp52 and ^{125}I-MMTV with a representative feral mouse serum are shown in Fig. 4. This serum precipitated approximately 50% of the ^{125}I-MMTV gp52 at a 1:10 dilution and had a 20% endpoint titer of 1:40. In contrast, the titer against intact ^{125}I-MMTV was appreciably higher, precipitating ≥ 80% of the virus at a 1:320 dilution with a titer of greater than 1:1,280. The ^{125}I-MMTV gp52 was 100% immunoprecipitable by rabbit anti-MMTV serum at a 1:100 dilution. These latter findings are consistent with the hypothesis that natural sera do not readily recognize gp52 in an altered configuration, whereas hyperimmune sera to the purified molecule do.

The specificity of the mouse serum binding of MMTV gp52 was determined by radioimmune competition assays (Fig. 5). MMTV from C3H or C3Hf tumor cells completely displaced the serum binding of ^{125}I-MMTV gp52, whereas no displacement occurred when G-MuLV of BALB/c lactating mammary gland extracts (data not shown) were used as competing antigens. In addition to the lack of immune recognition which may occur due to conformational changes in purified gp52, our inability to detect precipitating

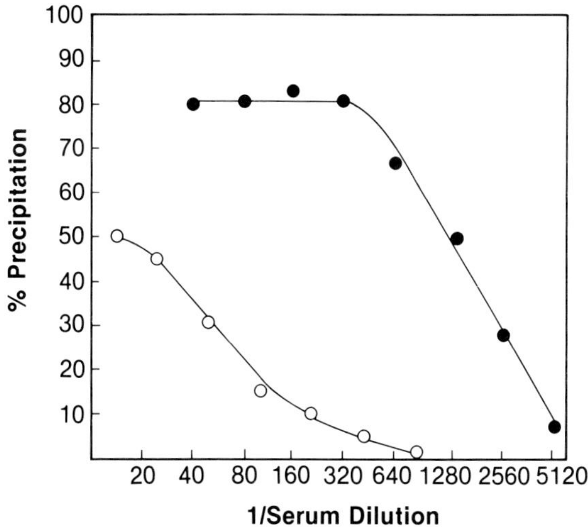

FIGURE 4. Titration of irradiated feral mouse serum against MMTV and MMTV gp52. Serum was titered against ^{125}I-MMTV (●—●) and ^{125}I-MMTV gp52 (O—O) in the direct radioimmunoprecipitation assay. Titration of a normal C57BL/6 serum against the same antigens was included as a control and was negative (data not shown).

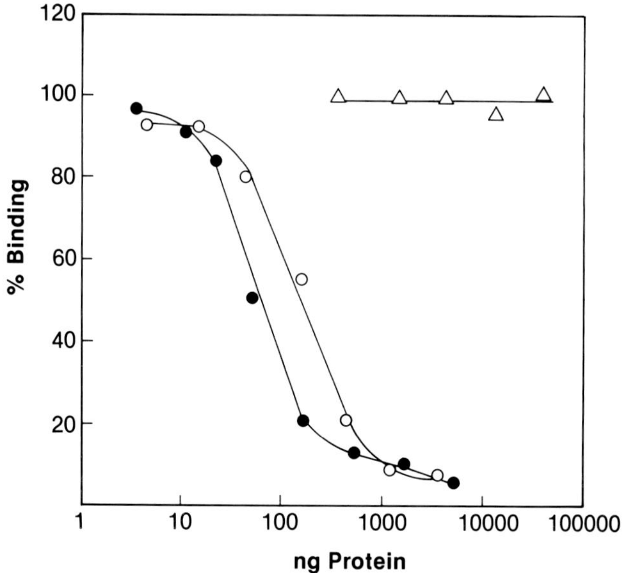

FIGURE 5. Demonstration of specificity for binding of a feral mouse serum to ^{125}I-MMTV gp52. Binding was displaced by unlabeled MMTV from C3Hf tumor cells (●——●), MMTV from C3H (Mm5mt/c_1) tumor cells (O——O), but not by G-MuLV (Δ——Δ).

antibodies to MMTV gp52 in the C3H and C3Hf strains may be the result of one or more of the following: (1) that the sera examined from these strains were generally of lower titer than those of the feral and BALB/c NIV mice and/or (2) that naturally occurring antibody is directed at a combination of group- and type-specific antigenic determinants, but the high degree of antigen expression which occurs in high tumor incidence mice consequently adsorbs out the natural reactivity to gp52.

VII. RECOGNITION OF MMTV VIRION PROTEINS BY SERA FROM MICE IMMUNIZED WITH MMTV

Although BALB/c and C57BL/6 mice have a low incidence of spontaneous mammary tumors, they are readily infected by MMTV and develop a high incidence of mammary tumors upon infection (Arthur *et al.*, 1978b). We previously reported that weanling BALB/c mice inoculated with MMTV derived from C3H mammary tumor cell cultures developed a high-titered MMTV-precipitating antibody but still succumbed to mammary tumors at an early age

(Ihle *et al.*, 1976). To determine whether the antibodies induced by MMTV inoculation were directed against the same MMTV polypeptides as naturally occurring antibodies, weanling BALB/c and C57BL/6 mice were immunized subcutaneously with 100 μg of intact MMTV in complete Freund's adjuvant followed four weeks later by a second subcutaneous inoculation with 50 μg of MMTV. Sera were collected at the time of the second immunization and four weeks later. Control mice were inoculated with Freund's adjuvant alone. Sera were incubated with lysed ^{3}H-leucine-labeled MMTV and the immunoprecipitates were analyzed by sodium dodecyl sulfate-polyacrylamide gel electrophoresis (SDS-PAGE) and fluorography (Fig. 6). The developed x-ray film was scanned and the radioactivity was quantitated. The results are expressed in Table III. All MMTV-immunized mice responded with a high-titered precipitating antibody to MMTV, whereas the sera from control mice showed no MMTV precipitating activity. Precipitation titers of the positive sera ranged from 1:800 to >1:12,800 despite the fact that each of the immunized mice received the same dose of virus. Sera from the MMTV-immunized C57BL/6 mice recognized gp52 and gp36, whereas sera from MMTV-immunized BALB/c mice recognized the same two antigens and p10. These results indicate that antibody responses in mice immunized with MMTV are predominantly against the viral envelope-associated polypeptides.

VIII. CELLULAR IMMUNE RECOGNITION OF MMTV AND MuLV IN NORMAL AND MAMMARY TUMOR-BEARING MICE

Naturally occurring cell-mediated immune (CMI) responses to MMTV have been previously demonstrated in both normal and mammary tumor-bearing mice (Blair *et al.*, 1975; Lopez *et al.*, 1976, 1978). For example, using BALB/c and BALB/cfC3H mice, Lopez *et al.* (1976) demonstrated CMI responses to MMTV antigens by both blastogensis and production of macrophage migration inhibition factors. These studies suggest that CMI responses are directed at MMTV antigens expressed in normal and tumor-bearing mice, but it is unclear against which antigen the cytotoxic lymphocytes are directed. As part of our model for studying immunity in C3H and C3Hf mice, we have examined spleen lymphocytes from normal and tumor-bearing mice of high, moderate, and low tumor inbred strains and from feral mice for their blastogenic responses to MMTV, MuLV, and the envelope glycoproteins of each virus. The results show that both C3H and C3Hf mice develop blastogenic responses to MMTV, which is dependent on the age of the animal (Table IV). This response is not seen in the low mammary tumor strain C57BL/6 but is evident in feral mice. This is the first evidence that lymphocytes from C3Hf

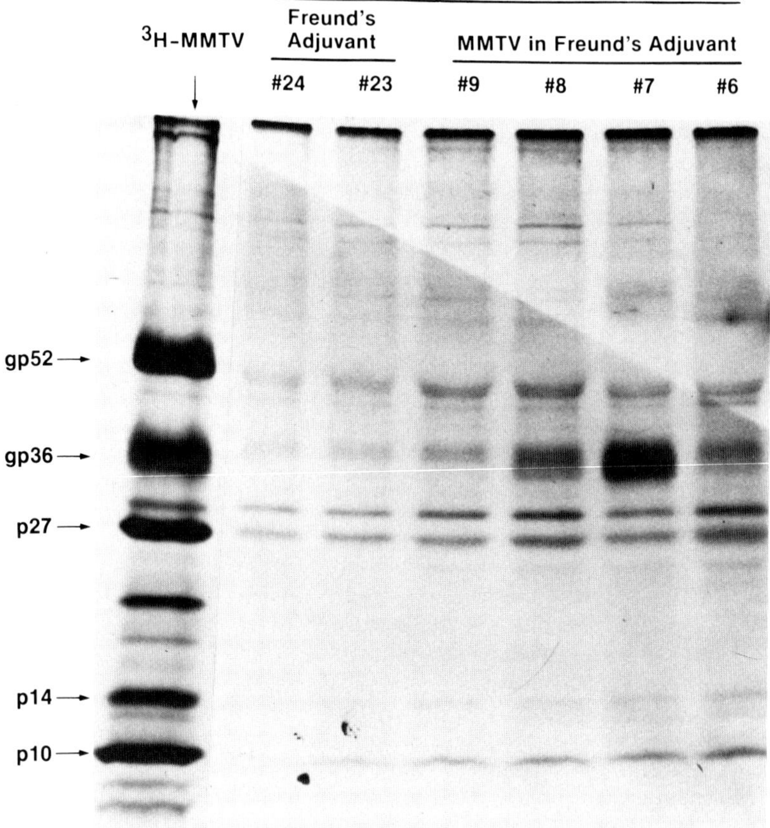

FIGURE 6. Recognition of MMTV polypeptides by sera from BALB/c mice immunized with MMTV. Sera were incubated with lysed ^{3}H-leucine labeled MMTV and the immune precipitates were analyzed by SDS-PAGE and fluorography. Control mice had been inoculated with complete Freund's adjuvant alone.

mice can be stimulated with MMTV. Consequently, this strain is capable of recognizing the endogenous MMTV by both CMI and humoral immune responses. This response persists in C3H and GR tumor-bearing animals; however, it should be noted that not all tumor-bearing mice respond to MMTV. It remains to be determined whether there is a correlation between tumor size and blastogenic responses, as has been previously suggested

TABLE III. *Mouse Mammary Tumor Virus Proteins Precipitated by the Sera of Mice Immunized with MMTV*

Mouse designation		MMTV proteins[a]						
		p10	p14	p27	p30	gp36	gp52	Anti-MMTV titer[b]
Inoculated with MMTV[c]								
C57BL/6	#2	0.6[d]	0.1	2.5	2.3	4.4(2)	7.5(4.2)	>12,800
	#3	0.5	0	1.5	1.2	1.1	5.5(3.1)	>12,800
	#4	1.9	0.2	2.2	2	2.4	1.4	800
	#5	0.5	0	1.2	1.4	22.6(10.3)	1.5	1,600
BALB/c	#6	3.8(2.2)	0.5	5	4	6.6(10.3)	0.4	3,200
	#7	3.4(2.0)	0.6	2	2	30.7(14.6)	1.5	3,200
	#8	1.8	0.2	3.4	3.8	10.6(5)	4.4(2.8)	6,400
	#9	3.1	0.8	3.4	4.2	4.1(2)	4(2.5)	1,600
Inoculated with Freund's adjuvant								
C57BL/6	#21	2.0	0.2	2.2	2.2	2.2	1.6	<20
	#22	1.6	0	2.5	2.2	2.2	2.0	<20
BALB/c	#23	2.2	0	2.8	2.2	2.7	2.1	<20
	#24	1.5	0.6	3.1	2.4	2.0	1.2	<20
	$25	1.5	1.0	1.8	1.1	1.5	1.4	<20

[a]MMTV proteins which were immunoreactive with mice sera were determined by incubating lysed ^{3}H-leucine labeled MMTV with mouse serum and analyzing immune precipitates by SDS-PAGE and fluorography.

[b]Reciprocal of the highest serum dilution capable of binding greater than 20% of the ^{125}I-MMTV.

[c]Mice were inoculated subcutaneously with 100 µg of MMTV in complete Freund's adjuvant followed four weeks later by a second subcutaneous inoculation with 50 µg of MMTV. Control mice were inoculated with Freund's adjuvant at same time intervals.

[d]Values represent area under peaks obtained by scanning exposed x-ray film and are in direct proportion to the radioactivity in the labeled polypeptide. Values given in parenthesis are the relative increases in precipitation for those activities which exceed the mean of the control sera by greater than two-fold.

TABLE IV. *Blastogenic Response*[a] *of Mouse Spleen Lymphocytes to MMTV and MuLV*

Mouse strain	Age (months)	Antigens			
		MMTV	MuLV	gp52	gp70
Mammary tumor bearing					
C3H/HeN	6	5/6[b]	3/6	3/3	2/3
GR/N	8	6/6	4/6	N.T.[b]	N.T.
Normal females					
C3H/HeN	1	0/3	0/3	N.T.	N.T.
	3	3/3	0/3	N.T.	N.T.
	6	4/6	1/6	2/3	2/3
GR/N	3	3/3	0/3	N.T.	N.T.
	8	5/6	3/6	N.T.	N.T.
C3H/HeNf	1	0/3	0/3	N.T.	N.T.
	3	5/6	1/6	N.T.	N.T.
	>8	4/6	2/6	N.T.	N.T.
C57BL/6	>8	0/6	1/6	N.T.	N.T.
Feral mice	>6	3/5	4/5	N.T.	N.T.

[a]*The blastogenic response was tested by incubating* 10^6 *mouse spleen lymphocytes with 0.1 ml of different concentrations of antigen for five days, pulsing with 3H-thymidine, and measuring the thymidine incorporation. A stimulation index was calculated based on the thymidine incorporation of lymphocytes incubated in medium without antigen. Stimulation indices were tested for statistical significance by a t-test. The results here are the number of animals with significant blastogenic responses/the number of animals tested.*

[b]*Not tested.*

(Creemers and Bentvelzen, 1977). Blastogenic responses to MuLV were also observed in all strains of mice tested and were most frequent in the older animals. Naturally occurring cellular immune responses to MuLV may also occur since we had previously observed precipitating antibodies to MuLV in sera of normal and tumor-bearing C3H mice (Ihle *et al.*, 1976). We examined the specificities of the reactions in the C3H/HeN strain with purified MMTV gp52 and MuLV gp70 and found responses to both. We can conclude that these proteins, which constitute the major envelope glycoproteins of MMTV and MuLV, stimulate both the humoral and cell-mediated immune responses in normal and tumor-bearing mice.

IX. EXPRESSION OF MMTV STRUCTURAL PROTEINS IN MOUSE MAMMARY TUMOR CELLS

The results presented above demonstrate that specific expression of MMTV antigens occur in select tissues of normal and mammary tumor-bearing mice. In mouse mammary tumors these antigens include MMTV gp52 and at least two MMTV polypeptides (p14 and p10) synthesized by the *gag* region of the MMTV genome (Arthur *et al.*, 1978c; Arthur and Fine, 1978). However, in order to understand antitumor immune responses it is necessary to determine which MMTV proteins are expressed on tumors as virus-specific cell surface antigens and as potential targets for immune recognition by the mouse. We have studied the appearance of virus-specific antigens on the surface of mammary tumor cells using combined techniques of cell-surface labeling and immunoprecipitation with monospecific antisera prepared against purified viral proteins.

Labeling of cell surface antigens (CSA) was performed by lactoperoxidase catalyzed iodination and labeling of glycoproteins with tritiated sodium borohydride by the galactose oxidase method on neuraminidase-treated cells. The presence of viral CSA was first studied on cultured mammary tumor cells producing MMTV and MuLV (clone 13D), and on nonvirus-producing cells (clone B9). B9 cells did, however, synthesize high levels of MMTV antigens. All the cells possessed the genomes of MMTV and MuLV when first placed in culture; they were not infected *in vitro*. Cells 13D and B9 are single-cell clonal isolates of Mm5mt/c_1. The cells were radioiodinated, extensively washed, and lysed. The virus-specific proteins were immunoprecipitated using (1) monospecific antisera to the MMTV glycoproteins gp52 and gp36; (2) monospecific antisera to the MMTV nonglycoproteins p27 and p10; (3) polyvalent anti-MMTV serum; (4) monospecific antiserum to the MuLV glycoprotein gp70; (5) monospecific antiserum to the MuLV nonglycoproteins p30, p12, and p10; and (6) preimmune normal rabbit serum (NRS). Figure 7 shows the cell surface labeling results obtained with the 13D cells and Fig. 8 shows the results obtained with B9 cells. The major iodinated MMTV antigen detected on the surface of 13D, B9, and Mm5mt/c_1 cells was gp52, which was precipitated by anti-MMTV and anti-gp52 sera. MMTV antisera to the internal viral proteins p27 and p10 did not precipitate significant levels of iodinated proteins. Although MMTV anti-gp36 did not precipitate gp36, it, as well as anti-MMTV, did occasionally precipitate a surface-iodinated protein with a molecular weight of about 65,000. No other antisera precipitated this protein and its significance remains to be determined, as it is present on numerous cells of different animal origin (Table V). The fact that gp52 was present on B9 cells which do not produce MMTV demonstrated that gp52 represents an integral membrane component and was not the result of surface labeling of budding or passively adsorbed virus. Furthermore, the fact that gp52 and not its precursor polyprotein gPr75 was iodinated on the cell surface indicated that gPr75 must be cleaved to its individual components, gp52 and gp36, prior to the appearance of gp52 on the cell surface. The inability to detect iodinated gPr75 on the cell surface is not due to proteolysis, because gPr75 can be readily detected in ^{3}H-leucine pulse-labeled cells (Schochetman *et al.*, 1977, 1978b). Furthermore, the inability to iodinate gp36 on the cell surface is consistent with the inability to iodinate gp36 on intact purified MMTV (Cardiff *et al.*, 1974; Schloemer *et al.*, 1976; Fig. 7), demonstrating that gp52 and gp36 are already properly oriented prior to the budding of a complete MMTV particle.

In addition to gp52 all three cell types possessed MuLV gp70, precipitated by MuLV anti-gp70 as a CSA (Figs. 7 and 8). Primary mammary tumor cells never placed in culture also possessed gp52 and gp70 on their surfaces, whereas lymphocytes from the same animals possessed only gp70 on their surfaces (Table V). The 13D cells producing both MMTV and MuLV also possessed as a CSA a protein with a molecular weight of 90,000 (gp70), which was precipitated only by MuLV anti-gp70. The gp70-related protein may represent the gp70 precursor polyprotein. An additional two iodinated proteins with molecular weights of 85,000 and 95,000 were precipitated from 13D cells by antisera to the p30s of AKR-MuLV and R-MuLV [Figs. 7 and 9(a)]. These two proteins were also precipitated by antiserum to the p12 of R-MuLV, whereas antiserum to the p10 of R-MuLV precipitated only the 95,000-dalton protein [Fig. 9(a)]. These proteins are analogous, if not identical, to the Gross cell surface antigen (GCSA) as shown by the fact that similar results are obtained with leukemic cells from AKR mice with thymomas [Fig. 9(b)]. Only 13D cells and AKR leukemic cells possessed GCSA and gp90. AKR preleukemic cells possessed only gp70 as a

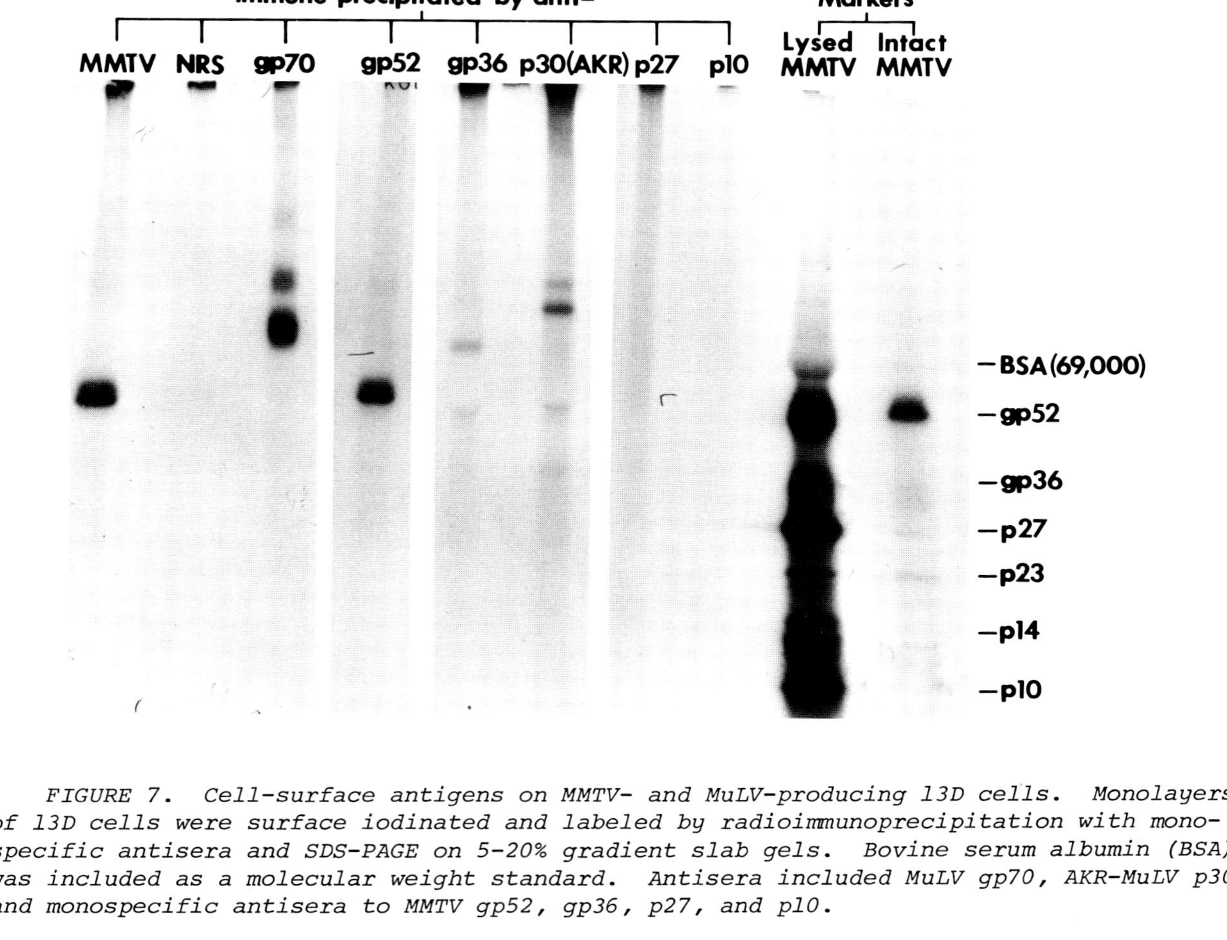

FIGURE 7. Cell-surface antigens on MMTV- and MuLV-producing 13D cells. Monolayers of 13D cells were surface iodinated and labeled by radioimmunoprecipitation with monospecific antisera and SDS-PAGE on 5-20% gradient slab gels. Bovine serum albumin (BSA) was included as a molecular weight standard. Antisera included MuLV gp70, AKR-MuLV p30, and monospecific antisera to MMTV gp52, gp36, p27, and p10.

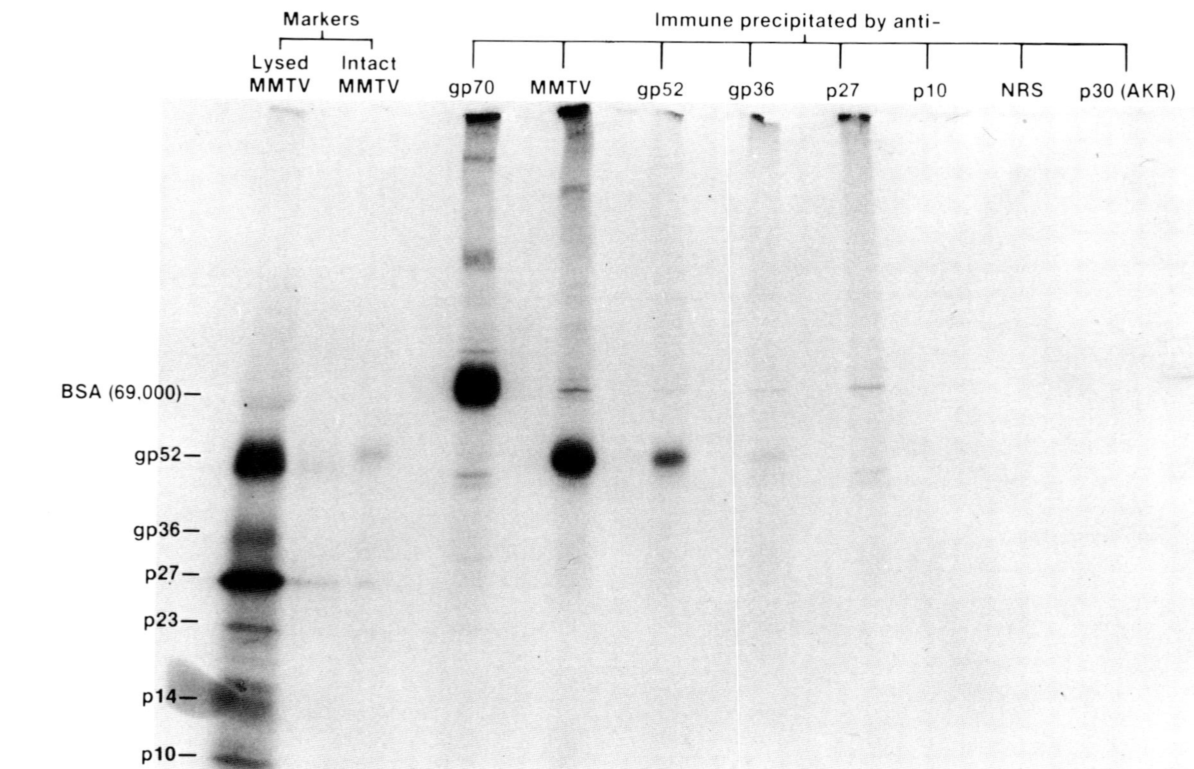

FIGURE 8. Viral cell-surface antigens on non-virus-producing B9 cells. Cells were surface iodinated and labeled surface antigens were analyzed as in Fig. 7.

TABLE V. Summary of MuLV and MMTV Antigens Present on the Surface of Various Cells as Determined by Cell-Surface Iodination

		Virus antigen				
		MuLV			MMTV	
Cells[a]	Virus production	gp70	gp90	GCSA	gp52	gp65
		Cultured Mouse Mammary Tumor Cells				
13D	B,C	+[b]	+	+	+	±
Mm5mt/c_1	B	+	-	-	+	±
C-21A	C	+	+	-	+	-
B-9	-	+	-	-	+	±
C3Hf-1	B (low level)	+	-	-	+	+
M9	B	+	-	-	+	+
RIII MT	B	+	-	-	+	+
		Mouse lymphocytes				
AKR-leukemic	C	+	+	+	-	-
AKR-preleukemic	C	+	-	-	-	-
C3H lymph	?	+	-	-	-	-
GR lymph	?	+	-	-	-	-
BALB/c lymph	?	+	-	-	-	-
		Miscellaneous cells				
A-MuLV (#292)	C	+	-	-	-	+
MCF	C	+	-	-	-	-
FRE	-	-	-	-	-	+
FRE(MMTV)	B	-	-	-	+	+
BALB/c	-	-	-	-	-	+
BALB/c(MMTV)	B	-	-	-	+	+
NIH	-	-	-	-	-	+
NIH(MMTV)	B	-	-	-	+	+
HESM	-	-	-	-	-	+
HESM(MMTV)	B	-	-	-	+	+
HBL-100	-	-	-	-	-	+

[a]Target cells used and brief descriptions include: Mm5mt/c_1 --- continuous cell line from mammary tumor of a C3H/Cgrl mouse; 13D, C-21A, B-9 --- single-cell clones of Mm5mt/c_1 cultured mammary tumor cells of a C3Hf mouse; RIIIMT --- cultured mammary tumor cell of a RIII mouse; AKR-leukemic/preleukemic --- thymocytes from thymuses of preleukemic and leukemic animals with thymonas; C3H-lymph/GR-lymph --- spleen lymphocytes from respective mammary tumor bearing mouse; BALB/c-lymph --- spleen lymphocytes from normal BALB/c mouse; A-MuLV (#292) --- mink lung (CCL-64) cells infected with amphotrophic feral mouse MuLV; MCF --- mink lung (CCL-64) cells infected with amphotrophic mink cell focus forming MuLV; FRE --- fisher rat embryo cells; BALB/c --- BALB/c mouse embryo cells; NIH --- NIH mouse embryo cells; HESM/HESM (MMTV) --- human embryonic skin and muscle uninfected (MMTV-infected); HBL-100 --- human mammary epithelial cells.

[b](+) = present; (-) = absent.

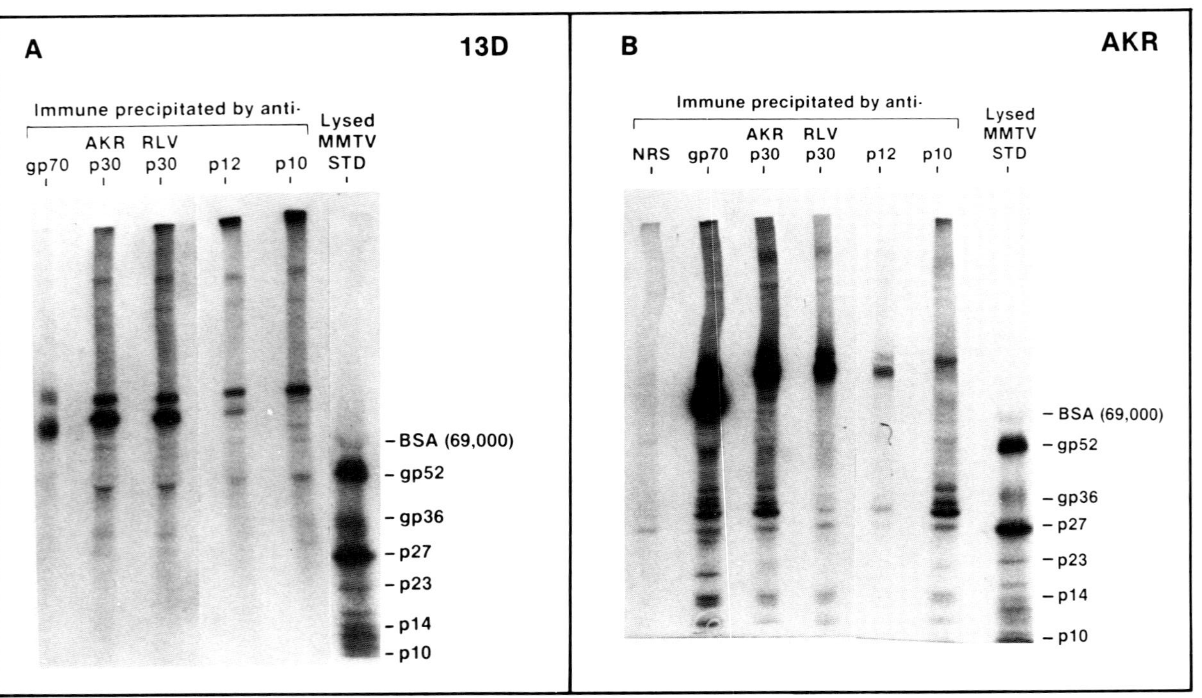

FIGURE 9. Comparison of viral cell surface antigens on 13D cells and AKR leukemic cells from AKR lymphomas. Cells were surface iodinated and labeled antigens were analyzed with MuLV antisera as in Fig. 7.

CSA (Table V). Galactose oxidase labeling of carbohydrates on neuramindase-treated 13D cells yielded labeled gp52, gp70, and gp90, demonstrating the cell surface location of these antigens and that gp90 was a glycoprotein (Fig. 10). However, MMTV gp36 was also labeled, indicating that at least its carbohydrate regions are exposed even though it could not be iodinated. The presence of additional CSA on mammary tumor cells propagated in culture, which were not present on the original cells (e.g., GCSA, gp90), dictates the need for extreme caution in studying host immune responses to surface antigens utilizing cells propagated in culture or serially transplanted in animals. A specific example of this is our observation that gp65 is recognized by MMTV gp36 antisera on a variety of virus- and non-infected mouse, rat, mink, and human cells, including HBL-100, an epithelial cell line derived from a human breast aspirate.

X. CYTOTOXICITY OF MONOSPECIFIC ANTISERA FOR VIRAL CELL SURFACE ANTIGENS

Additional antigens might be present on cell surfaces which would not be detected using cell-surface labeling with lactoperoxidase and galactose oxidase. Alternative approaches for identifying virus-specific cell-surface antigens include complement-dependent serum cytotoxicity and membrane immunofluorescence. The complement-dependent serum cytotoxicity assay is based on ^{51}Cr release and employs monospecific antisera to MMTV and MuLV proteins to test whether these antigens could function as targets for cytolysis. Target cells were the Mm5mt/c_1, 13D, and B9 cells, in addition to C3H10T1/2 cells which are normal C3H mouse embryo cells. The cytotoxicity results are summarized in Table VI. The antisera to MMTV, gp52, gp36, p10, and MuLV gp70 are specifically cytotoxic for the MMTV-producing Mm5mt/$_1$ cell and for the B9 cell, which did not produce detectable levels of MMTV or MuLV but continued to express MMTV antigens. This result suggested that these antigens were integral membrane components and that the reactions were not a result of passively absorbed or budding virus. The specificity of the serum cytotoxicity assay is clearly demonstrated by the lack of any significant cytotoxicity for C3H10T1/2 cells, which express little or no viral antigens based on gp52 RIA (Schochetman *et al.*, 1978a). Cytotoxicity tests were also run using 13D cells as targets since these were the only cells studied other than AKR leukemic cells, which contained GCSA. The serum cytotoxicity data for the 13D cells confirm our iodination results and demonstrate that gp52, gp70, and GCSA reside on the surface of the same cell. This finding, in conjunction with the observation that extracellular MMTV and MuLV

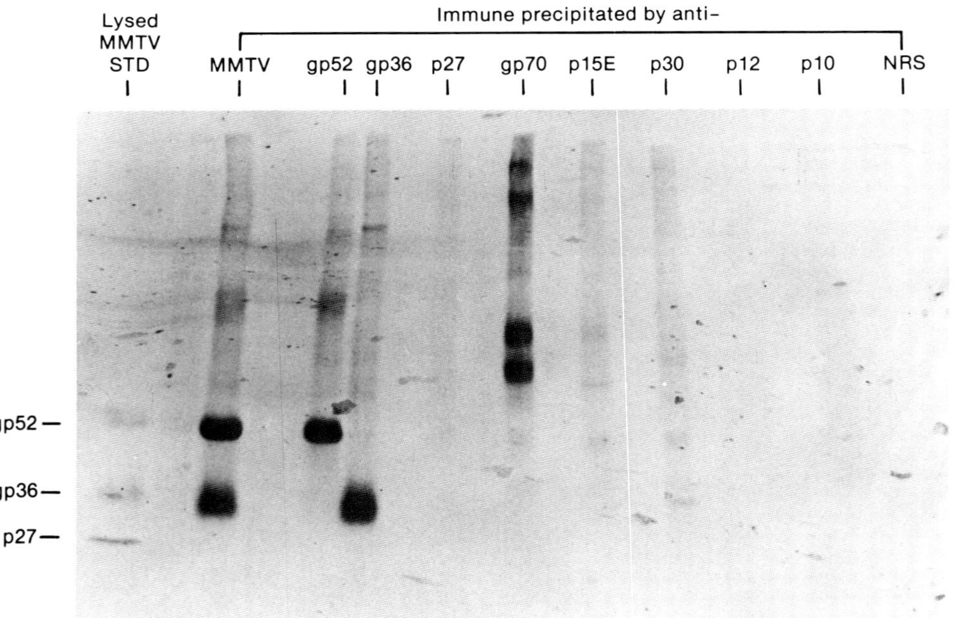

FIGURE 10. Viral glycoproteins on the surface of 13D cells. Monolayers of 13D cells were treated with neuraminidase followed by surface labeling with galactose oxidase and tritrated sodium borohydride. Labeled viral antigens were analyzed as described in Fig. 7. Antisera included MMTV gp52, gp36, and p27 sera and MuLV anti-gp70, p15E, p30, p12, and p10 sera.

TABLE VI. *Complement-Dependent ^{51}CR-Release Cytotoxicity[a] Assay with Antisera to MuLV and MMTV Antigens*

	Target cells expressing/nonexpressing virus			
	Mm5mt/c_1	B-9	C3H1OT1/2	13D
Cytotoxicity with antisera to MMTV	Type B	---	---	Type B, C
Whole virus	82 ± 4.5[a]	58 ± 5.0	10 ± 3.3	71 ± 8.7
gp52	24 ± 2.0	40 ± 0.2	- 3 ± 2.6	39 ± 3.5
gp36	39 ± 1.4	12 ± 2.3	-13 ± 1.2	14 ± 1.2
p27	-0.4 ± 0.3	3 ± 2.6	1 ± 1.7	3 ± 3.2
p10	24 ± 3.2	7 ± 0.4	-11 ± 1.7	41 ± 3.7
Antisera to MuLV				
gp70	89 ± 4.2	18 ± 3.0	10 ± 6.7	76 ± 12.4
p30	2 ± 3.0	3 ± 2.9	8 ± 3.6	77 ± 2.6
p12	3 ± 1.4	8 ± 7.5	8 ± 4.1	3 ± 2.6
p10	12 ± 2.3	6 ± 0.7	13 ± 4.6	17 ± 19.2
Normal rabbit serum	2 ± 0.4	1 ± 1.3	-12 ± 4.4	11 ± 2.9

[a]Percent cytotoxicity ± S.E. at 1:10 dilution of MuLV antisera and 1:20 dilution of MMTV antisera. Complement toxicity in these assays ranged from 3 to 10%. Titers for positive sera: 1:40 to 1:320 for MuLV antisera and 1:160 to 1:1,280 for MMTV antisera.

contained only gp52 and gp70, respectively (Schochetman *et al.*, 1978b), indicated that all three antigens must exist on mutually exclusive cell surface sites on a common cell.

We have investigated the reasons for the cytotoxicity of the antisera to gp36 and p10 because data from the cell-surface iodination experiments indicated that only gp52 and gp70 were on the cell surface. Because the cells used for the serum cytotoxicity assays were trypsinized and allowed to regenerate cell-surface antigens overnight at 37°C, we tested for the possibility that trypsinization affected the cell membranes. When cells were allowed to regenerate at 37°C for up to 48 hr, the only MMTV monospecific serum which was cytotoxic was antiserum to gp52. Versene was also employed to prepare the target cells and, using this procedure, the antisera to intact MMTV, gp52, gp36, and p10 were found to be cytotoxic. Similar results were observed using membrane immunofluorescence.

These results in conjunction with galactose-oxidase surface labeling (Fig. 10) indicate that gp52 is the most external MMTV antigen on the cell surface and that gp36 and p10 are presumably located within the cellular membrane. These results are in good agreement with the reported localization of viral proteins within the mature virion (Cardiff *et al.*, 1978).

XI. NATURAL REACTIVITY OF MOUSE SERA FOR VIRAL CELL SURFACE ANTIGENS

These results demonstrate that viral-specific CSA can act as targets for immune cytolysis with hyperimmune monospecific viral antisera. A more important consideration is whether these antigens actually serve as immune targets for either antibodies or lymphocytes in the mouse. To determine if natural sera contain antibodies capable of recognizing any of the viral CSA, we have reacted serum from a C3H mammary tumor-bearing animal with iodinated CSA derived from the mammary tumor cells of two different strains of mice. The results are presented in Fig. 11. The natural serum precipitated only iodinated gp70 from Mm5mt/c_1 cells even though these MMTV-producing cells also contain surface-iodinated gp52, which is presumably exogenous MMTV. Interestingly, the serum precipitated gp70 as well as gp52 from the M9 cell line, which was derived from a mammary tumor of a C3Hf mouse and presumably synthesized only endogenous MMTV. These results demonstrate the existence in tumor-bearing mice of an antibody population directed against the gp52 of the endogenous MMTV but not the gp52 of the exogenous MMTV. They further indicate the existence of type-specific reactivity for the two gp52s in natural sera. This result extends the finding of type-specific reactivity reported for the gp52s of exogenous

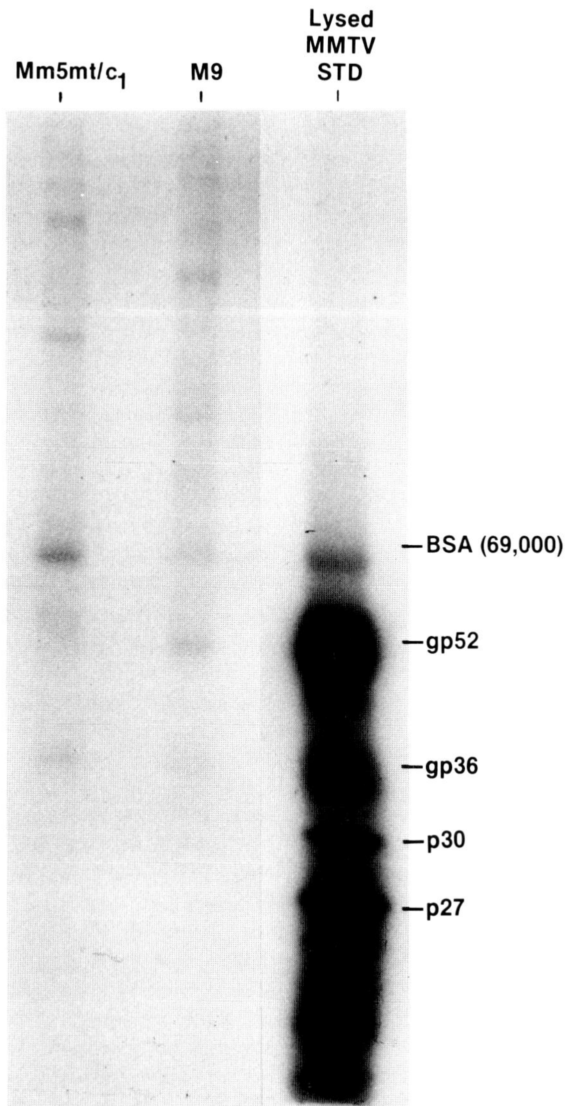

FIGURE 11. Viral cell surface antigens on mammary tumor cells recognized by antiserum from a C3H mammary tumor-bearing mouse. Monolayers of Mm5mt/c_1 (C3H tumor) cells and M9 (C3Hf tumor) cells were surface iodinated and labeled virus antigens were precipitated with the C3H tumor-bearing mouse serum. Immunoprecipitates were analyzed on 5-20% gradient slab gels. Lysed MMTV standard includes BSA (69,000) as a molecular weight marker.

and endogenous MMTV using hyperimmune rabbit sera (Teramoto *et al.*, 1977). However, we cannot exclude the possibility that the mouse did develop antibodies to the gp52 of the exogenous MMTV but that these antibodies were consumed in antigen-antibody complexes with intact exogenous MMTV or free gp52 of the exogenous MMTV (Arthur *et al.*, 1978a).

XII. NATURALLY OCCURRING CYTOTOXIC ANTIBODY TO MAMMARY TUMOR CELLS

Viral glycoproteins such as MMTV gp52, gp36, and MuLV gp70 present on the surface of mammary epithelial cells are of biological significance as antigenic targets, assuming that the mouse is capable of mounting an immune response against these proteins, which results in the lysis of cells expressing these antigens. Because sera from various strains of normal and tumor-bearing mice specifically precipitate MMTV (some sera also recognize MMTV gp52) and also react with MMTV-producing cells, as measured by immunoelectron microscopy and immunofluorescence (Miller *et al.*, 1977; Hoshino and Dmochowski, 1973), these same sera might be cytotoxic for cells expressing MMTV or MuLV antigens. Sera from a group of virgin and breeder C3H and C3Hf mice which had developed MMTV-precipitating antibody were tested *in vitro* for C'-mediated cytotoxicity on Mm5mt/c_1 cells. The data presented in Table VII show that sera from these groups were also cytotoxic for Mm5mt/c_1 target cells. Furthermore, because we found C3Hf sera which were cytotoxic, we can now conclude that mice develop cytotoxic antibodies to mammary tumor cells and precipitating antibodies to MMTV as a result of exposure to their endogenous MMTV. Several of the sera had neither precipitating antibody for MMTV nor cytotoxic activity for Mm5mt/c_1 cells. Other sera with MMTV precipitating antibody lacked cytotoxic activity. This latter group seemed to be age dependent, since other sera samples from the same animals had cytotoxic antibodies at an earlier age. Among the possible reasons that some sera have high precipitation titers and low cytotoxicity values are: (1) the antibodies responsible for the respective activities from different immunoglobulin classes and the high titered precipitating antibodies block the interaction of cytotoxic antibodies with cell-surface antigens; (2) cytotoxicity is dependent on the C' concentration and sera with no cytotoxic activity could be anticomplementary because of immune complexes in the serum; and (3) these responses are coincidental but are directed at different viruses or viral antigens.

To demonstrate that the *in vitro* cytotoxic activity of natural mouse sera was indeed C' dependent, serial dilutions of

TABLE VII. Cytotoxic Activity Against Mm5mt/c_1 Cells by Mouse Sera Positive for MMTV Precipitating Antibody

Mouse strain	Breeding status	Age (weeks)	Tumor status	Precipitation titer[a]	Mean percent cytotoxicity (±S.E.)[b,c]
C3H	Virgin #1	6	-	1,600	50 ± 3.4
		26	-	800	40 ± 0.5
	Virgin #2	20	-	200	- 8 ± 0.3
		21	-	50	32 ± 3.1
		25	-	800	-10 ± 0.2
		28	-	800	- 9 ± 1.8
		31	-	1,600	- 9 ± 0.2
	Breeder #1	15	-	200	57 ± 2.3
		19	+	1,600	64 ± 2.1
		23	+	1,600	51 ± 3.4
	Breeder #2	6	-	≤ 20	6 ± 2.1
	Breeder #3	26	-	3,200	38 ± 4.7
	Breeder #4	15	+	50	63 ± 7.0
		19	+	400	55 ± 1.9
C3Hf	Virgin #1	27	-	≤ 20	- 8 ± 2.0
		30	-	800	26 ± 1.0
		33	-	1,600	31 ± 0.8
	Virgin #2	26	-	200	35 ± 0.5
		30	-	200	43 ± 0.6
		34	-	400	52 ± 1.1
	Breeder #1	15	-	100	59 ± 5.6
		18	-	400	49 ± 0.5
		19	-	400	43 ± 0.4
		23	-	400	4 ± 4.4
		27	-	3,200	12 ± 1.4
		30	-	800	2.1 ± 3.9

[a]Reciprocal of highest titer binding 20% of the labeled MMTV.

[b]Sera were tested at a 1:20 dilution. Toxicity of complement was -5% cytotoxicity in these assays. Sera were also tested for cytotoxicity without complement and percent cytotoxicity ranged from -11 to 5%.

[c]These same sera were not cytotoxic for C3H10T1/2 cells, which do not express MMTV antigens. Cytotoxicity values ranged from 9.0 to 9.7%.

a tumor-bearer serum were incubated with Mm5mt/c_1 cells in the presence and absence of rabbit complement. The results (Table VIII) show that cytotoxicity is both dilution- and C'-dependent. No lysis was observed with serum from a C57BL/6 mouse in the presence or absence of complement. Sera from normal and tumor-bearing mice, which were cytotoxic for Mm5mt/c_1 cells, were not cytotoxic for C3H10T1/2 cells, which do not express MMTV antigens.

XIII. INDUCTION OF CYTOTOXIC AND PRECIPITATING IMMUNE RESPONSES IN MICE IMMUNIZED WITH INFECTIOUS MMTV

Based on the above results mice which have MMTV-precipitating antibody also express antibodies which are cytotoxic for mammary tumor cells. The naturally occurring antibody appears to be specifically cytotoxic for MMTV-expressing target cells but not MMTV-nonexpressing C3H derived cells. To determine if cytotoxic responses can be induced against virus antigens expressed on the cell membrane, mice were immunized with MMTV. Weanling C3H/HeNf mice were inoculated intramuscularly with 100 μg of MMTV. Control groups of mice were immunized with 100 μg of G-MuLV, 100 μg of BSA, or medium. At weekly intervals representative mice were exsanguinated and their sera used in RIP and serum cytotoxicity assays. At four weeks after the primary inoculation a subgroup were given a second intramuscular inoculation with 100 μg of MMTV. The virus inocula had been purified by double banding on sucrose gradients and by SDS-PAGE analysis contained only the MMTV structural proteins, previously described (Schochetman *et al.*, 1978a). Furthermore, this virus had been previously tested and was highly oncogenic in weanling BALB/c mice (Arthur *et al.*, 1978b).

One week following the primary inoculation all mice inoculated with MMTV but not G-MuLV, BSA, or medium had sera which precipitated MMTV and which were cytotoxic for Mm5mt/c_1 cells. The highest levels of cytotoxicity (50 - 100%) were found in sera of those mice bled one and two weeks after inoculation with MMTV. In subsequent weeks the cytotoxic activity decreased to levels ≤10%, whereas RIP titers increased to titers of >12,800. In the group of mice which received a second inoculation with MMTV only one animal responded with a heightened cytotoxic response one week following the booster. No differences in RIP titers were noted in these animals. Representative sera from mice receiving single or multiple MMTV inoculations were reacted with ^{3}H-leucine labeled MMTV and the immunoprecipitates were analyzed by SDS-PAGE. Only MMTV gp52 and gp36 were precipitated from the labeled virus lysate.

TABLE VIII. *Titration of Mouse Serum Cytotoxicity for Mammary Tumor Cells*[a]

Mouse strain	Tumor status	Serum dilution	% cytotoxicity ± S.E. to Mm5mt/c_1 cells	
			+C'	-C'
GR/N	Mammary tumor	1:10	65 ± 1.4	3 ± 1.4
		1:20	58 ± 1.6	1 ± 0.4
		1:40	40 ± 0.8	2 ± 0.8
		1:80	23 ± 0.8	4 ± 0.8
		1:160	6 ± 0.7	-2 ± 0.9
C57BL/6	Normal	1:10	7 ± 0.8	-1 ± 1.2
		1:20	5 ± 0.6	1 ± 0.3

[a]Mice were approximately eight months old and sera were pooled from 6 females of each strain. The sera were heat-inactivated at 56°C for 30 min and serial two-fold dilutions were tested with and without rabbit complement (C') for cytotoxicity against Mm5mt/c_1 cells. The cytotoxicity of the complement was tested by incubating the target cells in complement without the addition of mouse serum and was 5% ± 0.5.

These data indicate that both naturally occurring and induced cytotoxic antibodies are directed at MMTV proteins; however, the possibility exists that the reactivity is directed at mammary tumor antigens or MuLV expressed on the surfaces of mammary tumor cells. The specificity of the reaction was directly demonstrated using C3H sera which were cytotoxic for both Mm5mt/c_1 cells and MMTV-infected feline cells which expressed MMTV gp52 but not MuLV gp70. This is a direct demonstration that there are naturally occurring cytotoxic antibodies against MMTV-coded proteins.

These results indicate that mice develop cytotoxic antibodies to viral antigens which are expressed in the membrane of mammary tumor cells. As such, the naturally occurring cytotoxic antibody may serve as an important arm of the immune system, in addition to the previously reported cytotoxic lymphocyte response (Blair, 1976; Stutman, 1976). However, on the basis of *in vitro* cytotoxicity tests we cannot conclude whether the cytotoxic antibody is functioning *in vivo*. If it does function in the mouse to destroy mammary tumor cells it may be effective only when the tumor size is small and not when the tumor is large and the antigenic load excessive. It is also possible that classes of antibodies which are present in higher concentrations and are not cytotoxic may block the antigenic sites on mammary tumor cells to which the cytotoxic antibodies must bind.

XIV. DISTRIBUTION OF NATURAL CYTOTOXIC ANTIBODY TO MAMMARY TUMOR CELLS

Because naturally occurring cytotoxic antibodies are directed at tumor-associated viral antigens they may serve as important markers for detecting the expression of these antigens *in vivo*. Consequently, one would expect to find cytotoxic antibodies in those strains of mice, both normal and tumor-bearing, which express MMTV structural antigens such as MMTV gp52. Table IX summarizes the results showing strain distribution of naturally occurring cytotoxic antibodies. Cytotoxic antibodies were found only in strains with moderate to high mammary cancer incidence and their development appeared to be age dependent. More than 50% of the mice of the C3H and C3Hf strains had cytotoxic antibodies at about three months of age. Furthermore, the majority of the mammary tumor bearing animals had cytotoxic sera, indicating that production of these antibodies persisted in the presence of palpable tumors. Consequently, the development of cytotoxic antibody has potential as

TABLE IX. Complement-Dependent Serum Cytotoxicity to Mouse Mammary Tumor Cells: Antibody Distribution in Mice Based on Strain, Age, and Tumor Status

Mouse strain	Age (months)	Number of positive mice	Cytotoxicity titers[b] to	
		Number tested[a]	$Mm5mt/c_1$	C3H10T1/2
Mammary tumor bearing				
C3H/HeN	6	10/12	80 - 160	<10
GR/N	8	8/10	40 - 160	10 - 40
Normal females				
C3H/HeN	1 - 3	1/6	40	<10
	3 - 6	5/6	80 - 640	10 - 20
C3H/HeNf	1 - 3	4/24	10 - 40	<10
	3 - 6	4/6	10 - 160	<10
	6 - 8	4/6	10 - 640	<10
GR/N	3 - 8	5/6	80 - 160	10 - 40
BALB/c	6 - 8	0/6	<10	N.T.
C57BL/6	6 - 8	0/6	<10	N.T.

[a]Sera from individual mice were tested in duplicate at 1:10 dilution against $Mm5mt/c_1$. Each assay included a test of the toxicity of the serum by itself which ranged from -8% to 5% as well as the toxicity of the rabbit complement which ranged from -5% to 4%. Sera were scored positive if the complement-dependent cytotoxicity was greater than 10%.

[b]Representative positive sera were selected and titrated against $Mm5mt/c_1$ and C3H10T1/2 cells. The cytotoxicity titers represent the reciprocal of the highest dilution of serum resulting in significant cytotoxicity above the toxicity of the complement control. Significance was based on a Student's t-test with $p < 0.05$. Sera from BALB/c and C57BL/6 were not titrated because they were not cytotoxic at a 1:10 dilution.

a diagnostic marker for mammary tumor development in female mice. Experiments are in progress to attempt to correlate the kinetic of cytotoxic antibody development with the appearance and development of mammary tumors.

XIV. SUMMARY AND PROJECTIONS

Our studies have demonstrated that both moderate (i.e., C3Hf) and high (i.e., C3H, GR) mammary tumor incidence mouse strains express MMTV gene products (i.e., gp52) at high frequencies. Although this expression is not restricted to mammary gland and mammary tumor tissues, it is in these target tissues and sera of tumor-bearing mice that the antigens are found in the highest concentrations. Furthermore, in mammary tumors the MMTV glycoproteins are expressed as true viral-coded cell-surface antigens and are presented as immune targets for the host immune response. Expression of MMTV genes results in the development of both humoral and cell-mediated immune responses which are directed at the MMTV envelope-associated antigens in both particulate and cell-associated forms.

These studies also show that the interaction between MMTV antigens and the host immune response is compounded by the following: (1) gene sequences of the endogenous MMTV are also expressed in both normal and mammary tumor-bearing mice, which may yield multiple forms of the same antigen (such as exogenous and endogenous gp52) on tumor cell surfaces and result in immune responses that appear to be both group and type specific, and (2) MMTV gp52 and gp36 are not the only CSA on mammary tumor cells; they coexist with additional virus-coded CSA (i.e., MuLV gp70, GCSA) and CSA which appear to share immunological cross reactivities with MMTV (i.e., gp65).

Taken individually, each of the parameters studied here, such as MMTV gp52 and cellular and humoral immune responses, serve as diagnostic markers which demonstrate the expression of specific virus genes. The expression of these genes in turn appears to be necessary for ultimate mammary tumor development. By itself, a single marker such as the presence of gp52 cannot be used to predict clinical course. Collectively, however, markers such as antigen expression and immune responses provide an approach for detecting conversion of normal cells to neoplastic cells, for monitoring tumor development, and for predicting clinical status. The potential of this approach is shown here. The analysis of multiple markers, in addition, should lead to a better understanding of the processes involved in tumor progression and rejection. More important is to use this approach in understanding factors responsible for human mammary cancer.

ACKNOWLEDGMENTS

In these studies the technical assistance of R. Imming, R. Devine, L. Orme, R. Bauer, G. Clarke, H. O'Connell, H. Rager, and B. Brown is acknowledged. We express our thanks to J. Clarke and M. Loose for assistance in manuscript preparation. This work was supported by the Virus Cancer Program, Contract No. NO1-CO-75380, National Cancer Institute, NIH, Bethesda, Maryland.

REFERENCES

Andervont, H. B., and Dunn, J. B. (1948). *J. Natl. Cancer Inst. 8,* 227-233.

Arthur, L. O., and Fine, D. L. (1978). *Internat. J. Cancer 22,* 734-740.

Arthur, L. O., Bauer, R. F., Orme, L. D., and Fine, D. L. (1978a). *Virology 83,* 72-93.

Arthur, L. O., Fine, D. L., and Bentvelzen, P. (1978b). *J. Natl. Cancer Inst. 60,* 461-464.

Arthur, L. O., Long, C. W., Smith, G. H., and Fine, D. L. (1978c). *Internat. J. Cancer 22,* 433-440.

Bernard, W., Guerin, M., and Oberling, Ch. (1956). *Acta Internat. Cancer 12,* 545-554.

Bittner, J. J. (1936). *Science 84,* 162.

Blair, P. B., Lane, M. A., and Yagi, M. J. (1975). *J. Immunol. 115,* 190-194.

Blair, P. B. (1976). *Cancer Res. 36,* 734-738.

Cardiff, R. D., Puentes, M. J., Teramoto, Y. A., and Lund, J. K. (1974). *J. Virol. 14,* 1293-1303.

Cardiff, R. D., Puentes, M. J., Young, L. J. T., Smith, G. H., Teramoto, Y. A., Altrock, B. W., and Prett, T. S. (1978). *Virology 85,* 157-167.

Creemers, P., and Bentvelzen, P. (1977). *Eur. J. Cancer 13,* 503-510.

Dmochowski, L., Haagensen, C. D., and Moore, D. H. (1954). *Proc. Am. Assoc. Cancer Res. 1,* 12.

Deome, K. B., Young, L., and Nandi, S. (1967). *Proc. Am. Assoc. Cancer Res. 8,* 13, Abstract.

Fine, D. L., Arthur, L. O., Plowman, J. K., Hillman, E. A., and Klein, F. (1974). *Appl. Microbiol. 28,* 1040-1046.

Fine, D. L., Arthur, L. O., and Gardner, M. B. (1978). *J. Nat. Cancer Inst. 61,* 485-491.

Gardner, M. B., Henderson, B. E., Estes, J. D., Rongey, R. W., Casagrande, J., Pike, M., and Huebner, R. J. (1976). *Cancer Res. 36,* 574-581.

Hageman, P. C., Links, J., and Bentvelzen, P. (1968). *J. Natl. Cancer Inst. 40,* 1319-1324.

Heston, W. E., Deringer, M. K., Dunn, J. B., and Levillian, W. D. (1950). *J. Natl. Cancer Inst. 10,* 1139-1155.

Hoshino, M., and Dmochowski, L. (1973). *Cancer Res. 33,* 2551-2561.

Ihle, J. N., Hanna, M. G., Jr., Robertson, L. E., and Kenney, F. T. (1974). *J. Exp. Med. 139,* 1568-1581.

Ihle, J. N., Arthur, L. O., and Fine, D. L. (1976). *Cancer Res. 36,* 2840-2844.

Lopez, D. M., Ortiz-Muniz, D., and Sigel, M. (1976). *Proc. Soc. Exptl. Biol. Med. 151,* 225-230.

Lopez, D. M., Sigel, M. M., Ortiz-Muniz, G., and Parks, W. (1978). *Proc. Soc. Exptl. Biol. Med. 158,* 23-27.

Miller, M. F., Dmochowski, L., and Bowen, J. N. (1977). *Cancer Res. 37,* 2086-2091.

Noon, M. C., Wolford, R. G., and Parks, W. P. (1975). *J. Immunol. 115,* 653-658.

Owens, R. B., and Hackett, A. J. (1972). *J. Natl. Cancer Inst. 49,* 1321-1332.

Parks, W. P., Howk, R. J., Scolnick, E. M., Oroszlan, S., and Gilden, R. V. (1974). *J. Virol. 13,* 1200-1210.

Ritzi, E., Martin, D. S., Stolfi, R. L., and Spiegelman, S. (1976). *Proc. Natl. Acad. Sci. 73,* 4190-4194.

Schloemer, R. H., Schlom, J., Schochetman, G., Kimball, P., and Wagner, R. R. (1976). *J. Virol. 18,* 804-808.

Schochetman, G., Oroszlan, S., Arthur, L., and Fine, D. L. (1977). *Virology 83,* 72-93.

Schochetman, G., Arthur, L. O., Fine, D. L., and Massey, R. J. (1978a). In "Proceedings of the International Conference on Biological Markers of Neoplasia: Basic and Applied Aspects" (R. Ruddon, ed.), pp. 115-141. Elsevier, Holland.

Schochetman, G., Fine, D. L., and Massey, R. J. (1978b). *Virology 85,* 384-388.

Scolnick, E. M., Parks, W. P., Kawakami, T., Kohne, D., Okabe, H., Gilden, R. V., and Hatanaka, M. (1974). *J. Virol. 13,* 363-369.

Smith, G. H. (1966). *J. Nat. Cancer Inst. 36,* 685-701.

Strong, L. C. (1943). *Proc. Soc. Exptl. Biol. Med. 53,* 257-258.

Stutman, O. (1976). *Cancer Res. 36,* 739-747.

Teramoto, Y. A., Keefe, D., and Schlom, J. (1977). *J. Virol. 24,* 525-533.

Varmus, H. E., Bishop, J. M., Nowinski, R. C., and Sarkar, N. H. (1972). *Nature (London) 238,* 189-191.

Verstraeten, A. A., and Van Nie, R. (1974). In "Proceedings of the IXth Meeting on Mammary Cancer in Experimental Animals and Man," p. 34, Abstract 19. Pisa, Italy.

Witte, O. N., Weissman, J. L., and Kaplan, H. S. (1973). *Proc. Natl. Acad. Sci. 70,* 36-40.

Zangerle, P. F., Calberg-Bacq, C., Calin, C., Franchimont, P., Francois, C. Gosselin, L., Kozma, S., and Osterrieth, P. M. (1977). *Cancer Res. 37,* 4326-4331.

CELL-MEDIATED IMMUNITY TO MMTV ANTIGEN(S): ITS RELEVANCE TO HOST DEFENSES AGAINST MAMMARY TUMORS

Diana M. Lopez
*M. Michael Sigel**
Vijaya Charyulu
and
Gabriel Ortiz-Muniz

Department of Microbiology
University of Miami School of Medicine
Miami, Florida

Jeffrey Schlom

National Cancer Institute, NIH
Bethesda, Maryland

Bismarck B. Lozzio

University of Tennessee
Knoxville, Tennessee

I. GENERAL CONSIDERATIONS

Mouse mammary tumors have been proven to be useful and relevant models for the study of human breast cancer. The complexities of carcinogenesis and of host-tumor interactions can be easily analyzed in these defined systems. Genetic and hormonal factors play crucial roles in the mammary oncogenic

**Present address: Department of Microbiology and Immunology, University of South Carolina, School of Medicine, Columbia, South Carolina*

ISBN 0-12-131150-3

processes. There are many mouse strains, exhibiting high and low incidences of spontaneous mammary tumors. Within the high incidence strains the appearance of mammary tumors is increased in females with frequent matings.

Immunological analyses of spontaneous tumors are complicated by the coexistence of a multiplicity of antigens, i.e., tumor-specific, virus-induced, and virus-associated structural antigens. The presence of mouse mammary tumor virus (MMTV) has been assumed to be of etiological significance. Yet, the mere presence of virus does not lead to immediate tumorigenesis, and there are tumors induced by chemical agents where there is no evidence of participation of infectious MMTV in the host or in the tumor. While the etiologic role of Bittner virus in the genesis of certain tumors in mice has not been discounted, there exists the possibility that viruses may be only indirectly involved in the overall carcinogenic process. For example, MMTV antigens may be induced by the same putative factors that also activate host genes coding for malignant transformation. On the other hand, viruses may influence initiation and progression of neoplasia by modifying either tumor antigens and/or immunologic status of the host. Recently, several strains with low incidence mammary tumors have been found to contain genetic information for MMTV, which in some cases has been expressed in the appearance of virulent MMTV. (Reviewed by Hilgers and Bentvelzen, 1978).

The presence of MMTV in the case of high incidence mammary tumor strains conceivably would give rise to immunological tolerance to the virus. Indeed, several investigators provided some evidence of this effect (Vaage, 1968; Morton, 1969; Morton *et al.*, 1969). However, several studies have demonstrated lack of immunological tolerance. Müller *et al.* (1971) detected presence of antibodies toward MMTV in the sera of both tumor-bearing and tumor-free female mice. Ihle *et al.* (1976) found autogenous immunity of MMTV in mouse strains of high mammary tumor incidence by means of a specific radioimmune precipitation technique. Using a variety of cell-mediated reactions, different authors have reported positive responses against MMTV antigens in various high- and low-incidence mammary tumor mouse strains (Blair and Lane, 1975; Müller and Zotter, 1972; Creemers and Bentvelzen, 1977; Blair, 1976; Stutman, 1976; Gillette and Lowery, 1977; Tagliabue *et al.*, 1978). Blair *et al.* (1974) have demonstrated that both the MMTV-negative BALB/cCrgl and the MMTV-positive BALB/cfC3H possess spleen cells that are reactive in a cytotoxicity assay with antigens of MMTV-induced mammary tumors. These responses are qualitatively different since the latter can be blocked by pretreatment of target tumor cells with BALB/cfC3H serum, whereas the response of BALB/cCrgl cannot be blocked by such serum (Blair and Lane, 1974a).

In our laboratories we have demonstrated that despite freedom from MMTV and mammary tumors early in life, BALB/cCrgl mice possess lymphocytes sensitive to MMTV antigen(s). This sensitivity was manifested in blastogenic transformation and migration inhibition reactions using RIII milk and purified MMTV from RIII milk (Sigel *et al.*, 1976a,b; Lopez *et al.*, 1976). These reactions were not elicited with the MMTV-negative milk from NIH Swiss mice. Preincubation of MMTV with anti-MMTV antibody inhibited the blastogenic reaction. In contrast, antibody raised against a type C murine oncornavirus had no inhibitory effect and did not by itself induce blastogenic transformation (Lopez *et al.*, 1978a). The nature of the virus-related antigen responsible for the lymphocyte sensitivity has not been ascertained, nor has its location in the animals' tissue been determined. However, radioimmune assays for p14 antigen in multiple tissues of BALB/c mice have yielded insignificant values suggesting either incomplete expression of the genome and/or different levels of the diverse mouse mammary tumor virus antigenic components. MMTV-induced lymphocyte transformation is observed at low levels and in a small percentage of BALB/cCrgl mice as early as two weeks after birth in the blastogenic assay. At eight weeks of age the responses in the lymphocyte transformation and migration inhibition assays are intermediate in frequency and/or intensity; by 16 weeks essentially maximal responses are noted (Lopez *et al.*, 1978a).

In contrast with the findings in the BALB/cCrgl mice, we found that BALB/cfC3H mice that contain MMTV and develop high numbers of spontaneous mammary tumors, do not react significantly to MMTV except after transplantation with MMTV-positive tumors (Lopez *et al.*, 1976). Both lines of mice show a similar pattern of blastogenic reaction to their respective tumor antigens: No response prior to transplantation, peaked reactivities 2-3 weeks after transplantation, and loss of activity when tumors reach maximum size. This pattern was also seen with splenocytes of BALB/cfC3H exposed to MMTV *in vitro*, indicating that this was *de novo* sensitization (Lopez *et al.*, 1978b). In BALB/cCrgl mice there was a dissociation of responses to tumor antigen depending on tumor size as noted above, while the responses to MMTV were constant in normal and tumor-bearing animals at all stages. We interpret these results as a possible recognition by the lymphocytes of BALB/cCrgl of a viral antigen produced by a partially expressed virogene. Other investigators have entertained the hypothesis of horizontal transmission (Tagliabue *et al.*, 1978; Blair and Lane, 1974b), however, this could not be the case in our studies since we keep our colonies of mice in geographically separated animal facilities, and the animals are handled by entirely different personnel.

II. DETECTION OF DIFFERENCES IN MMTVs USING CELL MEDIATED IMMUNE ASSAYS

Molecular hybridization studies by Varmus *et al.* (1973) have indicated presence of MMTV sequences in the DNA of all mouse strains that have been examined. These findings were obtained using [^{3}H]cDNA probes that contained unequal representation of the MMTV genome (Varmus *et al.*, 1973). Thus, because only a portion of the viral genome was being followed, one could not conclude whether all the mouse strains studied contained the same kind of MMTV or whether actually there are different strains of the virus. Competitive molecular hybridization experiments by Michalides and Schlom (1975) using [^{3}H]- or [^{32}P]-labeled 60-70S RNAs indicated that there were no differences between the MMTVs obtained from early mammary tumors of the RIII, C3H, and GR mouse. The limits of the assay set the relatedness of these viruses at a 95% level of their nucleic acid sequences. However, using the same types of probes they could detect a 25% difference between the nucleic acid sequence of MMTV obtained from early and late mammary tumors from the C3H mouse strain.

The temperature required to dissociate the duplex formed between different nucleic acid sequences can be used as a measurement of relatedness. Using this technique (Schlom *et al.*, 1977), small but consistent differences (less than 5%) were found among the MMTVs from C3H, RIII, and GR mice.

More recently, Teramoto *et al.* (1977) have presented evidence that MMTV virions from C3H, RIII, and GR mice competed identically in "group-specific" radioimmunoassays, but either competed with altered slopes or competed incompletely using appropriate "type-specific" radioimmunoassays.

In addition to the nucleic acid and antigenic differences described above, Squartini and Bistocchi (1977) have recently reported that C3H and RIII mammary tumor viruses differ in their bioactivities. Using virgin female BALB/c mice foster-nursed either in RIII or C3H mice, they have found differences in the numbers of mammary hyperplastic alveolar nodules per mouse, in the incidence of spontaneous mammary tumors and the frequency of lung metastases: All these parameters seemed to be higher in MMTV-C3H as compared to MMTV-RIII.

Using lymphocyte transformation assays, we first observed different magnitudes of response when MMTV-RIII from milk and MMTV-C3H from tissue culture sources were used. Since these different responses could be due to the diverse background of the murine cellular antigens, MMTV-RIII, and MMTV-C3H grown in one common cell line, Crandall feline kidney cells (CrFK), were used as antigenic sources. Lymphocytes from normal BALB/cCrgl mice or from BALB/cCrgl mice bearing D1-DMBA-3 tumor were tested in blastogenesis assays. Culture fluids of noninoculated CrFK cells or extracts from disrupted CrFK cells failed to give any significant amounts of stimulation indicating that allogeneic reactions were not occurring in our experimental protocol. As seen in Fig. 1, both types of MMTVs, RIII, and C3H, were antigenic to the lymphocytes of normal and tumor-bearing mice. No significant differences were observed between the responses of lymphocytes from these two kinds of animals to the same antigen. However, significant higher responses were observed in all cases with lymphocytes stimulated with MMTV-C3H in comparison to MMTV-RIII antigen(s).

Teramoto *et al.* (1977) conducted competitive radioimmunoassays using MMTVs from RIII and C3H from CrFK cell cultures. They found that MMTV-C3H Fe (MMTV-C3H virus grown in feline cells) competed in the anti-MMTV-RIII vs. [^{125}I]-MMTV-RIII radioimmunoassay with reduced slopes and much more competing protein was required as compared to the complete competition observed with MMTV-RIII Fe preparations. With completely different techniques, i.e., cell-mediated immune assays, we have also demonstrated that the MMTV-RIII and the MMTV-C3H possess intrinsic viral coded antigenic differences.

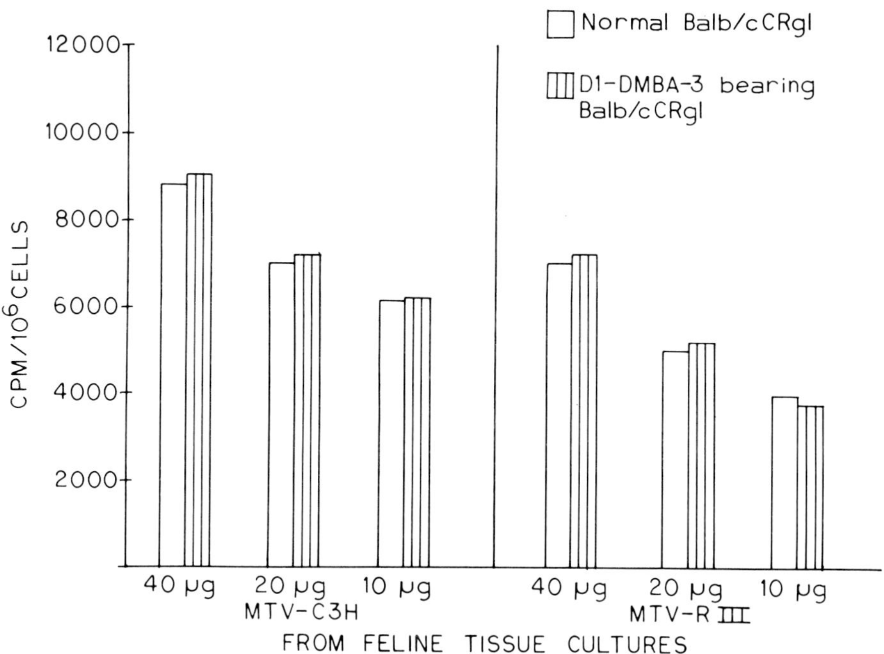

FIGURE 1. Differences of lymphocyte responses to MMTV-RIII and MMTV-C3H.

III. LYMPHOID CELLS INVOLVED IN THE NATURAL IMMUNITY TO MMTV IN BALB/cCrgl MICE

Migration inhibition and lymphocyte transformation reactions using lymphoid cells from BALB/cCrgl mice have demonstrated that these animals that are free of MMTV and have a low incidence of spontaneous mammary tumors display a natural reactivity to MMTV antigen(s) (Lopez *et al.*, 1976; Sigel *et al.*, 1976b).

A study was undertaken to determine the effector cells of this natural immunity. Spleen cells were separated into adherent and nonadherent by passing through nylon wool columns as described by Julius *et al.* (1973). The nonadherent cells are referred to as T cells and the nylon adherent cells are referred to as B cells. To remove macrophages, the splenocytes were incubated for 2 hr at 37°C on glass prior to nylon column fractionation in RPMI-1640 medium with 40% fetal bovine serum (FBS). The high concentration of serum prevents glass adherence of B cells. The resulting populations were analyzed by means of cell surface markers (presence of surface immunoglobulin, SIg, and of theta antigen, Thy 1) and with functional tests using T cell mitogens (phytohemagglutinin, PHA, and concanavalin A, Con A). The results of these studies are summarized in Table I. It is evident that the two cell populations obtained by the experimental protocol have the classic characteristics of T and B lymphocytes.

Stimulation of the nylon wool separated lymphocytes revealed that the effector cells operative in the natural immunity to MMTV antigen(s) seen in BALB/cCrgl mice belong to the B class of lymphocytes (Table II). Nylon nonadherent cells bearing the Thy 1 antigen (T cells) do not respond in the lymphocyte transformation assay when stimulated with MMTV. Since it can be argued that the lack of response of T cells after stimulation to MMTV may be due to absence of macrophages, parallel cultures were suplemented with peritoneal exudate cells. Addition of these macrophage-enriched populations to nylon column separated populations exerted no effect on the response of either B or T cells to MMTV antigen(s).

TABLE I. Surface Markers and Functional Studies in Nylon Column Separated Lymphocytes from Normal and D1-DMBA-3 Tumor Bearing BALB/cCrgl Mice[a]

	Normal animals		Tumor bearers	
	T cells	B cells	T cells	B cells
Cell surface markers[b]				
SIg+	1	88 ± 5	0	86 ± 8
Thy 1+	91 ± 3	1	90 ± 2	0
Responses in functional tests after stimulation with[c]				
PHA	55,789	4000	73,497	6139
(1:800)	±7,240	±397	±9243	±598
Con A	247,032	22,138	312,828	28,002
(1 μg)	±32,129	±1473	±40,901	±3912
Response to LPS (25 μg)	300	9932	571	10,235
	±97	±1007	±108	±1543

[a]Values represent mean results of six separate experiments.

[b]Results expressed in percentage of fluorescent cells.

[c]Results expressed in cpm of mitogen-stimulated lymphocytes minus cpm of nonstimulated lymphocytes.

TABLE II. Indirect Immunofluorescence of Lymphoid Cells from Normal BALB/cCrgl and BALB/cfC3H Mice[a]

	BALB/cCrgl		*BALB/cfC3H*	
	Spleen	*Thymus*	*Spleen*	*Thymus*
Rabbit anti-MMTV + FITC[b] *goat anti-rabbit IgG*	*23.5 ± 4*	*0*	*39.6 ± 5*	*0*
Normal rabbit serum + FITC goat anti-rabbit IgG	*3.1 ± 0.4*	*0*	*5.5 ± 1*	*0*
FITC goat anti-rabbit IgG alone	*0*	*0*	*0*	*0*

[a]*Results expressed in % fluorescent cells*
[b]*FITC: fluorescein isothiocyanate conjugated.*

IV. EXPRESSION OF MMTV ANTIGEN(s) ON THE SURFACE OF SPLEEN LYMPHOCYTES

An investigation was undertaken to elucidate the nature of the cells that express the putative antigen responsible for the sensitization of lymphocytes in BALB/cCrgl mice. Indirect immunofluorescence studies were performed with rabbit anti-MMTV and FITC (conjugated) goat anti-rabbit IgG. Using unseparated splenocyte populations (Table III), MMTV antigen(s) could be detected on the surface of the MMTV-negative BALB/cCrgl mice and of the MMTV-positive BALB/cfC3H mice. Normal rabbit serum in place of the rabbit anti-MMTV was used as a negative control. There was absence of MMTV antigen(s) from thymocytes of these two mouse strains as measured with the indirect immunofluorescence assay.

Investigations on the nature of the cells expressing MMTV antigen(s) were performed using nylon column separated lymphocytes. In Fig. 2 are the results of such studies. It can be seen that most of the fluorescence appeared on the nylon adherent population (B cells). Specificity of the reaction was ascertained by means of blocking experiments. *In vitro* neutralization of the rabbit anti-MMTV serum with purified MMTV prior to use in the indirect immunofluorescence assay reduced more than 50% of the amount of positive fluorescent cells. Recent double-label fluorescence studies in which rhodamine

TABLE III. Effector Cells Responsible for the Natural Immunity to MMTV Antigen(s)

Unseparated lymphocytes	GM	MMTV (1:200)	MMTV (1:800)
Normal BALB/cCrgl	2699 ± 371	25864 ± 3709	17221 ± 590
T cells	852 ± 120	720 ± 101	817 ± 93
T cells + macrophages	2765 ± 293	2594 ± 211	2927 ± 401
B cells	1450 ± 203	14457 ± 940	8709 ± 603
B cells + macrophages	5150 ± 429	16352 ± 837	8422 ± 437
Dl-DMBA-3 tumor-bearing BALB/cCrgl	4297 ± 563	21879 ± 1999	16241 ± 1227
T cells	2914 ± 225	2361 ± 201	2749 ± 309
T cells + macrophages	4981 ± 411	3527 ± 417	4110 ± 294
B cells	4181 ± 297	13207 ± 946	6129 ± 483
B cells + macrophages	5096 ± 377	10684 ± 1008	6364 ± 625

Results in cpm ± standard deviation.
Values represent mean results of 8 separate experiments.

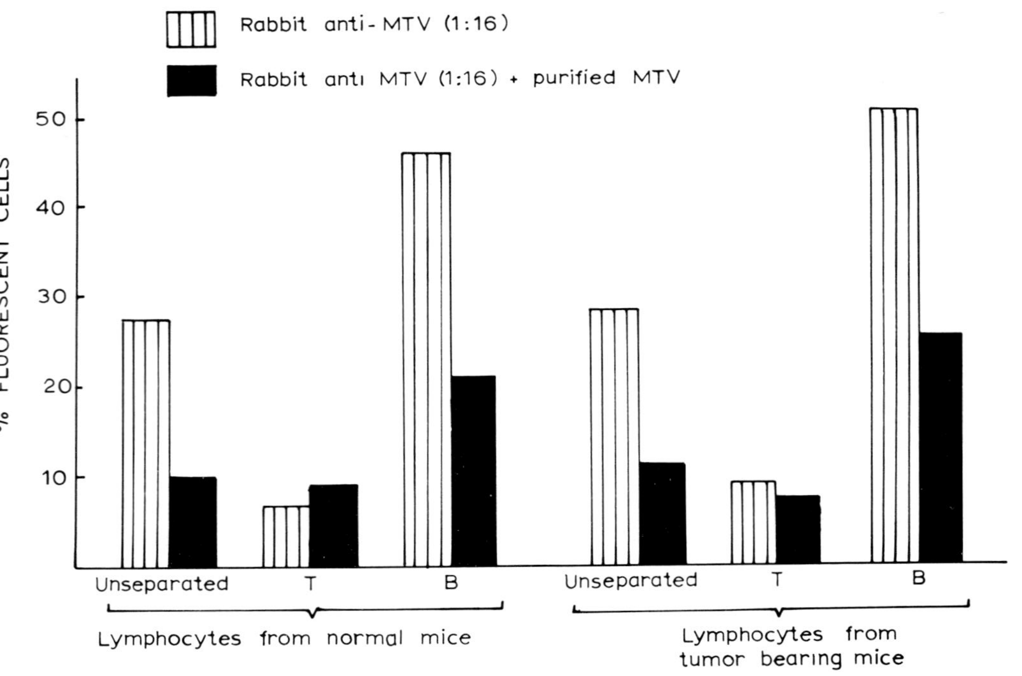

FIGURE 2. Detection of MMTV antigen(s) on the surface of nylon wool separated lymphocytes by means of an immunofluorescence assay.

conjugated Fab'2 rabbit anti-mouse IgG to detect directly surface immunoglobulin appeared simultaneously with the cells stained with the indirect fluorescence assay of rabbit anti-MMTV antibody and fluorescence conjugated Fab'2 goat anti-rabbit IgG reconfirmed the observation that the expression of viral antigen(s) is limited to the B lymphocytes.

Gillette *et al.* (1974) have found MMTV cell surface antigen(s) in all mouse strains examined including low expressor strains such as BALB/c NIH Swiss and C57BL1/Cum. They also observed a relative absence of MMTV expression in the thymus and suggested that the MMTV structural components were expressed on lymphoid cells associated primarily with bone marrow derived lymphocytes. In further studies by Gilette and Lowery (1976) using a cytostasis assay, it was found that the degree of reactivity to the MMTV-positive mammary tumor cells used as targets was greater in spleen cells from low MMTV expressors. Since depletion of splenic T lymphocytes by use of anti-θ serum plus complement did not significantly affect cytostasis, they concluded that the effector cells were not theta (θ) positive.

V. RELEVANCE OF THE NATURAL IMMUNITY TO MMTV TO THE ACTUAL HOST DEFENSE

A. *Resistance to Transplantation with MMTV-Positive Mammary Tumors*

In vivo studies explored the relevance to the host defense of the natural immunity to MMTV. BALB/cCrgl and BALB/cfC3H of 16 weeks of age were implanted with cell suspensions of a syngeneic spontaneous MMTV-positive mammary tumor arising in the BALB/cfC3H colony. Groups of animals were implanted with different tumor cell concentrations. As seen in Table IV, BALB/cCrgl demonstrated a lower incidence of tumors than BALB/cfC3H mice inoculated with the same numbers of tumor cells. Moreover, the time of appearance and the sizes the tumors attained during progression of the disease were delayed in the BALB/cCrgl mice. It should be emphasized that the MMTV-positive BALB/cfC3H possess splenocytes nonsignificantly reactive to MMTV in our experience at 16 weeks of age. Since these animals develop spontaneous mammary tumors at high incidence levels and the BALB/cCrgl mice do not, it appears that there is a strong correlation between the presence of natural immunity in spleen cells and a low incidence of breast tumors.

Another line of evidence supporting the importance of the natural immunity expressed by BALB/cCrgl mice comes from a new model system described below.

TABLE IV. *Resistance of BALB/c Mice to Cells of MMTV+ Spontaneous BALB/cfC3H Tumor*

Colony	No. of cells inoculated	Days after implantation[a] Day 7 A	Day 7 B	Day 12 A	Day 12 B	Day 17 A	Day 17 B	Day 24 A	Day 24 B	Day 32 A	Day 32 B	Day 41 A	Day 41 B
BALB/cCrgl	10^7	0/12	0	11/12	5.8	12/12	12.0	12/12	20.8	12/12	43.0	12/12	53.6
	10^6	0/24	0	1/24	4.0	2/24	4.8	6/24	10.8	18/24	20.8	22/24	24.0
	10^5	0/24	0	0/24	0	0/24	0	2/24	8.0	3/24	14.0	4/24	21.5
BALB/cfC3H	10^7	11/12	6.0	12/12	7.2	12/12	18.0	12/12	32.6	12/12	52.0	12/12	54.5
	10^6	2/24	3.0	7/24	6.0	9/24	9.5	19/24	18.4	24/24	28.6	24/24	38.4
	10^5	0/24	0	1/24	4.0	5/24	6.8	6/24	12.6	10/24	15.4	16/24	27.8

[a]A = Number of positive animals; B = Mean tumor size (millimeter of sum of two diameters).

B. *Hereditarily Asplenic BALB/c Mice with a High Incidence of Spontaneous Mammary Tumors*

A mutant strain suffering from hemimelia and asplenia was discovered by (Searle, 1959; Searle, 1964) among the breeding stock of luxoid mice (Green, 1955). The abnormalities that include skeletal anomalies, mainly of the hind limbs, and visceral defects in homozygous (Dh/Dh) mice result in death within a few days after birth. Thus, only heterozygous (Dh/+) mice are available for breeding and research. As a result of the absence of the embryonic epithelial anlage from which the spleen develops (Green, 1967), these mice are the only mammals known to have a true inherited asplenia. A breeding colony of mice with dominant hemimelia (Dh) and asplenia has been maintained for more than seven years at the Memorial Research Center of the University of Tennessee, Knoxville by Dr. Bismarck Lozzio and colleagues (Lair *et al.*, 1974; Lozzio and Wargon, 1974; Lozzio and Machado, 1975; Machado and Lozzio, 1976).

A mutant strain of hairless (nude) mice was discovered by Flanagan (1966) and was subsequently shown to be characterized by congenital athymia (Pantelouris, 1968; Pantelouris and Hair, 1970), which is inherited via an autosomal recessive gene (nu). In addition to a marked deficiency of thymus-derived lymphocytes and depressed humoral immunity toward thymus-dependent antigens, nude mice fail to reject grafts of normal and neoplastic xenogeneic tissues due to their lack of cellular immunity. By crossing nude mice having a BALB/c background with asplenic mice, it has been possible to produce a new mutant colony of mice that is heterozygous for both the nu and Dh genes. Since the nude trait is recessive, the phenotype expresses only the characteristics of hemimelia and asplenia. To demonstrate that these asplenic (nu/+,Dh/+) mice have mainly a BALB/c background after many generations of inbreeding, 2-month old siblings have been transplanted with an allogeneic skin graft from a stock of BALB/c mice that had never been bred with any other strains of mice. The transplanted asplenic mice did not reject the skin grafts, hence indicating that their genetic makeup is mostly that of BALB/c mice. Female littermates heterozygous for the nu gene and with spleen (nu/+,+/+) have a moderate incidence (13%) of spontaneous mammary tumors, whereas asplenic BALB/c breeders (nu/+,Dh/+) have a drastic increase in the incidence of spontaneous mammary tumor to 51% when bred under identical conditions (Table V). Female (nu/+, Dh/+) BALB/c breeder mice were observed to develop spontaneous mammary tumors as early as six months of age and had a maximum incidence at ten months. In contrast, littermate sister breeders (nu/+,+/+) developed no tumors prior to 10 months of age and the maximum incidence occurred at 15 months. No spontaneous mammary tumors were observed in (nu/+,Dh/+), (nu/+,+/+), and

TABLE V. *Comparison of Incidence and Age Distribution of Spontaneous Mammary Tumors (SMT) in Normal (nu/+) Breeder Females and that of Asplenic (nu/+,Dh/+) Breeder Females*

	Normal (nu/+)			*Asplenic (nu/+,Dh/+)*		
Age (months)	*Total number of mice*	*With SMT*	*%*	*Total number of mice*	*With SMT*	*%*
6	228	0	0	254	5	2.0
7	216	0	0	222	13	5.9
8	206	0	0	188	17	9.0
9	189	0	0	163	17	10.4
10	173	1	0.6	135	28	20.7
11	167	2	1.2	89	11	12.4
12	157	1	0.6	66	12	18.2
13	131	1	0.8	44	9	20.5
14	117	2	1.7	33	11	33.3
15	103	5	4.9	17	2	11.8
16	67	4	6.0	10	0	0
17	39	3	7.7	10	3	30.0
18	24	4	16.7	6	0	0
19	11	3	27.3	6	2	33.3

(+/+,Dh/+) virgins maintained in the same specific pathogen-free environment for up to 14 months. Similarly, no spontaneous mammary tumors were seen in nu/nu,Dh/+ virgins of 1 to 4 months of age. The latter are termed lasat mice and are very poor breeders and do not survive long enough to make adequate comparisons.

Immunofluorescence studies were performed to detect the possible presence of MMTV antigens on the cells of the spontaneous mammary tumors from the BALB/c breeder (nu/+,Dh/+) asplenic mice. Dl-DMBA-3 tumors (MMTV-negative) transplanted in BALB/c mice were used as negative controls. MMTV-positive spontaneous mammary tumors arising in BALB/cfC3H mice were used as positive controls. Dl-DMBA-3 tumors did not express MMTV antigen(s) on their cell surfaces (Fig. 3), whereas the

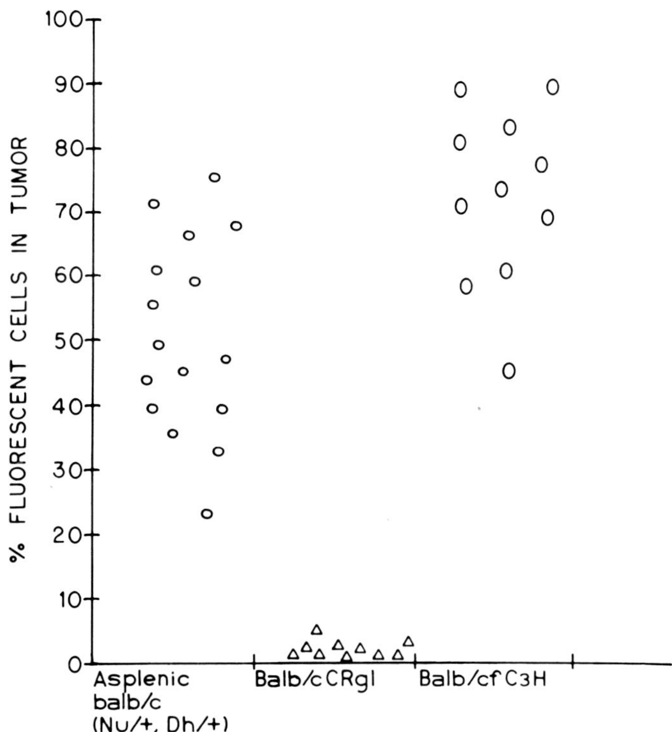

FIGURE 3. Presence of MMTV antigen(s) on cells from spontaneous mammary tumors arising in asplenic (nu/+,Dh/+) BALB/c mice.

MMTV-positive spontaneous mammary tumors from BALB/cfC3H strain had high percentages of fluorescent cells. All the spontaneous mammary tumors from the asplenic mice had positive fluorescent cells ranging from 29 to 81%, indicating presence of viral antigen(s) in these mammary tumors.

Our study suggests that the introduction of the nu gene in BALB/c increases slightly but significantly the incidence of spontaneous mammary tumors. However, it should be cautioned that other or multiple *loci* may be responsible for the increase. If the nu gene is involved, it should be possible to demonstrate an increased spontaneous mammary tumor incidence when other mouse strains carrying the gene such as NIH Swiss or C57Bl/10 are mated to nu/+ mice. The number of spontaneous mammary tumors in BALB/c nu/+ mice may indicate that these mice have impaired immunocompetence even though we cannot demonstrate immunological alterations with the available methodology. Since an increase of the incidence of spontaneous mammary tumors in nu/+ mice with a strain background other than BALB/c has not yet been reported, it appears that the agenesis of the spleen rendered nu/+, Dh/+ mice immunodeficient, thus enhancing the incidence of spontaneous mammary tumors expressing MTV antigen(s).

Since all parent strains (CBA, C57Bl, and BALB/c) have a very low incidence of spontaneous mammary tumors, it appears that the lack of spleen is a major factor accounting for an earlier and higher incidence of these tumors in hereditarily asplenic (nu/+,Dh/+) mice than in normal (nu/+,+/+) siblings.

In our studies with BALB/cCrgl and BALB/cfC3H mice, there was a strong correlation between the presence of natural immunity in spleen cells and a low incidence of mammary tumors. These results coupled with the high incidence of spontaneous mammary tumors in hereditarily asplenic BALB/c mice heterozygous for the nu gene suggest that one of the important functions of the spleen is the regulation of cellular and/or humoral immune reactions controlling the onset and progression of malignant growth in mammals. The availability of these asplenic mice with a high incidence spontaneous mammary tumors is an important tool for experiments designed to investigate the function of the spleen in the development of solid tumors in general and of mammary tumors in particular.

VI. DISCUSSION AND CONCLUDING REMARKS

The perennial problem facing immunologists and oncologists is the continuous growth of tumors in the presence of detectable cell-mediated immunity. One of the current hypotheses is that the lymphoreticular system performs a diversity of functions, some of which are antagonistic to the host's defense mechanisms. There is no longer any doubt that the various constituents of the lymphoreticular system interact, but the exact nature of these interactions and the identity of individual cellular subpopulations are not completely understood.

Studies by several investigators have revealed that it is possible to detect cell-mediated immune responses to MTV antigen(s) in mice strains with low and high incidence of spontaneous mammary tumors (Blair and Lane, 1975; Müller and Zotter, 1972; Creemers and Bentvelzen, 1977; Ihle *et al.*, 1976; Gillette and Lowery, 1976; Sigel *et al.*, 1976a; Lopez *et al.*, 1976). However, no universal conclusions can be deduced from such investigations. The problem is complicated not only by the wide range of mouse strains used, but also by the variety of *in vitro* parameters employed. Even when the same mouse strains and assay systems have been employed, each laboratory has utilized different modifications of the various techniques. Furthermore, it has become evident that a mouse strain undergoes certain variations after it has been maintained for some generations in a laboratory. Thus, for the BALB/c strain, the incidence of spontaneous mammary tumors varies from less than 1% up to 40% after the first year of life in the colonies maintained in various laboratories within the United States and Europe. All these factors contribute to the difficulty of making generalizations in this field.

Despite these variabilities, the relevance of the mouse system as a model for the study of human breast cancer has been amply documented. Recently, there have been many suggestions of an association between MMTV and human carcinoma of the breast. Moore *et al.* (1971) have described viruslike particles in human milk and in fresh human breast carcinomas with characteristics similar to MMTV. McGrath *et al.* (1974) found oncornavirus like particles replicating in a human breast carcinoma cell line. Schlom *et al.* (1971, 1972) described the presence of RNA-dependent DNA polymerase activity in viruslike particles isolated from human milk. Serologic studies by Hoshino and Dmochowski (1973) suggested a relationship between MMTV and human breast cancer. Cell-mediated immune assays have given further support to this contention. Black *et al.* (1974, 1975, 1976) reported *in vitro* responsiveness of breast carcinoma patients' leukocytes to MMTV protein(s) using a migration inhibition assay. Cunningham-Rundles *et al.* (1976) obtained similar results using the lymphocyte transformation assay. In contrast, McCoy *et al.* (1978) found that breast carcinoma patients react to MMTV gp52 and gp70 antigens; however, responses were also observed in patients with benign breast disease. All these studies point to the relevance of the mouse model to the actual human situation and further attest to the importance of research in the field. The understanding of the cancer process that will be obtained could be the basis for the ultimate goal of immunoprevention of mammary tumors.

ACKNOWLEDGMENTS

This work was supported under Contract NO1-CP-53532 within the Virus Cancer Program of the National Cancer Institute, NIH, U.S.P.H.S. We thank Mr. Mantley Dorsey, Jr., and Mrs. Lynn Herbert for their able technical assistance.

REFERENCES

Black, M. M., Moore, D. H., Shore, B., Zachrau, R. E., and Leis, R. E. (1974). *Cancer Res. 34,* 1054-1060.

Black, M. M., Zachrau, R. E., Shore, B., Moore, D. H., and Leis, H. P., Jr. (1975). *Cancer Res. 35,* 121-128.

Black, M. M., Zachrau, R. E., Dion, A. S., Shore, B., Fine, D. L., Leis, H. P., Jr., and Williams, C. J. (1976). *Cancer Res. 36,* 4137-4142.

Blair, P. B. (1976). *Cancer Res. 36,* 734-738.

Blair, P. B., and Lane, M. A. (1974a). *J. Immunol. 112,* 439-443.

Blair, P. B., and Lane, M. A. (1974b). *J. Immunol. 113,* 1446-1449.

Blair, P. B., and Lane, M. A. (1975). *J. Immunol. 114,* 17-23.

Blair, P. B., Lane, M. A., and Yage, M. J. (1974). *J. Immunol. 112,* 693-705.

Creemers, P., and Bentvelzen, P. (1977). *Eur. J. Cancer 13,* 503-510.

Cunningham-Rundles, S., Feller, W. F., Cunningham-Rundles, C., DuPont, B., and Wanebo, H., O'Reilly, R., and Good, R. A. (1976). *Cell. Immunol. 25,* 322-327.

Flanagan, S. P. (1966). *Genet. Res., Camb. 8,* 295-309.

Gillette, R. W., Robertson, S., Brown, R., and Blackman, R. E. (1974). *J. Natl. Cancer Inst. 53,* 499-505.

Gillette, R. W., and Lowery, L. T. (1976). *Cancer Res. 36,* 4008-4014.

Gillette, R. W., and Lowery, L. T. (1977). *J. Reticulo. Soc. 21,* 1-6.

Green, M. C. (1955). *J. Hereditary 46,* 91-99.

Green, M. C. (1967). *Developmental Biol. 15,* 62-89.

Hilgers, J., and Bentvelzen, P. (1978). *In* "Advances in Cancer Research" (G. Klein and S. Weinhouse, eds.), pp. 143-195. Academic Press, Inc., New York.

Hoshino, M., and Dmochowski, L. E. (1973). *Cancer Res. 33,* 2551-2561.
Ihle, J. N., Arthur, L. O., and Fine, D. L. (1976). *Cancer Res. 36,* 2840-2844.
Julius, M. H., Simpson, E., and Herzenberg, L. A. (1973). *Eur. J. Immunol. 3,* 645-649.
Lair, S. V., Brown, A., and Lozzio, B. B. (1974). *Proc. Soc. Exp. Biol. Med. 146,* 475-477.
Lopez, D. M., Ortiz-Muniz, G., and Sigel, M. M. (1976). *Proc. Soc. Exp. Biol. Med. 151,* 225-230.
Lopez, D. M., Sigel, M. M., and Ortiz-Muniz, G., and Parks, W. (1978a). *Proc. Soc. Esp. Biol. Med. 158,* 23-27.
Lopez, D. M., Ortiz-Muniz, G., and Sigel, M. M. (1978b). Abstracts of the Annual Meeting of the American Society for Microbiology, p. 50.
Lozzio, B. B., and Wargon, L. B. (1974). *Immunology 27,* 167-178.
Lozzio, B. B., and Machado, E. A. (1975). *Exp. Haematol. 3,* 156-168.
Machado, E. A., and Lozzio, B. B. (1976). *Am. J. Pathol. 85,* 515-518.
McCoy, J. L., Dean, J. H., Cannon, G. B., Alford, T. C., Parks, W. P., Gilden, R. V., Onoszlan, S. T., and Herberman, R. B. (1978). *J. Natl. Cancer Inst. 60,* 1259-1267.
McGrath, C. M., Grant, P. M., Soale, H. D., Glana, T., and Rich, M. A. (1974). *Nature 252,* 247-250.
Michalides, R., and Schlom, J. (1975). *Proc. Natl. Acad. Sci. 72,* 4635-4639.
Moore, D. H., Charney, J., Kramarsky, B., Lasfargues, E. Y., Sarkar, N. H., Brennan, M. J., Burrows, J. H., Sirsat, S. M., Paymaster, J. C., and Vaidya, A. B. (1971). *Nature 229,* 611-615.
Morton, D. L. (1969). *J. Natl. Cancer Inst. 42,* 311-320.
Morton, D. L., Miller, G. F., and Wood, D. A. (1969). *J. Natl. Cancer Inst. 42,* 289-299.
Müller, M., Hageman, P. C., and Deams, J. H. (1971). *J. Natl. Cancer Inst. 47,* 801-805.
Müller, M., and Zotter, S. (1972). *Eur. J. Cancer. 8,* 495-500.
Pantelouris, E. M. (1968). *Nature 217,* 370-371.
Pantelouris, E. M., and Hair, J. (1970). *J. Embryol. Exp. Morph. 24,* 615-623.
Schlom, J., Colcher, D., Drohan, W., Kettmann, R., Michalides, R., Vlahakis, M. A., and Young, J. (1977). *Cancer 39,* 2727-2733.
Schlom, J., Spiegelman, S., and Moore, D. H. (1971). *Nature, 231,* 97-100.

Schlom, J., Spiegelman, S., and Moore, D. H. (1972). *J. Natl. Cancer Inst. 48,* 1197-1203.

Searle, A. G. (1959). *Nature 184,* 1419-1420.

Searle, A. G. (1964). *Genet. Res., Camb. 5,* 171-197.

Sigel, M. M., Lopez, D. M., and Ortiz-Muniz, G. (1976a). *Annu. N.Y. Acad. Sci. 276,* 358-368.

Sigel, M. M., Lopez, D. M., and Ortiz-Muniz, G. (1976b). *Cancer Res. 36,* 748-752.

Squartini, F., and Bistocchi, M. (1977). *J. Natl. Cancer Inst. 58,* 1845-1847.

Stutman, O. (1976). *Cancer Res. 36,* 739-747.

Tagliabue, A., Herberman, R. B., Arthur, L. O., and McCoy, J. L. (1979). *Cancer Res. 39,* 35-41.

Teramoto, Y . A., Kufe, D., and Schlom, J. (1977). *Proc. Natl. Acad. Sci. 74,* 3564-3568.

Vaage, J. (1968). *Cancer Res. 28,* 2477-2483.

Varmus, H. E., Quintrell, N., Mediras, E., Bishop, J. M., Nowinski, R. C., and Sarkar, N. H. (1973). *J. Mol. Biol. 79,* 663-679.

8107826
3 1378 00810 7826